Brain Imaging
Case Review Series

THIRD EDITION

SUYASH MOHAN, MD, PDCC

Associate Professor of Radiology & Neurosurgery
Director, Neuroradiology Clinical Research Division
Division of Neuroradiology
Department of Radiology
Perelman School of Medicine at the University of Pennsylvania
Pennsylvania
United States

LAURIE A. LOEVNER, MD

Chief, Division of Neuroradiology
Professor of Radiology
Otorhinolaryngology: Head & Neck Surgery Neurosurgery, and
Ophthalmology
Division of Neuroradiology
Department of Radiology
Perelman School of Medicine at the University of Pennsylvania
Pennsylvania
United States

ELSEVIER

Elsevier
1600 John F. Kennedy Blvd.
Ste 1800
Philadelphia, PA 19103-2899

Content Strategist: Melanie Tucker
Senior Content Development Specialist: Priyadarshini Pandey
Content Development Manager: Somodatta Roy Choudhury
Publishing Services Manager: Shereen Jameel
Project Manager: Haritha Dharmarajan
Design Direction: Amy Buxton

Printed in India

Last digit is the print number: 9 8 7 6 5 4 3 2 1

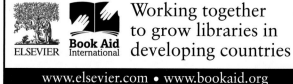

Series Foreword

I am very happy to announce the publication of *Brain Imaging*, third edition of the Case Review Series. Just as *Neuroradiology: The Requisites* was the anchor and most popular subspecialty volume of "The Requisites" Series, so too has *Brain Imaging* by Laurie Loevner been the anchor of the Case Review Series. It has always been the best seller and received the highest reviews and gold stars on Amazon and elsewhere.

Laurie Loevner and I have been friends for 30 years, and she has reigned as a top educator in all of radiology for many years. Her prowess in clinical care and interventional head and neck procedures has made her a stalwart as Division Chief of Neuroradiology at the University of Pennsylvania and highly respected for her patient care acumen by clinicians and fellow neuroradiologists alike. Laurie's research has been fundamental in understanding MRI's role in many head and neck diseases, but she has also published extensively on brain, spine, and leadership topics. She is truly at the top of her field, and in this latest volume she shares some of those insights on brain imaging. Her partner in this latest edition, Suyash Mohan, has published extensively on neoplasms and infections in the brain, and he too brings the perspective of an interventionalist in neuroradiology. The combined fund of knowledge of Drs. Loevner and Mohan goes unmatched in our field.

I have been very gratified by the popularity and positive feedback that the authors of the Case Review Series have received on the publication of their volumes. Reviews in journals and word-of-mouth comments have been uniformly favorable. The authors have done an outstanding job in filling the need for an affordable, easy-to-read, case-based learning tool that is fun to use.

Although some students learn best in a noninteractive study book mode, others need the anxiety or excitement of being quizzed—being put on the hot seat. The Case Review format—a limited number of images needed to construct a differential diagnosis presented with a few clinical and imaging questions—was designed to simulate the (1) Core exam, (2) Diagnostic Radiology Boards, (3) Neuroradiology Subspecialty Boards, and (4) online longitudinal assessment (OLA) of the American Board of Radiology for maintenance of certification. The main difference is that the Case Review books give you the correct answer and immediate feedback! A brief commentary for each case and up-to-date references also are provided. It's a great way to learn a subspecialty field in a case-based approach even if there is no examination looming ahead.

I am pleased to present for your imminent pleasure the latest volume of *Brain Imaging: Case Review* by Laurie Loevner and Suyash Mohan.

David M. Yousem, MD, MBA

Acknowledgment

Every day each of us work toward providing the highest level of care to our patients—and to serve as a source of hope and inspiration for them. This book reflects collective efforts to bring together these concepts as they apply to the practice of neuroradiology, especially *brain imaging*.

When we reflect upon the process of writing this book, we realize this is very similar to solving a complex radiology puzzle. Each image and clinical clue are vital pieces in the overall puzzle, without which the whole picture would be incomplete. While selecting cases for the book, we made sure that all recent concepts, new entities, new techniques, current guidelines, classification systems, and cutting-edge topics were covered in an easy-to-understand "bottom-up" approach.

We would like to express our gratitude and appreciation to the many individuals who have contributed throughout this journey to complete the book. Their support has added color, depth, and "meaning" to the process.

Our heartfelt gratitude is extended to our amazing research assistants Samantha Guiry and Morgan Burke. Samantha was instrumental in the early phases, maintaining a robust foundational structure for this book, and when she moved to attend medical school, Morgan very effectively took over.

We would also like to take this opportunity to acknowledge "each and every" member of our terrific "Neuroradiology Dream Team," which undoubtedly is one of the best neuroradiology departments in the world! Each of you is a star in the radiology constellation. Your support, encouragement, wisdom, and knowledge that you have shared reflects brightly throughout this book!

We would also like to thank the entire publishing team from Elsevier for their expertise, dedication, and patience. Without your support, this book would not have been possible.

On a personal note from Laurie, the third edition of this book would *not* have been possible without my colleague and friend Dr. Suyash Mohan who worked tirelessly, burning the midnight oil. I could not have selected a better partner for this journey, and this will now be his journey to carry forward. He is a shining star—eager, focused, dedicated, intelligent, creative, and detail oriented. Each image selected is like a sip of fine wine, and each case individually and meticulously crafted so that in the end you can never get enough. I also want to thank my family and friends for their endless love and support, my late husband and life mentor Steve Berger, and most importantly my two wonderful sons Ben and Alex, who are now young men raising me!

On a personal note from Suyash, first and foremost, a very special thanks to my lovely boss, my esteemed mentor, Prof. Laurie A. Loevner, aka "the Love-Train" who has been my guiding star, illuminating the path not just for this book but also throughout this vast radiology landscape—and *above all* for giving me this opportunity! When she first asked me to write this third edition with her, I was filled with pride, joy, excitement, and a *lot* of trepidation, as the prior editions of this book have been true masterpieces, a landmark for radiologists across the globe, strengthening core concepts in neuroimaging in addition to preparing trainees for their certifying examinations. Now seeing this book come to a completion—like individual tiles in a mosaic that come together to create a beautiful radiology image—gives me a tremendous sense of accomplishment!

I would like to thank my parents, my father, late Madan Mohan, and my mother, Sushila Varshney, who raised me and has been my pillar of strength. To my beautiful wife of 28 years (officially 21☺), Rashmi Tondon, for her unwavering love and affection, and for keeping me grounded, and my lovely kids, Aadi and Aanya, who have made it all worthwhile. In the famous lines from Rudyard Kipling that my father always quoted,

> If you can fill the unforgiving minute,
> With sixty seconds' worth of distance run,
> Yours is the Earth and everything that's in it,
> And. . . .what's more you'll be a Man, my son!

We hope you enjoy this book and the many lessons inside its covers. Academic medicine and radiology are a wonderful journey. We will remain forever indebted to the many mentors who encouraged us to pursue this path and for their guidance *to practice medicine, not just to make a living but to make a difference*, and pass this wisdom to future generations.

Contents

Case 1

History: A 48-year-old man with mitral valve endocarditis presents with new speech changes.

1. Which condition are these imaging findings most consistent with?
   A. Right ACA territory infarction
   B. Left MCA territory infarction
   C. Left PCA territory infarction
   D. Left ACA territory infarction
2. The recurrent artery of Heubner, or medial striate artery, arises from which of the following?
   A. A2 segment of the ACA
   B. M2 segment of the MCA
   C. P2 segment of the PCA
   D. M1 segment of the MCA
3. Which of the following structures are supplied by the recurrent artery of Heubner?
   A. Posterior limb of the internal capsule
   B. Head of the caudate nucleus, anterior portion of the lentiform nucleus, and anterior limb of the internal capsule
   C. Corpus callosum
   D. Olfactory tracts and bulbs
4. The medial lenticulostriate arteries generally arise from which of the following?
   A. A1 segment of ACA
   B. A2 segment of ACA
   C. M1 segment of MCA
   D. M2 segment of MCA

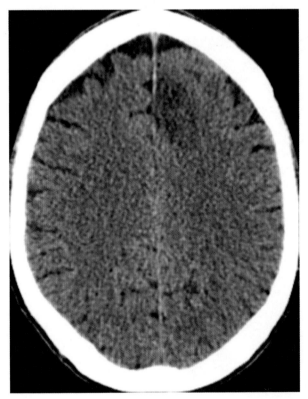

Fig. 1.1

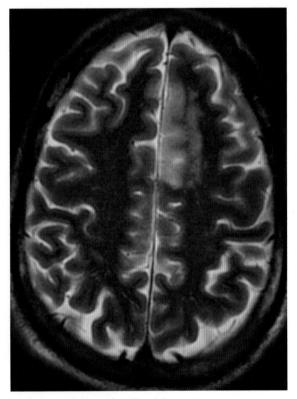

Fig. 1.2

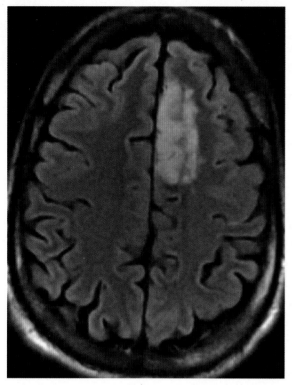

Fig. 1.3

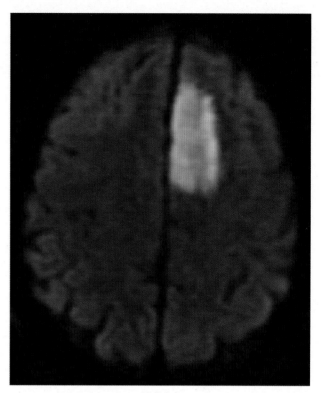

Fig. 1.4

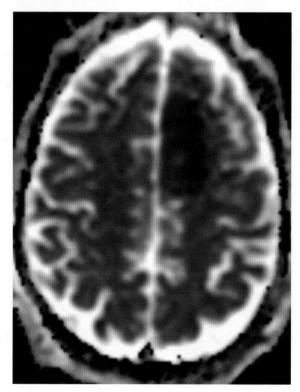

Fig. 1.5

Case 2

History: This is a 51-year-old man with seizures.

1. What is the most likely diagnosis?
   A. Hemangioblastoma
   B. Hemorrhagic metastases
   C. Pilocytic astrocytoma
   D. Glioblastoma

2. What factors may contribute to a lesion appearing hyperdense on an unenhanced CT and hypointense on a T2W MR image?
   A. Acute hemorrhage, high cellularity, high protein concentration, and the presence of calcification
   B. Fat
   C. Edema
   D. Extracellular methemoglobin

3. Which of the following primary tumors are associated with hemorrhagic metastases?
   A. Renal cell carcinoma
   B. Melanoma
   C. Choriocarcinoma
   D. All of the above

4. What is the most common posterior fossa mass in adults?
   A. Hemangioblastoma
   B. Hemangiopericytoma
   C. Medulloblastoma
   D. Metastases

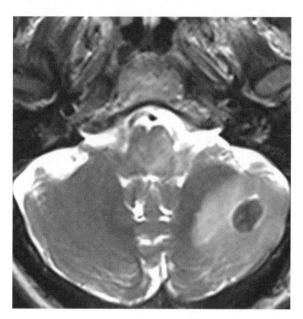

Fig. 2.1

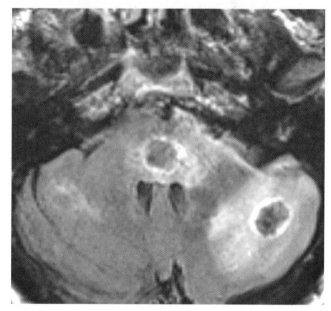

Fig. 2.2

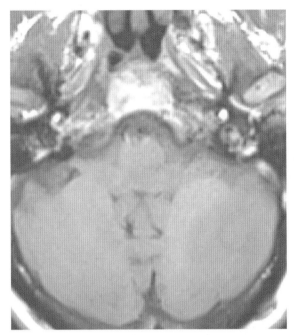

Fig. 2.3

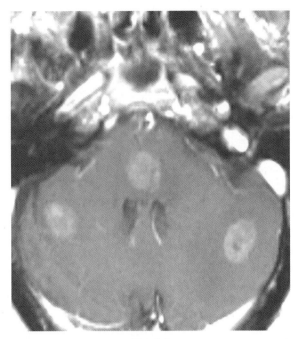

Fig. 2.4

Case 3

History: This 31-year-old male was found down.

1. What are the imaging findings? (Choose all that apply.)
   A. Intracranial hemorrhage with metallic artifact on bone window images
   B. Penetrating injury to the head, with frontal lobe intraparenchymal hemorrhage and intraventricular extension, and there is a retained bow and arrow
   C. Epidural hematoma
   D. Subdural hematoma
2. What is the most likely mode of this injury?
   A. Anoxic brain injury
   B. Drug overdose
   C. Aneurysmal rupture
   D. A self-inflicted injury, with likely entrance under the mandible (submental) and then through the anterior cranial fossa
3. What is the most effective and efficient way to work up a penetrating head injury?
   A. Plain radiography
   B. MRI
   C. Noncontrast head CT
   D. Conventional angiography
4. What are the potential causes of the intracranial air?
   A. Mechanical trauma with communication with the extracranial compartment
   B. Calvarial fracture involving both anterior and posterior tables of the frontal sinus
   C. Calvarial fracture through the adjacent temporal bone
   D. All of the above

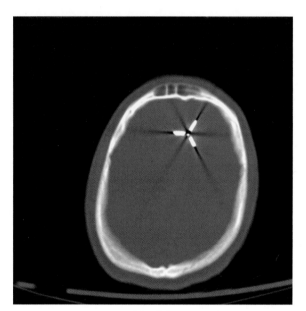

Fig. 3.1

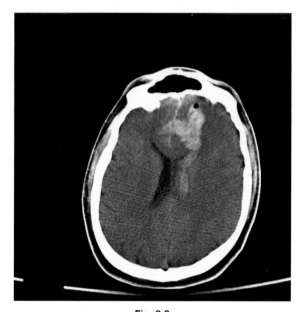

Fig. 3.2

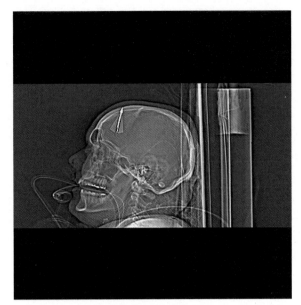

Fig. 3.3

Case 4

History: This is a 29-year-old injured in a bike crash.

1. Which of the following is true regarding heterogeneous or "swirling" appearance of an acute extra-axial hematoma? (Choose all that apply.)
   A. It represents unclotted fresh blood, which is of lower attenuation than the clotted blood
   B. It represents acute extravasation of blood into the hematoma
   C. Leakage of serum from the epidural clot or active bleeding. This may also be seen in coagulopathic patients or in patients receiving anticoagulation therapy
   D. All of the above
2. What type of extra-axial hematoma is most commonly associated with a skull fracture?
   A. Subdural hematoma
   B. Epidural hematoma
   C. Subarachnoid hemorrhage
   D. Intraventricular hemorrhage
3. What type of extra-axial hematoma runs between the periosteum of the inner calvarium and the dura mater?
   A. Epidural hematoma
   B. Subdural hematoma
   C. Subarachnoid hemorrhage
   D. Subgaleal hemorrhage
4. What is the most common cause of an epidural hematoma?
   A. Arterial injury, most commonly to the middle meningeal artery.
   B. Injury to bridging cortical veins.
   C. Rupture of a saccular aneurysm.
   D. Rupture of intradiploic venous channels.

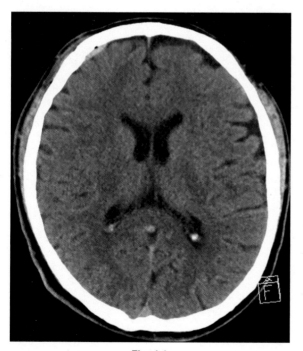

Fig. 4.1

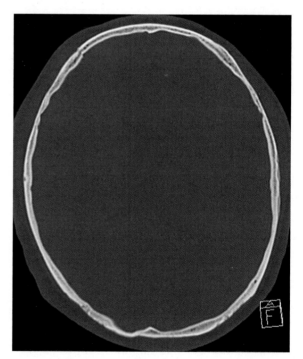

Fig. 4.2

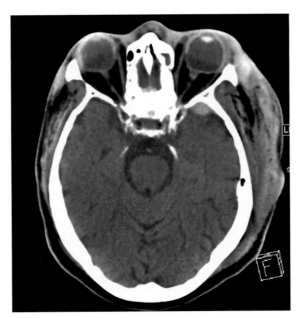

Fig. 4.3

Case 5

History: This is a 59-year-old with a history of lung cancer presenting with headache, nausea, and vomiting.

1. What is the primary imaging finding?
   A. Acute obstructive hydrocephalus
   B. Communicating hydrocephalus
   C. Pineal cyst
   D. Normal pressure hydrocephalus
2. What secondary imaging findings in this case indicate that this condition is acute?
   A. Prominent lateral ventricles
   B. Prominent cerebellar folia
   C. Hypodensity in the periventricular white matter consistent with transependymal edema
   D. Lack of midline shift
3. Transependymal edema represents?
   A. Cytotoxic edema
   B. Vasogenic edema
   C. Interstitial edema
   D. Combination of cytotoxic and vasogenic edema
4. What is the management of obstructive hydrocephalus?
   A. No management is needed; it is a self-limiting condition.
   B. Typically, shunting and management of the underlying etiology of the hydrocephalus. In this case, the patient has leptomeningeal carcinomatosis.
   C. IV fluids
   D. IV antibiotics

Case 6

History: This 21-year-old female was hit in the head with a soccer ball and had subsequent nausea and headache.

1. What is the finding on these MR images?
   A. Pineocytoma
   B. Cyst of the pineal gland
   C. Pineal apoplexy
   D. Cyst of velum interpositum
2. The vast majority of pineal cysts are small (<1 cm) and asymptomatic. Larger pineal cysts can present with which of the following symptoms?
   A. Parinaud syndrome
   B. Obstructive hydrocephalus
   C. Pineal apoplexy
   D. All of the above
3. What are the symptoms and signs of Parinaud's syndrome?
   A. Paralysis of upward gaze caused by compression of the superior tectal plate
   B. Bilateral small pupils that constrict briskly with accommodation but do not constrict when exposed to light
   C. Ophthalmoparesis with nystagmus, ataxia, and confusion
   D. Ptosis, miosis, and anhidrosis

4. What is the anatomic relationship of the pineal gland relative to the velum interpositum?
   A. The pineal gland is directly above the velum interpositum.
   B. The pineal gland is directly anterior to the velum interpositum.
   C. The velum interpositum is a small membrane containing a potential space just above and anterior to the pineal gland directly below the splenium of the corpus callosum.
   D. The pineal gland is situated inside the velum interpositum.

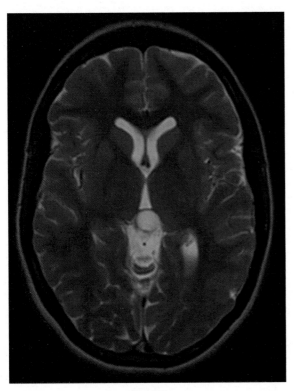

Fig. 6.1

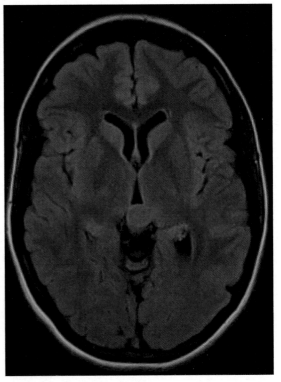

Fig. 6.2

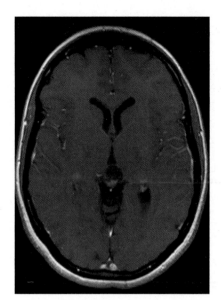

Fig. 6.3

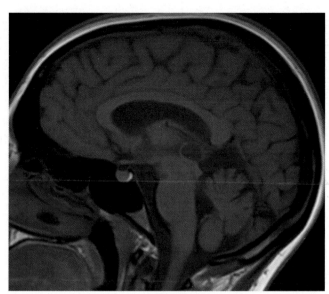

Fig. 6.4

Case 7

History: This 65-year-old male with a history of alcohol and polysubstance abuse presented to the ED after he was found down on a sidewalk.

1. What is the most likely diagnosis?
   A. Hemorrhagic metastases
   B. Multiple cavernomas
   C. Diffuse axonal injury
   D. Multiple parenchymal hemorrhagic contusions with surrounding edema
2. What are the characteristic locations of cortical contusions in the setting of acceleration–deceleration injuries?
   A. Anterior and inferior temporal and frontal lobes
   B. Posterolateral temporal lobes and the occipital poles
   C. Coup and contrecoup pattern
   D. All of the above
3. Which of the following locations of intracranial hemorrhage is not common in closed head injury?
   A. Parenchymal hemorrhagic contusions along the floor of the anterior cranial fossa
   B. Basal ganglia hemorrhage
   C. Subarachnoid hemorrhage
   D. Subdural hemorrhage

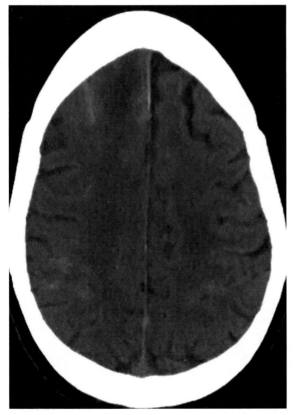

Fig. 7.1

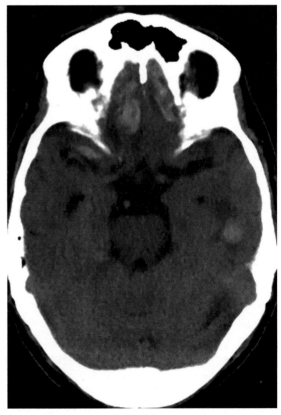

Fig. 7.2

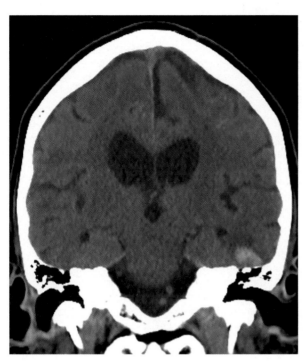

Fig. 7.3

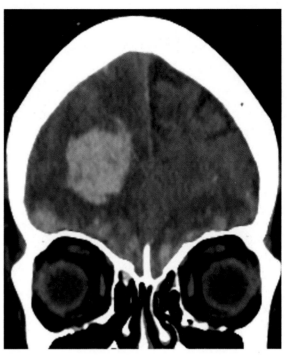

Fig. 7.4

Case 8

History: A 47-year-old with a history of Type A aortic dissection and repair presents with new-onset right upper extremity weakness.

1. What are the imaging findings?
   A. Multiple sclerosis
   B. Multiple embolic infarcts
   C. Multiple myeloma
   D. Metastatic melanoma
2. Which of the following indicate a high risk for a cardioembolic stroke?
   A. Left atrial thrombus with atrial fibrillation
   B. Left ventricular thrombus with acute myocardial infarction
   C. Type A aortic dissection
   D. Prosthetic valve vegetation
   E. All of the above

3. Within minutes of an acute ischemic stroke, diffusion-weighted imaging demonstrates increased DWI signal and reduced ADC values. ADC values returning to normal approximately 1 week after an ischemic infarct is known as which of the following?
   A. ADC pseudonormalization
   B. T2 shine through
   C. DWI pseudoreversal
   D. Fogging phenomenon
4. What are some hypercoagulable conditions that can cause thrombotic strokes?
   A. Antiphospholipid antibody syndrome
   B. Factor V Leiden mutation
   C. Oral contraceptives
   D. Protein C or S deficiency
   E. All of the above

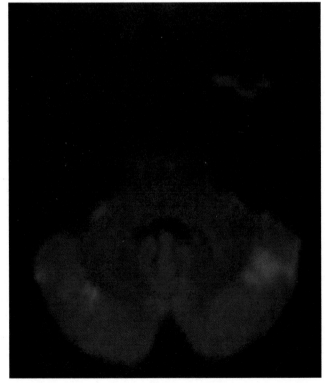

Fig. 8.1

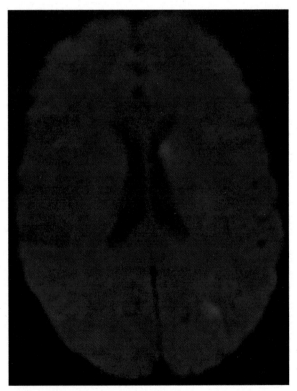

Fig. 8.2

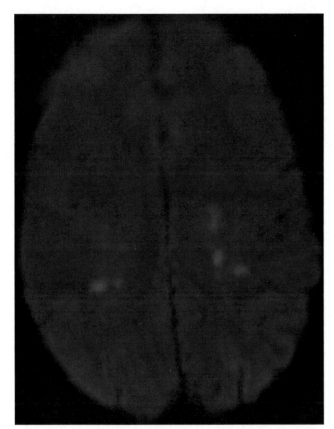
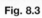

Fig. 8.3

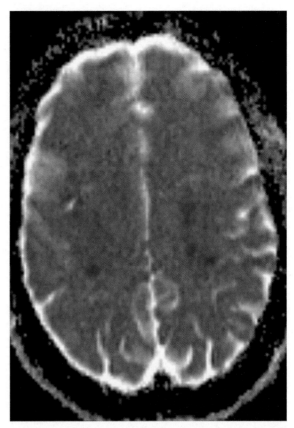

Fig. 8.4

Case 9

History: This is a 35-year-old female with hearing loss, left facial numbness, and tinnitus.

1. Bilateral vestibular schwannomas are diagnostic of which of the following conditions?
   A. Neurofibromatosis type 1
   B. Neurofibromatosis type 2
   C. Sturge Weber syndrome
   D. Von Hippel–Lindau disease
2. Vestibular schwannomas are tumors arising from which cranial nerve (CN)?
   A. CN VI
   B. CN VII
   C. CN VIII
   D. CN IX

3. What structure separates the internal auditory canal into superior and inferior portions?
   A. Crista falciformis
   B. Crista galli
   C. Crista terminalis
   D. Crista ampullaris

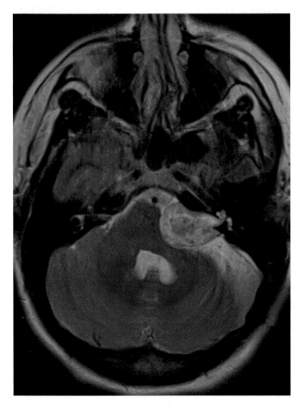

Fig. 9.1

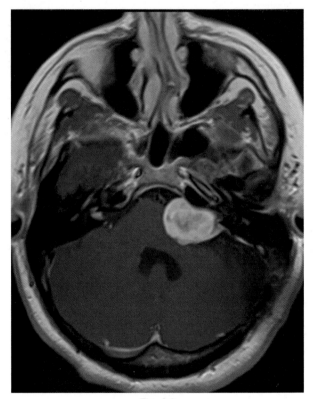

Fig. 9.2

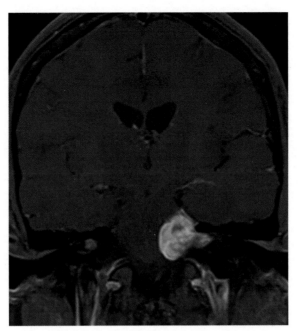

Fig. 9.3

Case 10

History: A 69-year-old male with a history of hypertension, hyperlipidemia, chronic kidney disease, paroxysmal atrial fibrillation, and cardioembolic CVA on Coumadin and aspirin presents with unresponsiveness.

1. What is the most common cause of acute nontraumatic intraparenchymal hemorrhage in adults?
   A. Hypertension
   B. Hyperlipidemia
   C. Chronic kidney disease
   D. Aspirin use
2. Which radiographic feature(s) predict a poor outcome?
   A. Bleed in the posterior fossa
   B. Significant mass effect
   C. Intraventricular extension and hydrocephalus
   D. All of the above
3. Which of the following MRI sequences can be used to maximize blooming artifacts?
   A. Susceptibility-weighted imaging (SWI)
   B. Gradient-Recalled Echo (GRE)
   C. Low B-value diffusion-weighted imaging
   D. All of the above
4. What are Duret hemorrhages?
   A. Putaminal hemorrhage from ruptured microaneurysms of perforating arteries (Charcot-Bouchard aneurysms)
   B. Small hemorrhages that develop within the pons or medulla due to rapidly developing brain herniation
   C. Subarachnoid hemorrhage from a ruptured berry aneurysm
   D. Hemorrhage in a venous infarct

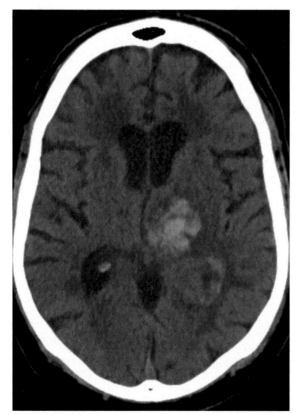

Fig. 10.1

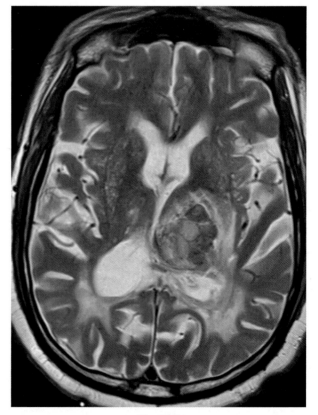

Fig. 10.2

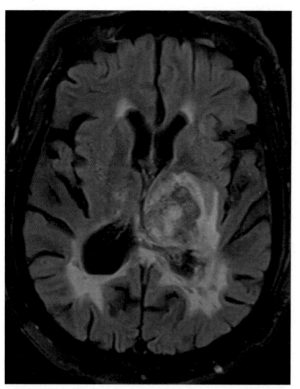

Fig. 10.3

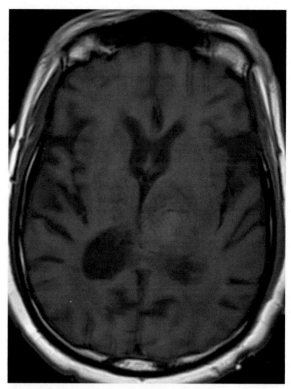

Fig. 10.4

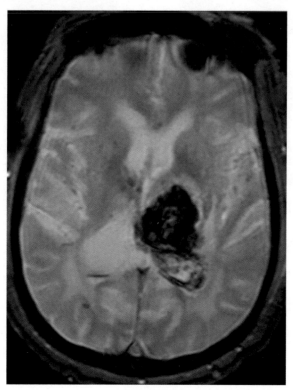

Fig. 10.5

Case 11

History: A 57-year-old man presents with an episode of dizziness, nausea, and vomiting associated with diaphoresis while working in the yard.

1. What is the most likely diagnosis?
   A. Epidermoid cyst
   B. Arachnoid cyst
   C. Cystic schwannoma
   D. Mega cisterna magna
2. Which MRI sequence can best differentiate an arachnoid cyst from an epidermoid cyst?
   A. T2
   B. FLAIR
   C. DWI
   D. GRE
3. Which is the most common location of arachnoid cysts in the central nervous system?
   A. Middle cranial fossa
   B. Posterior fossa
   C. Suprasellar cisterm
   D. Spinal canal

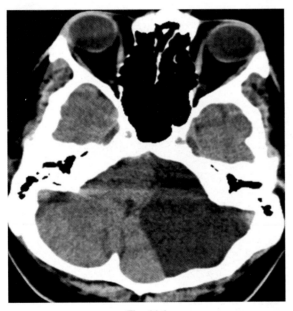

Fig. 11.1

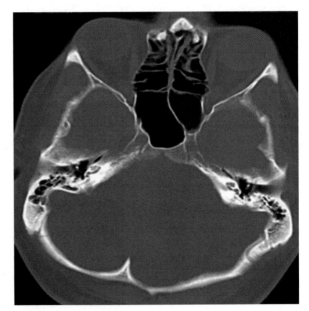

Fig. 11.2

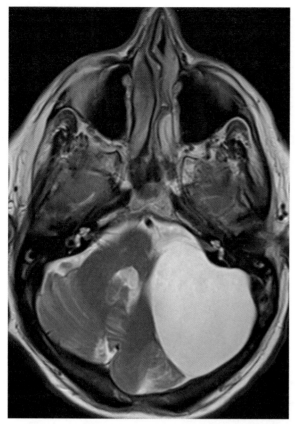

Fig. 11.3

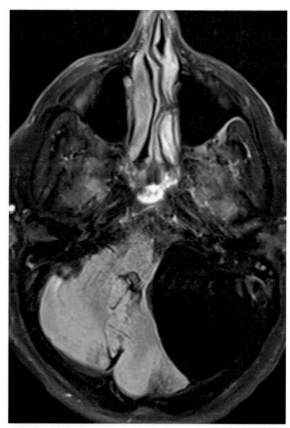

Fig. 11.4

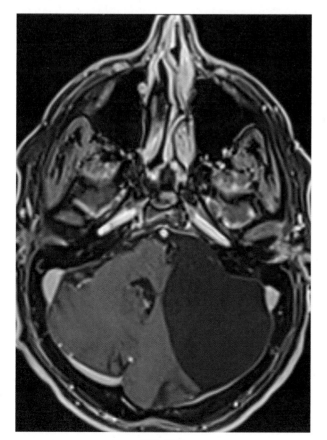

Fig. 11.5

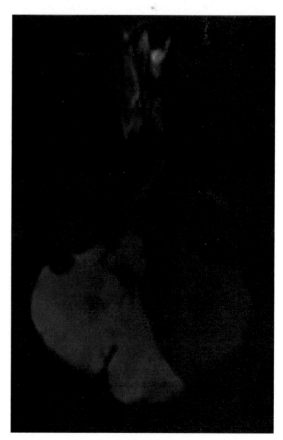

Fig. 11.6

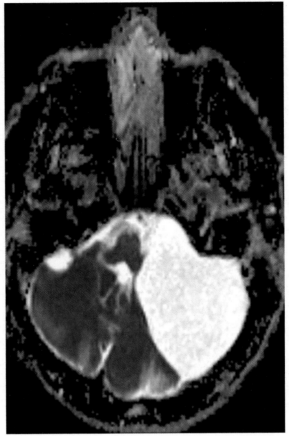

Fig. 11.7

Case 12

History: This is a 56-year-old patient with productive cough, upper respiratory symptoms, confusion, and aphasia.

1. What is the diagnosis?
   A. Epidural hematoma
   B. Subdural effusion
   C. Subdural empyema
   D. Subdural hematoma
2. Which MRI sequence can differentiate a subdural effusion from a subdural empyema?
   A. T2
   B. FLAIR
   C. DWI
   D. GRE

3. What is the most common cause of a subdural empyema?
   A. Sinusitis
   B. Otitis media
   C. Superficial infections of the scalp
   D. Subdural hematoma
4. What is the standard treatment for subdural empyema?
   A. Observation
   B. Oral antibiotics
   C. Craniotomy/surgical drainage and antibiotic therapy
   D. Embolization

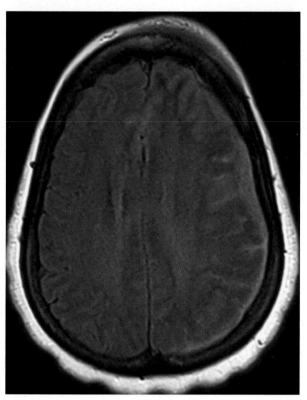

Fig. 12.1

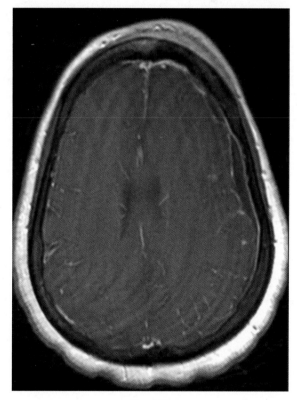

Fig. 12.2

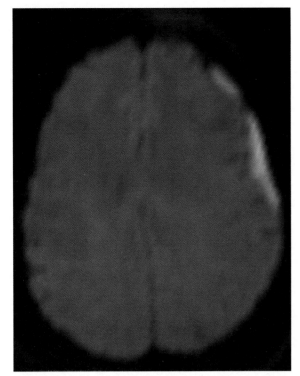

Fig. 12.3

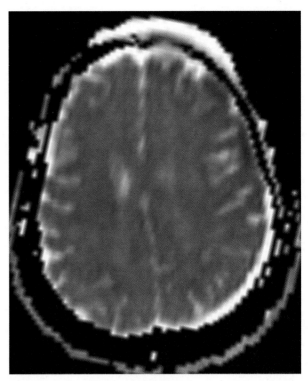

Fig. 12.4

Case 13

History: Patient A (Fig. 13.1): A 62-year-old female status post assault. Patient B (Fig. 13.2): A 36-year-old male with a right facial laceration from GSW.

1. What is the diagnosis for patient A?
   A. Globe rupture
   B. Extraocular muscle entrapment
   C. Ectopia lentis
   D. Hyphema
2. What is the most common cause of lens subluxation or dislocation?
   A. Spontaneous
   B. Trauma
   C. Marfan syndrome
   D. Homocystinuria

3. What is the diagnosis for Case B?
   A. Globe rupture
   B. Extraocular muscle entrapment
   C. Ectopia lentis
   D. Hyphema

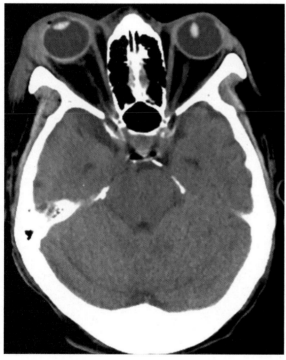

Fig. 13.1

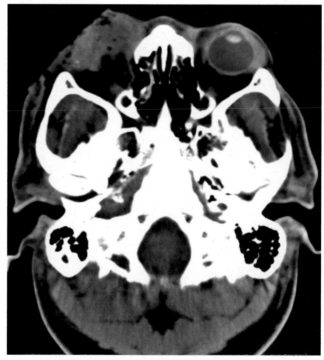

Fig. 13.2

Case 14

History: A 77-year-old male presents with headache, blurred vision, and poor memory.

1. What vascular anatomic variant is demonstrated in this case: axial TOF MRA (A), AP DSA (B)?
   A. Persistent otic artery
   B. Persistent hypoglossal artery
   C. Persistent proatlantal artery
   D. Persistent trigeminal artery
2. What are the other intracranial embryologic anastomoses between the carotid (anterior) and vertebrobasilar (posterior) circulations?
   A. Persistent otic artery
   B. Persistent hypoglossal artery
   C. Persistent proatlantal artery
   D. All of the above

3. What other intracranial vascular abnormalities have been associated with persistent trigeminal artery?
   A. Aneurysms and arteriovenous malformations
   B. Cavernomas
   C. Capillary telangiectasias
   D. Persistent falcine sinus
4. What percentage of cerebral arteriograms reveal a persistent trigeminal artery?
   A. 0.1% to 0.6%
   B. 1% to 6%
   C. 10% to 16%
   D. 16% to 26%

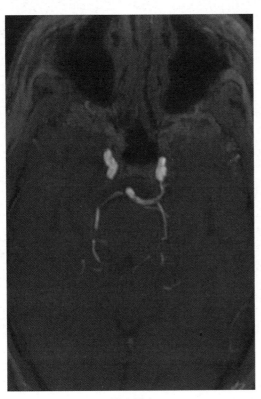

Fig. 14.1

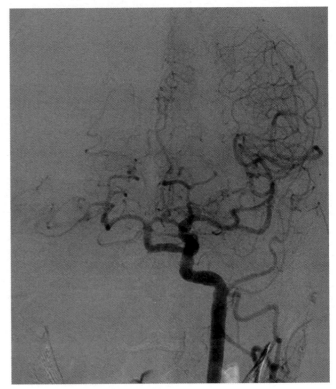

Fig. 14.2

Case 15

History: This 59-year-old patient presents with memory difficulty.

1. What normal anatomic variant is demonstrated in this case: axial T2 (A), FLAIR (B), coronal T2 (C)?
   A. Velum interpositum
   B. Dilated third ventricle
   C. Cavum septum pellucidum
   D. Cavum septum pellucidum and vergae
2. Development of the corpus callosum is intimately associated with the development of what other structure?
   A. Optic nerves
   B. Septum pellucidum
   C. Brain stem
   D. Thalamus
3. What structures traverse the cistern of the velum interpositum?
   A. Corpus callosum
   B. The internal cerebral veins and the medial posterior choroidal arteries
   C. Fornix
   D. Pineal gland
4. What is the normal volume of CSF in the entire CNS in adults?
   A. 1500 mL
   B. 15 mL
   C. 1.5 mL
   D. 150 mL

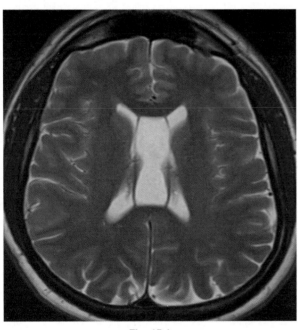

Fig. 15.1

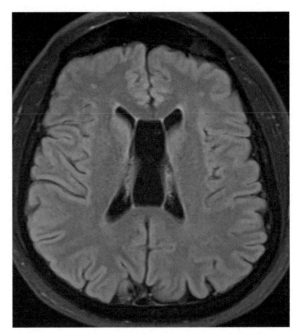

Fig. 15.2

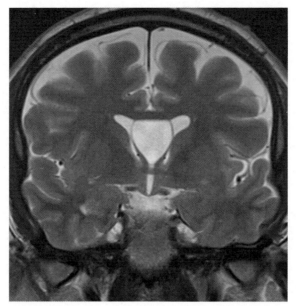

Fig. 15.3

Case 16

History: This is a 38-year-old woman with right ear pain and bilateral lower extremity numbness.

1. What is the most likely diagnosis?
   A. Developmental venous anomaly
   B. Cavernoma
   C. Arteriovenous malformation
   D. Dural AV fistula
2. What is the major vascular supply to the lesion in this case?
   A. Right anterior choroidal artery
   B. Parieto-occipital branches of the right posterior and middle cerebral arteries
   C. Right anterior cerebral artery
   D. Right middle meningeal artery

3. Where is the venous drainage in this case?
   A. Superficial
   B. Deep
   C. Superficial and deep
   D. Basilar cistern
4. What are the causes of false-negative findings on angiograms in patients with surgically proven arteriovenous malformations (AVMs)?
   A. Very small AVM
   B. Thrombosed AVM
   C. Compressed from mass effect related to an associated parenchymal hemorrhage
   D. All of the above

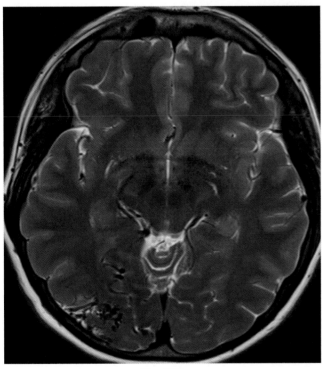

Fig. 16.1

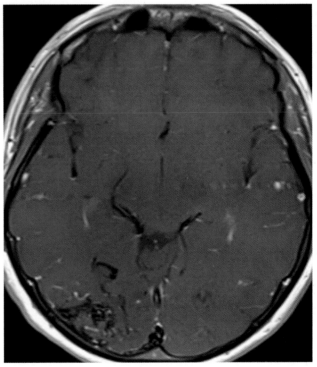

Fig. 16.2

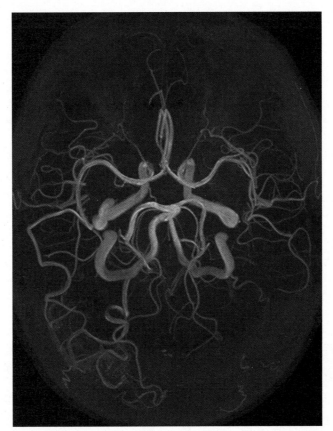

Fig. 16.3

Case 17

History: This is a 47-year-old-male with seizures.

1. What is the most likely diagnosis in this case?
   A. Acute infarction
   B. Acute hemorrhage
   C. Abscess
   D. Aneurysm
2. Regarding necrotic metastases, what is the most common cell type to result in this appearance?
   A. Metastatic adenocarcinoma
   B. Metastatic squamous cell carcinoma
   C. Metastatic adenoid cystic carcinoma
   D. Metastatic mucoepidermoid carcinoma
3. Which imaging feature distinguishes a fungal abscess from a pyogenic brain abscesses?
   A. Irregular walls with intracavitary projections
   B. Dual-rim sign on SWI
   C. Presence of amino acids, acetate, and succinate on MR spectroscopy
   D. Presence of acid fast bacillus in the walls of the abscess
4. What are the most common cerebral locations for pyogenic brain abscesses?
   A. Gray–white matter junction in the distribution of the anterior or middle cerebral arteries
   B. Gray–white matter junction in the distribution of the posterior cerebral artery
   C. Brain stem
   D. Cerebellar hemispheres

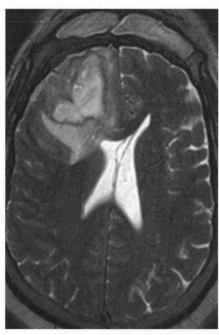

Fig. 17.1

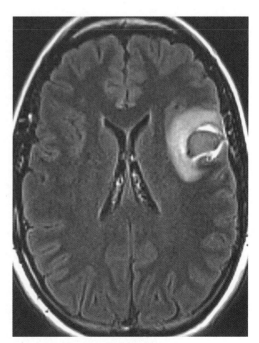

Fig. 17.2

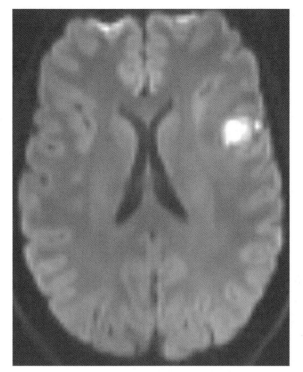

Fig. 17.3

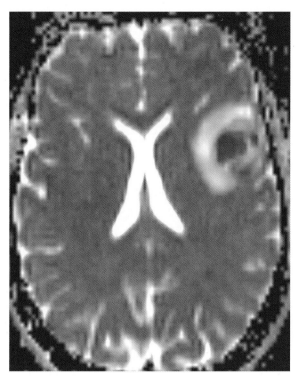

Fig. 17.4

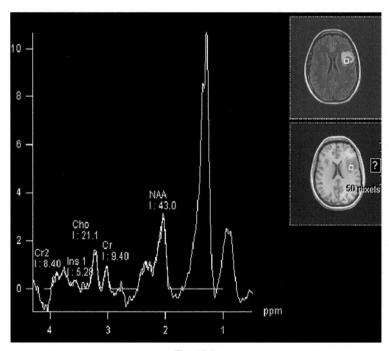

Fig. 17.5

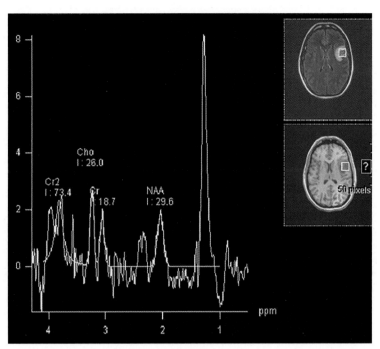

Fig. 17.6

Case 18

History: This is a 38-year-old male (Jehovah's Witness) with a past medical history of migraine who presented with sudden-onset aphasia.

1. Which is the most commonly affected vascular territory in cerebral infarction?
   A. Anterior cerebral artery (ACA)
   B. Middle cerebral artery (MCA)
   C. Posterior cerebral artery (PCA)
   D. Basilar artery
2. Which of the following are early signs of acute ischemia on an unenhanced head CT?
   A. Dense MCA sign
   B. MCA dot sign
   C. Insular ribbon sign
   D. Lentiform nucleus sign
   E. All of the above

3. Which of the following clinical signs would be expected in a patient with acute right middle cerebral artery territorial infarction?
   A. Right hemiplegia
   B. Aphasia
   C. Ataxic gait
   D. Left hemiplegia
4. Modified Treatment in Cerebral Infarction (mTICI) grading system is frequently used for patients who have undergone endovascular revascularization. What does Grade 3 reperfusion indicate?
   A. No perfusion
   B. Minimal perfusion
   C. Partial perfusion
   D. Complete perfusion

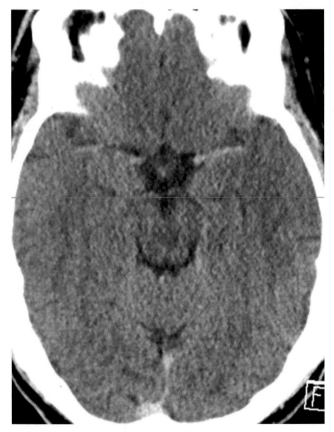

Fig. 18.1

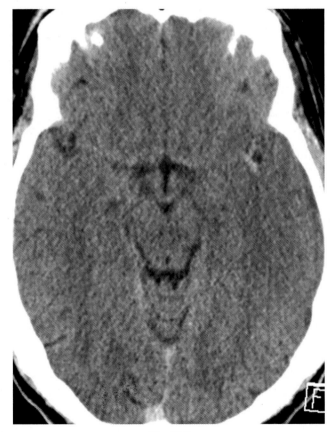

Fig. 18.2

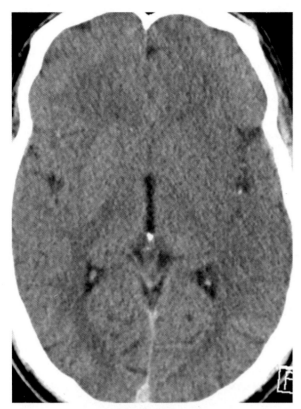

Fig. 18.3

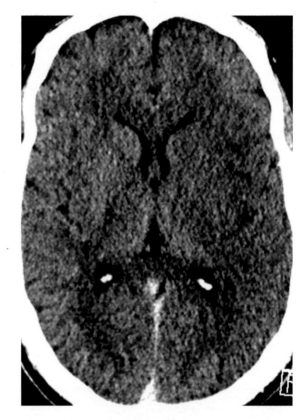

Fig. 18.4

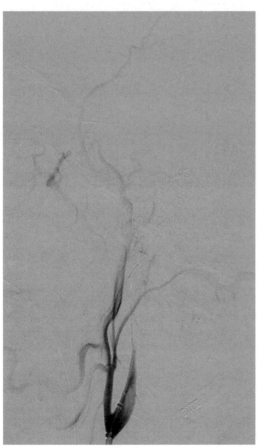

Fig. 18.5

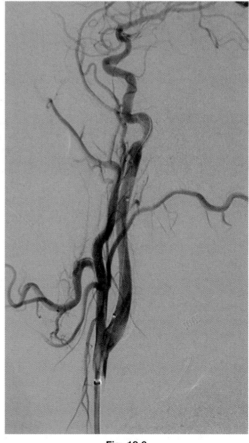

Fig. 18.6

Case 19

History: A 29-year-old female presents with intermittent dizziness and imbalance.

1. What is the most likely diagnosis?
   A. Acute disseminated encephalomyelitis
   B. Pyogenic abscess
   C. Balo's concentric sclerosis
   D. Acute infarction
2. According to the revised McDonald criteria for multiple sclerosis (2017 version), which of the following is not considered one of the four regions when assessing MRI scans for dissemination in space?
   A. Infratentorial
   B. Cortical and/or juxtacortical
   C. Periventricular
   D. Optic nerve

3. What percentage of patients with multiple sclerosis have isolated spinal cord disease?
   A. 1% to 5%
   B. 8% to 12%
   C. 40% to 50%
   D. 50% to 60%
4. Which of the following is true regarding "anti-MOG-associated encephalomyelitis"?
   A. Inflammatory disease characterized by the presence of IgG antibodies to myelin oligodendrocyte glycoprotein (MOG)
   B. No specific imaging features of anti-MOG-associated disease
   C. More common in children presenting with ADEM-like picture and young adults presenting with an NMO-like syndrome
   D. All of the above

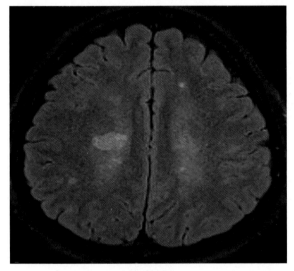

Fig. 19.1

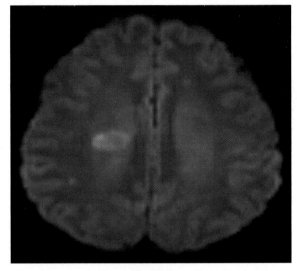

Fig. 19.2

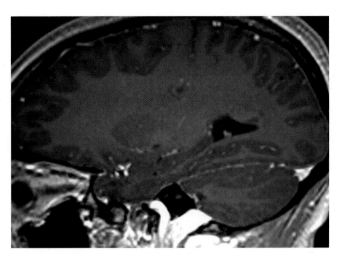

Fig. 19.3

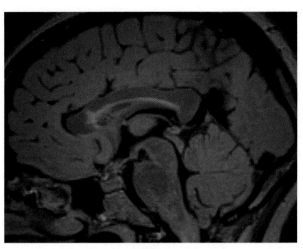

Fig. 19.4

Case 20

History: A 40-year-old male presents with a history of AML s/p chemotherapy and cranial irradiation with visual loss in the right eye.

1. What is the most likely diagnosis in this case?
   A. Pituitary macroadenoma
   B. Meningioma
   C. Chordoma
   D. Schwannoma
2. Which MR spectroscopy feature helps in distinguishing a meningioma from other dural-based mass lesions?
   A. Alanine peak at 1.48 ppm
   B. Acetate peak at 1.9 ppm
   C. 2-hydroxyglutarate at 2.25 ppm
   D. Taurine peak at 3.4 ppm
3. The dural tail sign occurs as a result of thickening and enhancement of the dura and can be seen with which of the following entities?
   A. Meningioma
   B. Pleomorphic xanthoastrocytoma (PXA)
   C. Dural plasmacytoma
   D. All of the above
4. Which of the following lesions tends to narrow arteries in the cavernous sinus?
   A. Pituitary macroadenoma
   B. Meningioma
   C. Chordoma
   D. Schwannoma

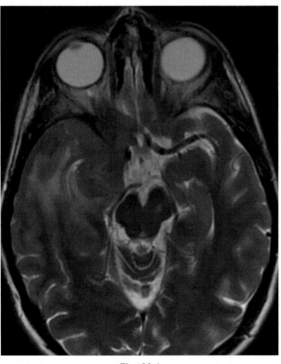

Fig. 20.1

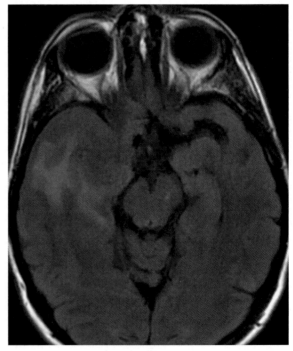

Fig. 20.2

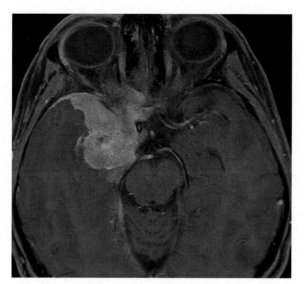

Fig. 20.3

Case 21

History: This 55-year-old male was injured in a motor vehicle crash.

1. What are the most important imaging findings in this patient's presenting head CT?
   A. Large left convexity subdural hematoma with mass effect
   B. Large acute on chronic SDH
   C. Large epidural hematoma
   D. Large, actively bleeding left convexity subdural hematoma with mass effect including left-to-right subfalcine herniation, hydrocephalus, and acute left ACA infarction
2. Which important radiological sign in the provided images represents active bleeding within the hematoma?
   A. Spot sign
   B. Swirl sign
   C. Dot sign
   D. Fluid levels
3. What are the complications of subfalcine herniation?
   A. Hydrocephalus
   B. Anterior cerebral artery (ACA) territory infarction
   C. Both
   D. None
4. Which of the following is true regarding subdural hematomas (SDHs)?
   A. Isolated interhemispheric fissure SDHs are seen more frequently in children and are common in cases of nonaccidental trauma.
   B. Vast majority of SDHs in adults are bilateral.
   C. In a SDH, the source of bleeding is usually arterial, most commonly from a ruptured middle meningeal artery.
   D. SDHs are typically biconvex in shape with mass effect and herniation.

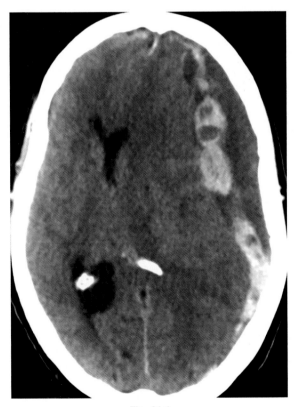

Fig. 21.1

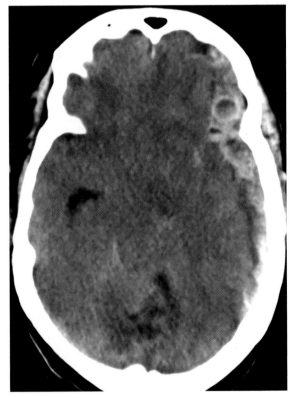

Fig. 21.2

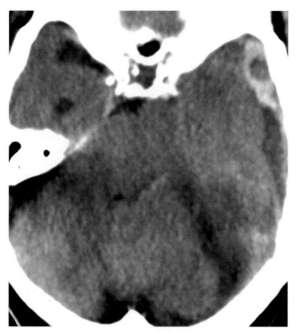

Fig. 21.3

Case 22

History: A 46-year-old female status-post unwitnessed syncopal fall.

1. What is the diagnosis?
   A. Acute multicompartment hemorrhage from a ruptured arteriovenous malformation
   B. Acute subarachnoid hemorrhage from a ruptured posterior communicating artery aneurysm
   C. Acute intraparenchymal hemorrhage from syncope and fall
   D. Acute subarachnoid hemorrhage from a ruptured anterior communicating artery aneurysm
2. What is the most common presenting symptom of aneurysmal subarachnoid hemorrhage?
   A. Syncope
   B. Fall
   C. Dizziness and giddiness
   D. Worst headache

3. Which of the following statements is correct regarding symptomatic vasospasm after aneurysmal subarachnoid hemorrhage (aSAH)?
   A. Vasospasm after aSAH is seen as narrowing of the large and medium-sized arteries most often in the anterior circulation.
   B. Presents within 3–7 days after aSAH but can occur at any time within the 21-day window following the initial hemorrhage.
   C. Hunt–Hess grade III–IV subarachnoid hemorrhages are associated with a much higher risk of subsequent severe vasospasm.
   D. All of the above
4. Aneurysms arising from which arteries may be associated with an acute-onset pupil involving third nerve palsy?
   A. Basilar tip aneurysm
   B. Posterior inferior cerebellar artery aneurysm
   C. Posterior cerebral artery aneurysm
   D. Posterior communicating artery aneurysm

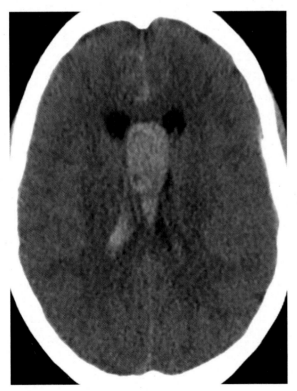

Fig. 22.1

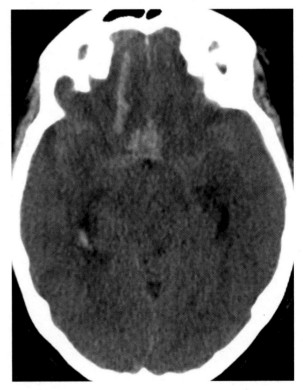

Fig. 22.2

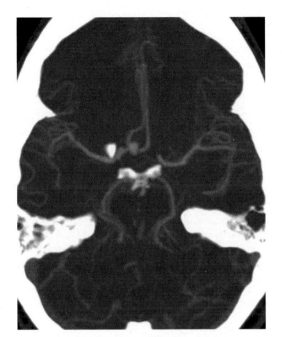

Fig. 22.3

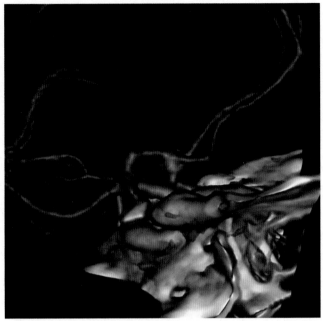

Fig. 22.4

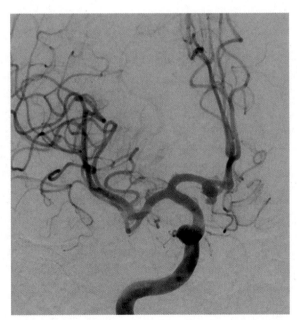

Fig. 22.5

Case 23

History: This 69-year-old female with a past medical history of malignant melanoma (left cheek, 19 years ago), hyperlipidemia, and hypertension presented with disorientation and lethargy for the past six days.

1. What is the most likely diagnosis?
   A. Metastatic melanoma
   B. Lymphoma
   C. Cerebral abscess
   D. Glioblastoma
2. What entities have a predilection for involving the corpus callosum?
   A. Lymphoma
   B. Demyelinating disease
   C. Glioblastoma
   D. All of the above
3. The patient underwent maximal safe resection, and postoperative integrated analysis of the tumor specimen revealed IDH wild-type, MGMT promotor methylated and EGFR VIII negative glioblastoma (GBM). After completing a course of external beam radiation to 6000 cGy with daily temozolomide (TMZ), she presents to the clinic to discuss the standard of care treatment options for her tumor. Standard treatment includes which of the following?
   A. Bevacizumab alone
   B. Bevacizumab plus temozolomide
   C. Temozolomide plus TTFields
   D. Immunotherapy
4. According to the revised 2016 WHO classification, GBMs are formally subdivided by the presence or absence of which mutation?
   A. Isocitrate dehydrogenase (IDH) gene
   B. 1p19q codeletion
   C. Methylation of the O6-methylguanine-DNA methyltransferase (MGMT) promoter
   D. P53

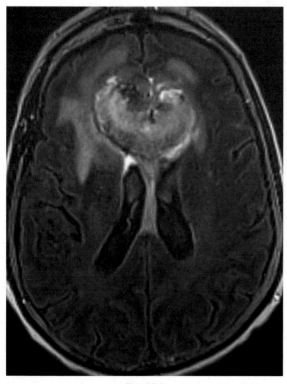

Fig. 23.1

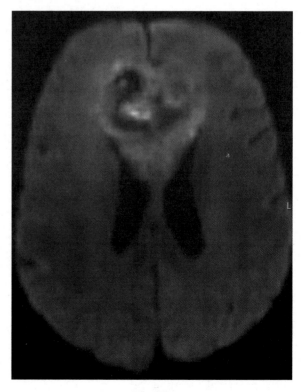

Fig. 23.2

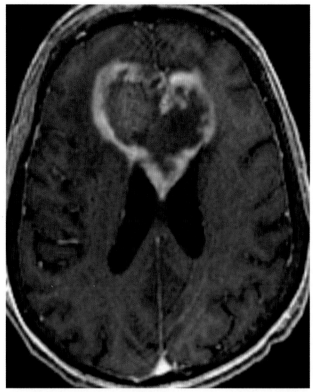

Fig. 23.3

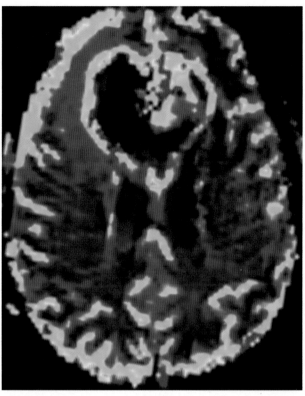

Fig. 23.4

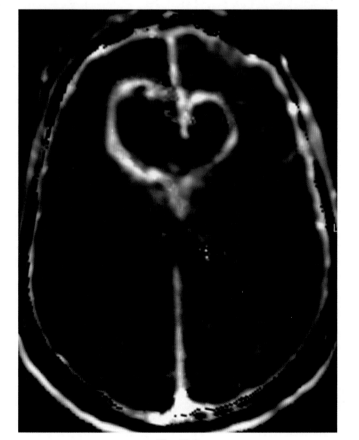

Fig. 23.5

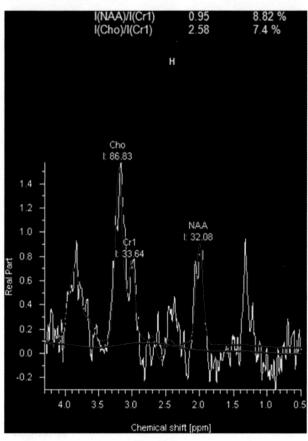

Fig. 23.6

Case 24

History:

Case 1: A 2-year-old boy was found pulseless at the scene, unknown downtime, status post prolonged CPR (Figures 24.1 to 24.4).

Case 2: A 2-month old boy presents with nonbloody, nonbilious emesis and refusal to eat which began after his father lost control of the baby, causing him to hit the kitchen countertop (Figures 24.5 and 24.6).

1. In the absence of a known significant head trauma, the radiologist must be highly suspicious of what diagnosis in Case 1?
   A. Acute leukemia
   B. Abusive head trauma
   C. Anemia
   D. Von Hippel–Lindau (VHL)

2. What are the imaging findings in Case 2?
   A. Benign enlargement of the subarachnoid spaces (BESS)
   B. Acute subdural hemorrhage
   C. Chronic subdural hemorrhage
   D. Subdural hygroma
   E. Subdural hemorrhages of different ages

3. Besides the skeletal survey, what imaging study of the head is recommended in suspected cases of child abuse in a 6-month-old baby?
   A. None. Only neurological examination is sufficient.
   B. CT head
   C. MRI head and spine
   D. Skull X-ray (four views)

4. Which of the following are included in the differential diagnosis for retinal hemorrhages in an infant?
   A. Coagulopathy
   B. Thrombocytopenia
   C. Acute leukemia
   D. Terson syndrome
   E. Bacterial meningitis
   F. Cytomegalovirus infection
   G. Accidental head trauma
   H. Abusive head trauma
   I. All of the above

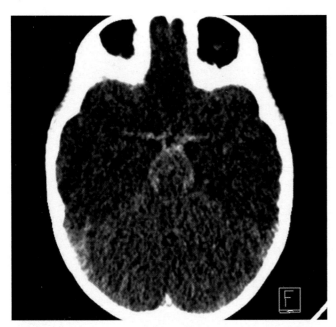

Fig. 24.1

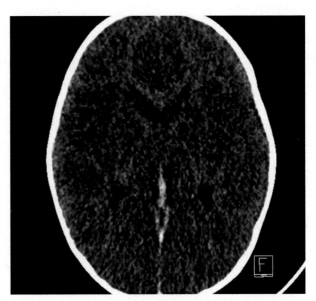

Fig. 24.2

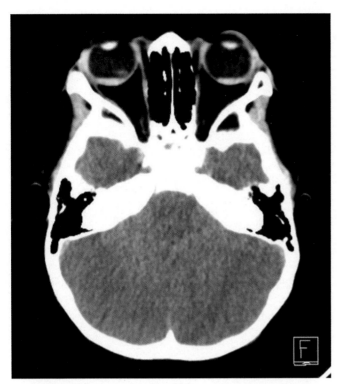

Fig. 24.3

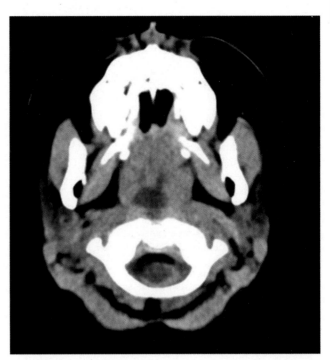

Fig. 24.4

Case 25

History: This 25-year-old male presents with dizziness.

1. What is the diagnosis?
   A. Cortical vein thrombosis
   B. Balo's concentric sclerosis
   C. Cavernous malformation
   D. Developmental venous anomaly
2. What is a mixed vascular malformation?
   A. A developmental venous anomaly and a cavernous malformation
   B. A developmental venous anomaly and a nevus flammeus
   C. A developmental venous anomaly and an arteriovenous malformation
   D. A developmental venous anomaly and a dural AF fistula

3. Thrombosed DVAs may occur under rare circumstances and can lead to which of the following?
   A. Venous congestive edema and infarction
   B. Parenchymal hemorrhage
   C. Subarachnoid hemorrhage
   D. All of the above
4. What neurocutaneous syndrome is associated with a diffuse venous malformation?
   A. Neurofibromatosis type 1
   B. Neurofibromatosis type 2
   C. Sturge–Weber syndrome
   D. Von Hippel–Lindau syndrome

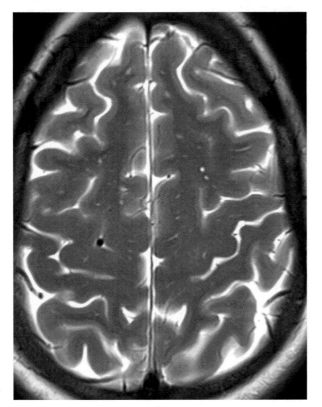

Fig. 25.1

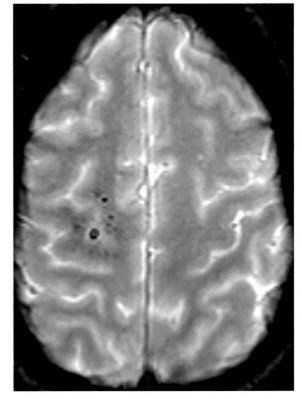

Fig. 25.2

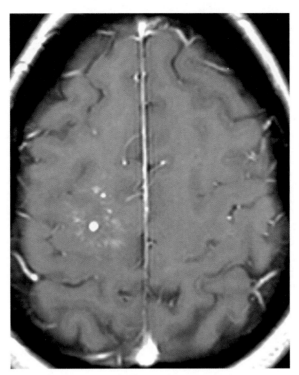

Fig. 25.3

Case 26

History: This 26-year-old female presents with irregular menses and galactorrhea.

1. What is the diagnosis?
   A. Normal pituitary gland
   B. Pituitary apoplexy
   C. Pituitary microadenoma
   D. Pituitary macroadenoma
2. Dynamic contrast-enhanced imaging improves the detection of small adenomas that demonstrate delayed enhancement compared to the rest of the pituitary gland. During dynamic contrast-enhanced imaging of the pituitary gland, which part of the anterior pituitary enhances first?
   A. Posterior
   B. Periphery
   C. Inferior
   D. Superior

3. Which of the following is true regarding pituitary apoplexy?
   A. Acute headache, ophthalmoplegia, and altered mental state in a patient with a hemorrhagic macroadenoma
   B. Bitemporal hemianopsia in a patient with macroadenoma
   C. Sudden headache with normal visual acuity in a patient with a microadenoma
   D. Asymptomatic patient with a macroadenoma with areas of high T1 signal suggesting blood or proteinaceous material
4. What treatment is associated with an increased incidence of hemorrhage within an adenoma?
   A. Bromocriptine
   B. Octreotide
   C. Steroids
   D. Ketoconazole

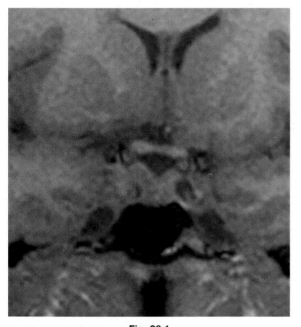

Fig. 26.1

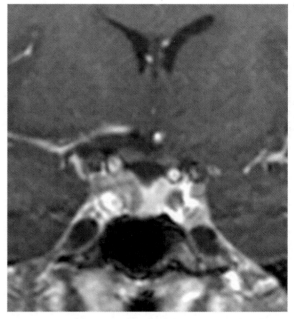

Fig. 26.2

Case 27

History: This is a 48-year-old male with unspecified epilepsy.

1. What is the most likely diagnosis?
   A. Hemorrhagic metastases
   B. Cavernous malformations
   C. Amyloid angiopathy
   D. Diffuse axonal injury
2. What do the central regions of T1W and T2W hyperintensity represent?
   A. Hemosiderin
   B. Methemoglobin
   C. Oxyhemoglobin
   D. Deoxyhemoglobin

3. Which imaging sequence is most sensitive for detecting small cavernous malformation?
   A. Magnetization-Prepared RApid Gradient Echo (MP-RAGE)
   B. Fluid-attenuated inversion recovery (FLAIR)
   C. Gradient Recalled Echo (GRE)
   D. Susceptibility-weighted imaging (SWI)
4. Multiple cavernous malformations can be seen in which of the following conditions?
   A. Mutations in KRIT1 gene
   B. Mutations in CCM2 gene
   C. Mutations in PDCD10 gene
   D. All of the above

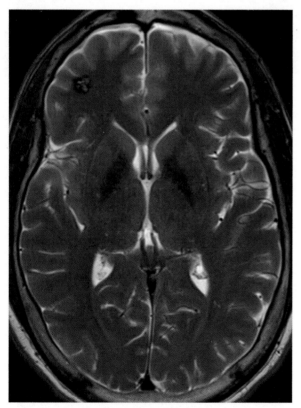

Fig. 27.1

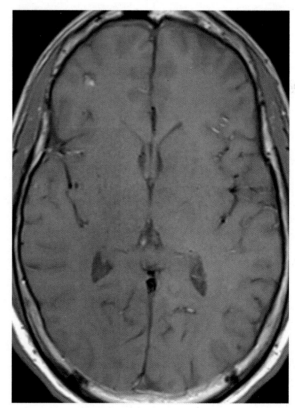

Fig. 27.2

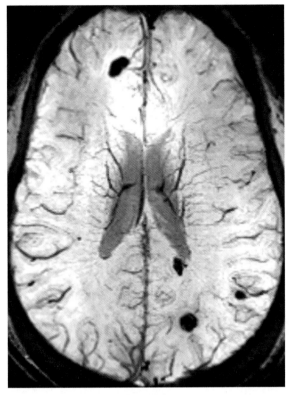

Fig. 27.3

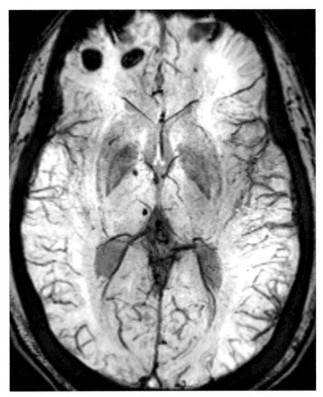

Fig. 27.4

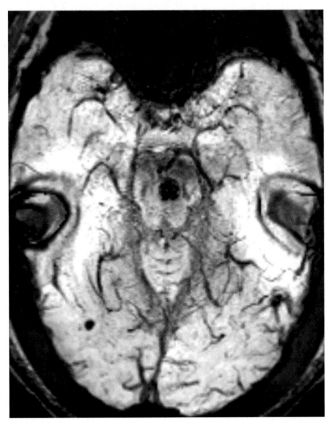

Fig. 27.5

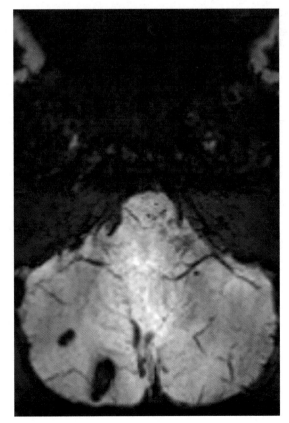

Fig. 27.6

Case 28

History: A 48-year-old man presents with a history of NF1 with worsening ataxia.

1. What is the differential diagnosis of a nonneoplastic cystic mass in the posterior fossa?
   A. Arachnoid cyst
   B. Dandy–Walker malformation
   C. Mega cisterna magna
   D. All of the above
2. Which of these cystic masses is associated with supratentorial developmental anomalies?
   A. Arachnoid cyst
   B. Dandy–Walker malformation
   C. Mega cisterna magna
   D. Blake's pouch cyst
3. What is the diagnosis in this case?
   A. Arachnoid cyst
   B. Dandy–Walker malformation
   C. Mega cisterna magna
   D. Blake's pouch cyst
4. Dandy–Walker malformation (DWM) is characterized by which of the following triad?
   A. Hypoplasia of the vermis
   B. Cystic dilatation of the fourth ventricle
   C. Enlarged posterior fossa with torcular-lambdoid inversion
   D. All of the above

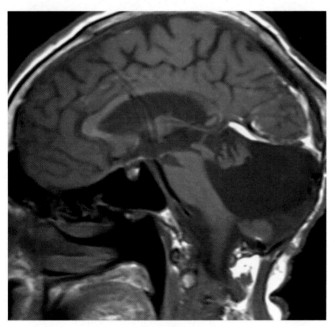

Fig. 28.1

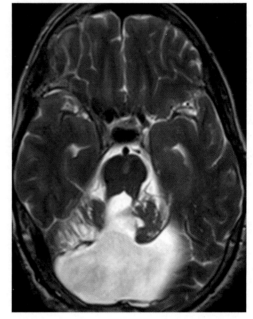

Fig. 28.2

Case 29

History: This is a 25-year-old patient with refractory epilepsy.

1. What is the most likely diagnosis?
   A. Neurofibromatosis type 1 (NF1)
   B. Neurofibromatosis type 2 (NF2)
   C. Tuberous sclerosis
   D. Von Hippel–Lindau syndrome
2. What benign neoplasm is associated with this syndrome?
   A. Juvenile pilocytic astrocytoma
   B. Optic nerve glioma
   C. Diffuse brainstem glioma
   D. Subependymal giant cell astrocytoma

3. What is the CNS imaging hallmark seen in 90% of patients with tuberous sclerosis?
   A. Cortical and subcortical tubers
   B. Subependymal hamartomas
   C. Subependymal giant cell astrocytomas
   D. Cerebellar atrophy
4. Which organ systems in addition to the CNS are affected in patients with tuberous sclerosis?
   A. Heart
   B. Lungs
   C. Kidneys
   D. All of the above

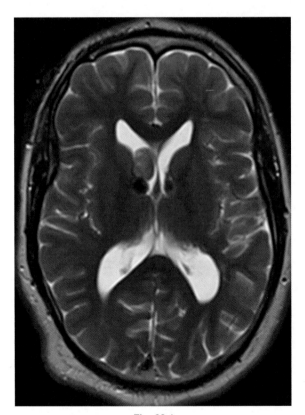

Fig. 29.1

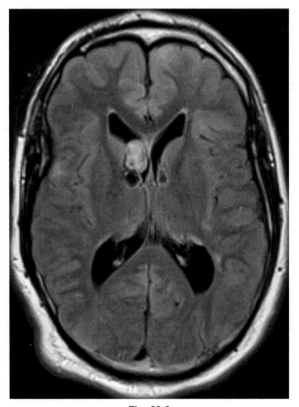

Fig. 29.2

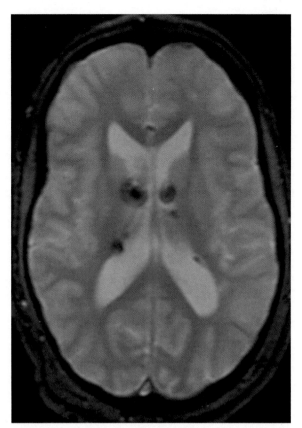

Fig. 29.3

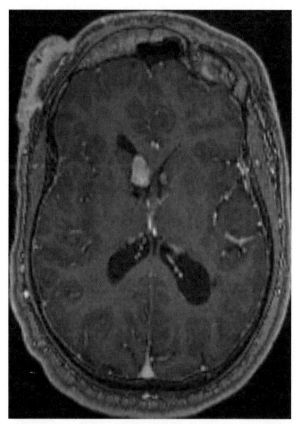

Fig. 29.4

Case 30

History: This 35-year-old male presents with congenital hydrocephalus and seizures.

1. What is the most likely diagnosis?
   A. Porencephalic cysts
   B. Schizencephaly
   C. Arachnoid cyst
   D. Holoprosencephaly
2. Which tissue lines the CSF-filled open-lip schizencephaly?
   A. Normal white matter
   B. Gliotic white matter
   C. Normal gray matter
   D. Polymicrogyric gray matter
3. Which tissue lines the porencephalic cyst?
   A. Normal white matter
   B. Gliotic white matter
   C. Normal gray matter
   D. Polymicrogyric gray matter
4. Porencephalic cysts are thought to occur from focal encephalomalacia due to a localized cerebral insult most frequently during early gestation. Which of the following can be potential causes of this entity?
   A. Cerebral ischemia and hemorrhage
   B. Trauma
   C. Infection
   D. Familial porencephaly with mutations in the COL4A1 gene
   E. All of the above

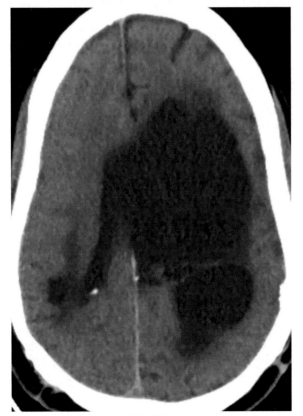

Fig. 30.1

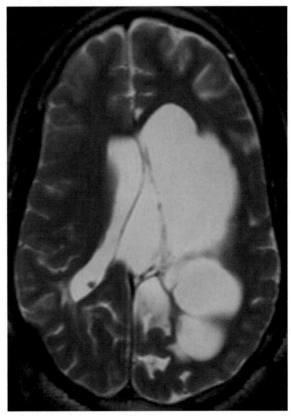

Fig. 30.2

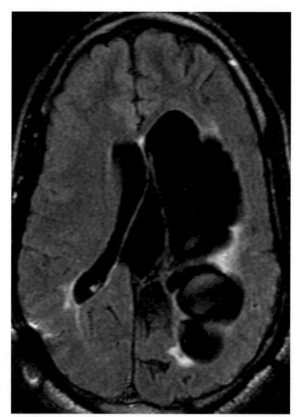

Fig. 30.3

Case 31

History: This 26-year-old woman with a history of bilateral renal cell carcinoma, pheochromocytoma, and Whipple's resection for pancreatic neuroendocrine tumors presents with worsening occipital headache associated with nausea and vomiting.

1. What is the most likely diagnosis in this patient?
   A. Metastasis
   B. Hemangioblastoma
   C. Pilocytic astrocytoma
   D. Glioblastoma
2. What is the most common cerebellar "mass" in adults?
   A. Metastasis
   B. Hemangioblastoma
   C. Pilocytic astrocytoma
   D. Subacute infarct

3. What imaging feature/s helps to distinguish a hemangioblastoma from a pilocytic astrocytoma?
   A. Presence of flow voids
   B. Lack of enhancement in the cyst wall
   C. Both
   D. None
4. What neurocutaneous syndrome is associated with multiple hemangioblastomas?
   A. Neurofibromatosis type 1 (NF 1)
   B. Neurofibromatosis type 2 (NF 2)
   C. Tuberous sclerosis
   D. Von Hippel–Lindau syndrome

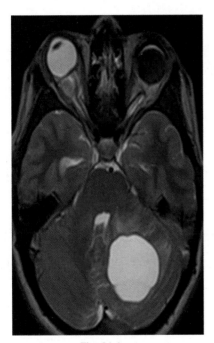

Fig. 31.1

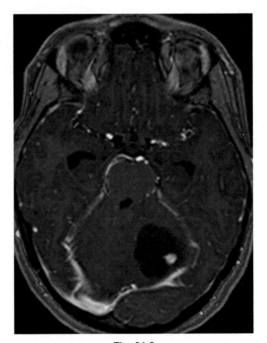

Fig. 31.2

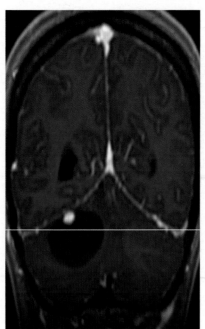

Fig. 31.3

Case 32

History: This is a 78-year-old patient with a history of shuffling gait, bradykinesia, and incontinence.

1. What is the diagnosis?
   A. Parkinson's disease
   B. Normal-pressure hydrocephalus (NPH)
   C. Alzheimer's disease
   D. Lewy body disease
2. The callosal angle has been proposed as a useful imaging marker for idiopathic normal-pressure hydrocephalus (iNPH). Which of the following is correct regarding callosal angle in iNPH?
   A. It is helpful in distinguishing ex-vacuo ventriculomegaly from central brain atrophy.
   B. It is measured on a coronal image perpendicular to the level of the posterior commissure.
   C. Patients with iNPH have acute callosal angles less than 90 degrees, while those with atrophy have callosal angles greater than 90 degrees.
   D. All of the above

3. Disproportionately enlarged subarachnoid space hydrocephalus (DESH) is a recently described pattern of communicating hydrocephalus classically seen in which of the following conditions?
   A. Parkinson's disease
   B. Normal-pressure hydrocephalus
   C. Alzheimer's disease
   D. External hydrocephalus
4. Treatment of established NPH involves CSF shunting, usually a ventriculoperitoneal shunt (VP shunt). Which of the following are favorable prognostic factors for identifying patients who will benefit from shunting?
   A. Short duration of symptoms
   B. Gait disturbance as a primary symptom
   C. Symptom relief from a CSF tap test
   D. Absence of significant cerebral vascular disease
   E. All of the above

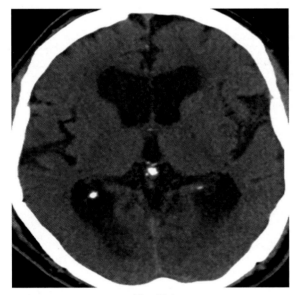

Fig. 32.1

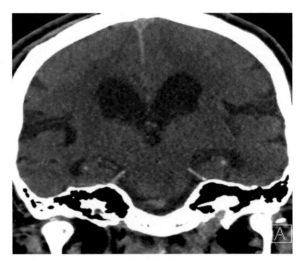

Fig. 32.2

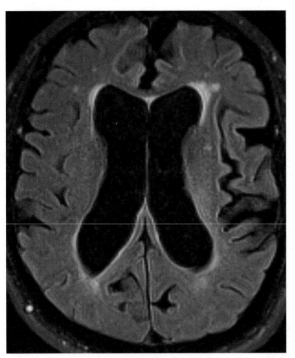

Fig. 32.3

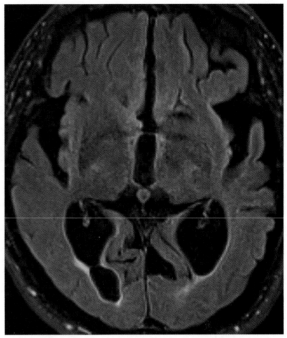

Fig. 32.4

Case 33

History: A 72-year-old female with stage IV serous fallopian tube cancer, staging studies.

1. What is the most likely diagnosis?
   A. Hemorrhagic metastasis
   B. Thrombosed inferior sagittal sinus
   C. Lipoma of corpus callosum
   D. Craniopharyngioma
2. What is the most common presenting symptom?
   A. Seizures
   B. Headache
   C. Dizziness
   D. Recurrent syncopal episodes

3. What other MR imaging finding(s) are helpful in confirming that the intracranial mass is composed of fat?
   A. Diffusion-weighted imaging (DWI)
   B. Fat-suppressed T1-weighted images
   C. Chemical shift artifact on T2-weighted image
   D. All of the above

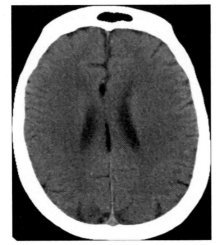

Fig. 33.1

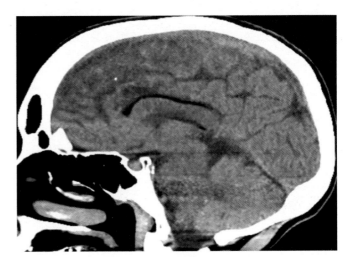

Fig. 33.2

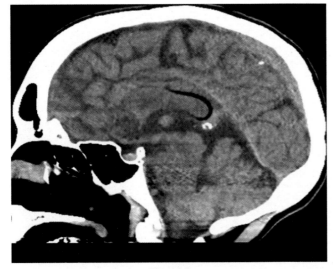

Fig. 33.3

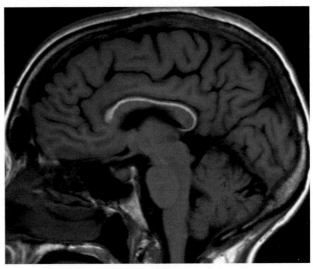

Fig. 33.4

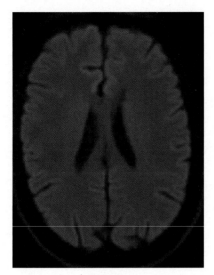

Fig. 33.5

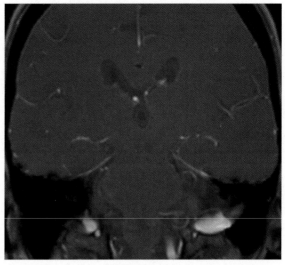

Fig. 33.6

Case 34

History: A 44-year-old with polycystic kidney disease. TOF MRA screening for berry aneurysm.

1. What is the diagnosis?
   A. Intracranial arterial fenestration
   B. Basilar tip aneurysm
   C. Intracranial arterial dissection
   D. Normal MRA
2. Which of the following is true regarding basilar artery fenestration?
   A. Increased incidence of basilar artery aneurysm formation at the site of fenestration
   B. Increased incidence of basilar artery dissection at the site of fenestration
   C. Increased risk of midbrain stroke
   D. Increased risk of pontine stroke
3. Which branch of the basilar artery may extend into the internal auditory canal?
   A. Anterior inferior cerebellar artery
   B. Posterior inferior cerebellar artery
   C. Posterior cerebral artery
   D. Superior cerebellar artery
4. What aneurysm may rupture into the fourth ventricle?
   A. Anterior inferior cerebellar artery
   B. Posterior inferior cerebellar artery
   C. Posterior cerebral artery
   D. Superior cerebellar artery

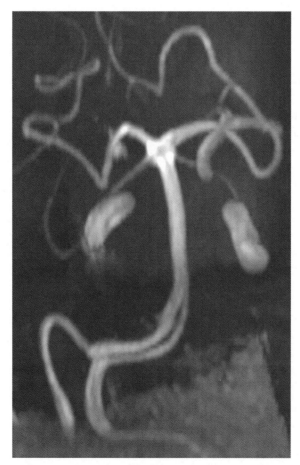

Fig. 34.1

Case 35

History: This is a 55-year-old patient with a history of sinus pressure and headaches.

1. What is the diagnosis in this patient?
   A. Acute right maxillary sinusitis
   B. Chronic left maxillary sinusitis
   C. Chronic right maxillary sinusitis
   D. Acute left maxillary sinusitis
2. What is the most common cause of new-onset acute sinusitis?
   A. Viral upper respiratory tract infection
   B. Dental caries
   C. Cystic fibrosis
   D. Seasonal allergies
3. Which of the following can be a manifestation of coronavirus infection?
   A. Fever
   B. Headache
   C. Cough
   D. Loss of taste and smell
   E. All of the above
4. Which of the following is true regarding concha bullosa of the middle turbinate?
   A. The air space within the turbinate is susceptible to the same pathologies as other sinuses, and may become infected, obstructed, or be the site of malignancy.
   B. Associated with deviation of the nasal septum away from the concha bullosa
   C. One of the most common variations of sinonasal anatomy
   D. All of the above

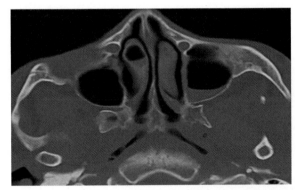

Fig. 35.1

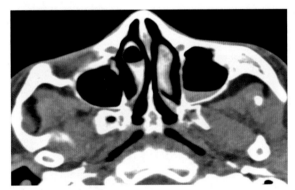

Fig. 35.2

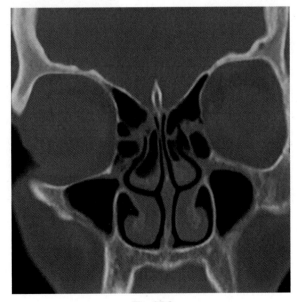

Fig. 35.3

Case 36

History: This 56-year-old female attempted suicide by beta-blocker overdose.

1. Which of the following conditions can present with basal ganglia calcification?
   A. Idiopathic
   B. Fahr disease
   C. Mineralizing microangiopathy
   D. Hypoparathyroidism
   E. Pseudohypoparathyroidism
   F. Pseudopseudohypoparathyroidism
   G. Hyperparathyroidism
   H. Hypothyroidism
   I. Down syndrome
   J. All of the above
2. Which TORCH infection is typically associated with periventricular calcification?
   A. Toxoplasmosis
   B. Other (syphilis, varicella-zoster, parvovirus B19)
   C. Rubella
   D. Cytomegalovirus (CMV)
   E. Herpes simplex virus (HSV)
3. Carbon monoxide poisoning classically affects which deep gray matter nucleus?
   A. Caudate nucleus
   B. Globus pallidus
   C. Putamen
   D. Subthalamic nucleus
4. What is the characteristic pattern of calcium deposition in Fahr disease?
   A. Basal ganglia
   B. Basal ganglia and dentate nuclei
   C. Basal ganglia, dentate nuclei, and white matter
   D. Basal ganglia, cerebellar dentate nuclei, white matter, and cortical gray matter

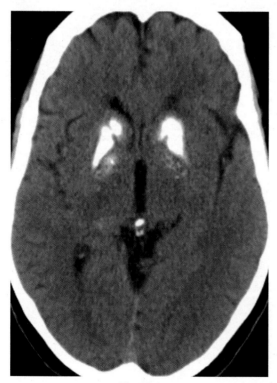

Fig. 36.1

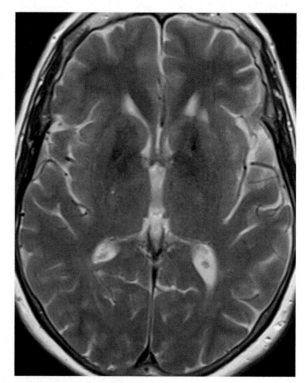

Fig. 36.2

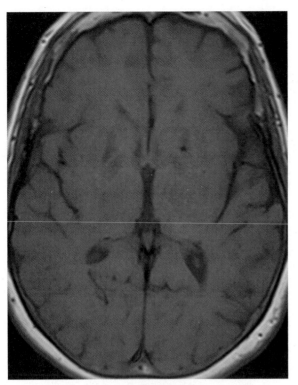

Fig. 36.3

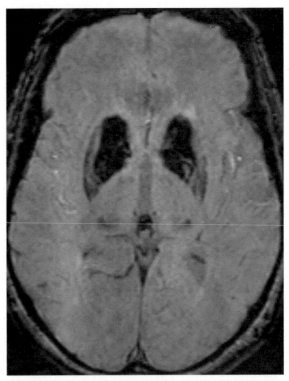

Fig. 36.4

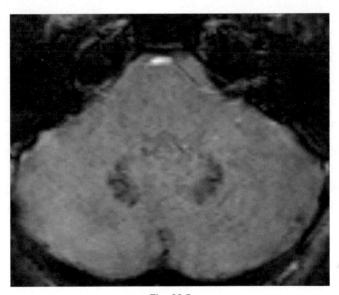

Fig. 36.5

Case 37

History: This 49-year-old female presents with a right facial skin lesion with new-onset vertigo with nausea, but no vomiting.

1. What is the most likely diagnosis?
   A. Neurofibromatosis type 1 (NF 1)
   B. Neurofibromatosis type 2 (NF 2)
   C. Tuberous sclerosis
   D. Sturge–Weber syndrome
   E. Von Hippel–Lindau syndrome
2. What is the classic cutaneous manifestation of this phakomatosis, and in what distribution does it typically occur?
   A. Nevus flammeus
   B. Café au lait spots
   C. Shagreen patch
   D. Ash-leaf spots

3. What is the inheritance pattern of this neurocutaneous disorder?
   A. Sporadic
   B. Autosomal dominant
   C. Autosomal recessive
   D. X-linked dominant
   E. X-linked recessive

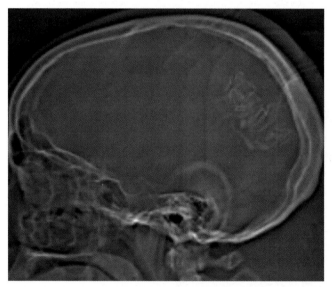

Fig. 37.1

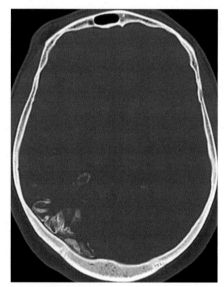

Fig. 37.2

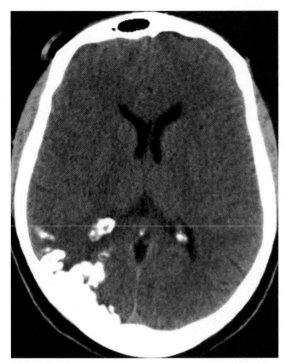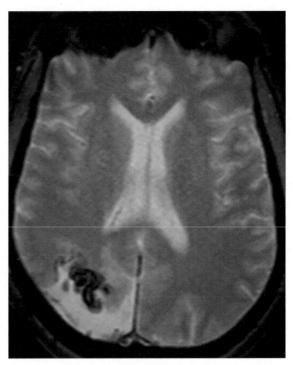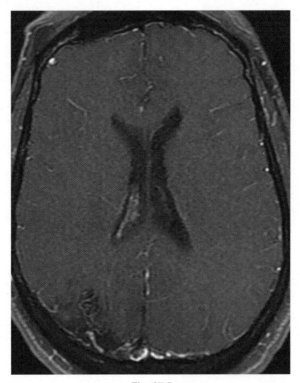

Fig. 37.3

Fig. 37.4

Fig. 37.5

Case 38

History: This is a 24-year-old female with increasing headaches and behavioral abnormalities.

1. What is the most likely diagnosis?
   A. Optic neuritis and likely multiple sclerosis
   B. Optic glioma and likely NF1
   C. Optic neuritis and likely neuromyelitis optica
   D. Optic glioma and likely NF2
2. What are common locations in which nonneoplastic T2W lesions may be identified in neurofibromatosis type 1?
   A. Basal ganglia
   B. Brainstem
   C. Cerebellar peduncles
   D. Dentate nuclei
   E. All of the above
3. What is the histologic subtype of optic pathway gliomas associated with neurofibromatosis type 1?
   A. Ganglioglioma
   B. Pilocytic astrocytoma
   C. Diffuse midline glioma
   D. Glioblastoma
4. RASopathies are a class of disorders caused by germline mutations in genes encoding for components of the RASs/mitogen-activated protein kinase (MAPK) pathway. Which of the following is not a RASopathy?
   A. Costello syndrome
   B. Neurofibromatosis type 1
   C. Neurofibromatosis type 2
   D. Noonan syndrome

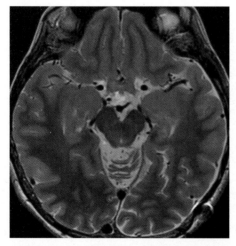

Fig. 38.1

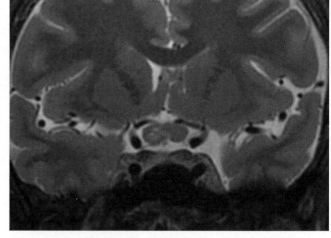

Fig. 38.2

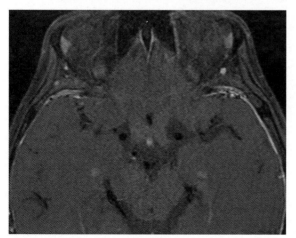

Fig. 38.3

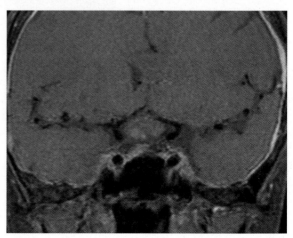

Fig. 38.4

Case 39

History: A 54-year-old man with a history of hypertension, hyperlipidemia, and alcohol use presents with acute liver and renal failure, and persistent altered mental status.

1. What is the most likely diagnosis?
   A. Superior sagittal sinus thrombosis
   B. Posterior reversible encephalopathy syndrome
   C. Brain stem encephalitis
   D. Osmotic demyelination
2. What is most common imaging abnormality in patients with PRES?
   A. Reversible cerebral edema
   B. Vasogenic edema
   C. Cytotoxic edema
   D. Interstitial edema
3. Severe PRES is characterized by which of the following?
   A. Frontal lobe involvement
   B. Presence of hemorrhage on GRE
   C. Presence of diffusion restriction
   D. Vasogenic edema extending from the cortex to the periventricular white matter with midline shift and involvement of cerebellum, brain stem, and basal ganglia

4. Hypertensive microangiopathy, also known as chronic hypertensive encephalopathy, presents with which of the following conditions?
   A. Microhemorrhages in the basal ganglia, brain stem, and cerebellum
   B. Microhemorrhages in the parietal and occipital lobes
   C. Superficial siderosis
   D. Subarachnoid hemorrhage

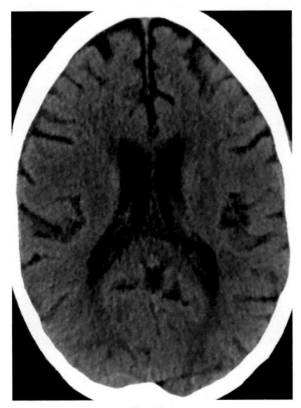

Fig. 39.1

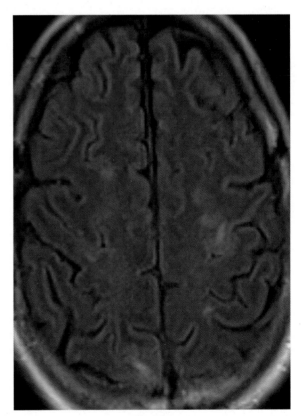

Fig. 39.2

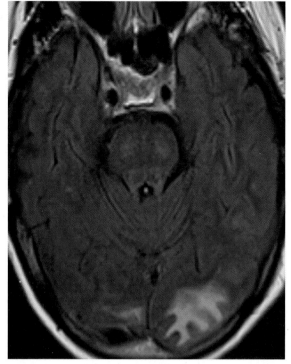

Fig. 39.3

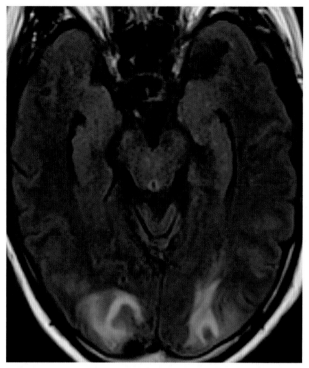

Fig. 39.4

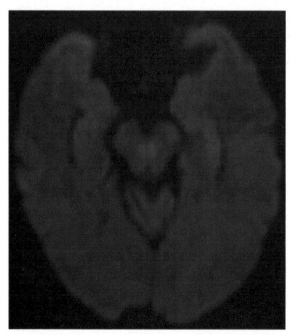

Fig. 39.5

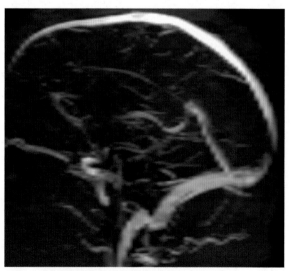

Fig. 39.6

Case 40

History: This 42-year-old patient with a history of polysubstance abuse presents with persistent dizziness and nausea.

1. What would be your recommendation based on these imaging findings?
   A. Stroke alert, page neuro IR for emergent thrombectomy
   B. Visual field testing and workup for possible multiple sclerosis
   C. Start heparin drip for deep cerebral vein thrombosis
   D. Administer vitamin B1
2. What is the diagnosis?
   A. Artery of Percheron infarction
   B. Deep cerebral vein thrombosis
   C. Osmotic demyelination
   D. Wernicke encephalopathy

3. Atypical imaging findings of Wernicke encephalopathy which include the cerebral cortex, corpus callosum, basal ganglia, cerebellum, and dorsal medulla (lower cranial nerve nuclei), are described in patients with:
   A. History of prolonged alcohol abuse
   B. Nonalcoholic patients
   C. Long-standing malnutrition secondary to malignancy
   D. All of the above
4. What of the following conditions can result in bilateral thalamic signal abnormalities?
   A. Artery of Percheron infarction
   B. Deep cerebral vein thrombosis
   C. Variant Creutzfeldt–Jakob disease
   D. Wernicke encephalopathy
   E. All of the above

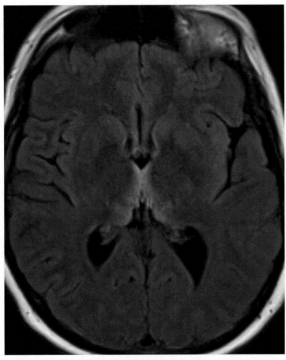

Fig. 40.1

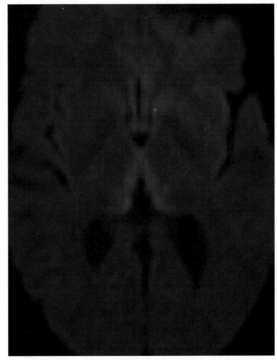

Fig. 40.2

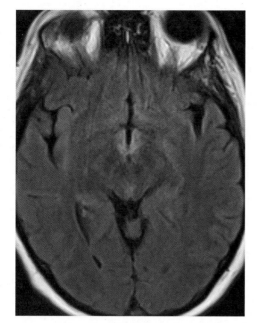

Fig. 40.3

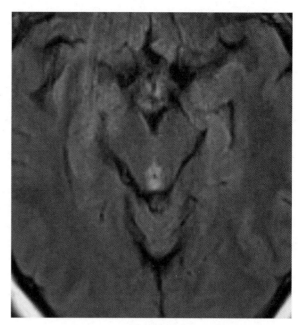

Fig. 40.4

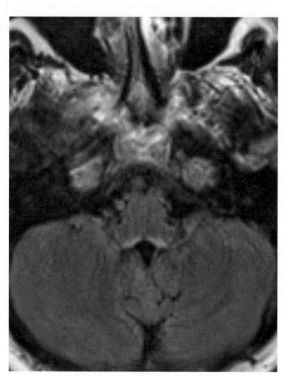

Fig. 40.5

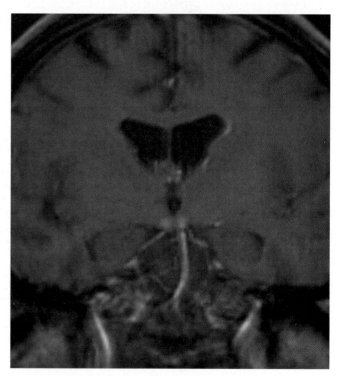

Fig. 40.6

Case 41

History: A 72-year-old female with ETOH abuse presents with gait unsteadiness, imbalance, and pseudobulbar affect.

1. What is the most likely diagnosis?
   A. Artery of Percheron infarction
   B. Deep cerebral vein thrombosis
   C. Osmotic demyelination syndrome
   D. Wernicke encephalopathy
2. Pseudobulbar palsy results from bilateral upper motor neuron brainstem lesions and is clinically characterized by which of the following?
   A. Dysarthria
   B. Dysphagia
   C. Hyperactive gag reflex
   D. Labile emotional responses
   E. All of the above

3. This condition is frequently associated with overzealous correction of what electrolyte abnormality?
   A. Sodium
   B. Potassium
   C. Magnesium
   D. Calcium
4. What other finding is seen on the axial T1-weighted images?
   A. Extrapontine myelinolysis
   B. Acute hemorrhage
   C. Physiologic calcification
   D. Manganese deposition from chronic liver disease

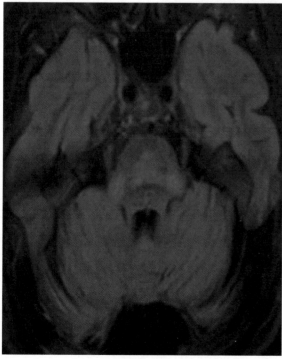

Fig. 41.1

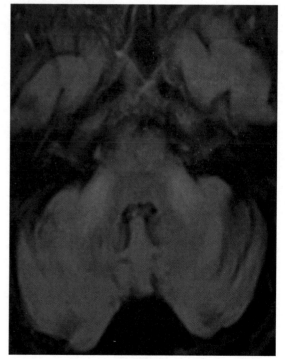

Fig. 41.2

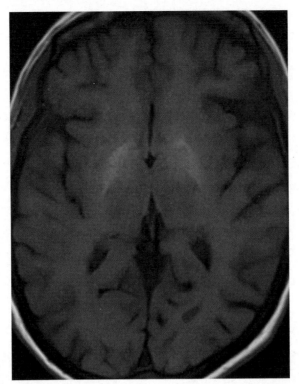

Fig. 41.3

Case 42

History: This is a 35-year-old patient with headache.

1. What is the diagnosis?
   A. Acute intraventricular hemorrhage
   B. Pituitary apoplexy
   C. Rathke's cleft cyst
   D. Colloid cyst
2. The arrow on image 42.2 points to what structure?
   A. Colloid cyst
   B. Mammillary body
   C. Pineal gland
   D. Anterior commissure
3. What is the precise anatomic location of these lesions?
   A. Interventricular foramen of Monro
   B. Anterosuperior portion of the third ventricle
   C. Posteroinferior portion of the third ventricle
   D. Frontal horn of the lateral ventricle
4. What would be your management recommendation in this case?
   A. Observation
   B. Stereotactic radiosurgery
   C. Neurosurgical resection
   D. CSF shunting

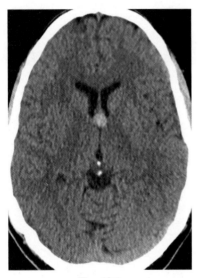

Fig. 42.1

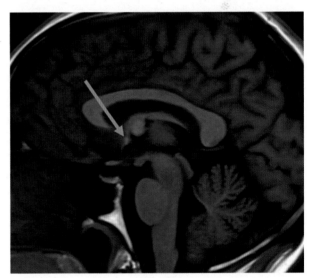

Fig. 42.2

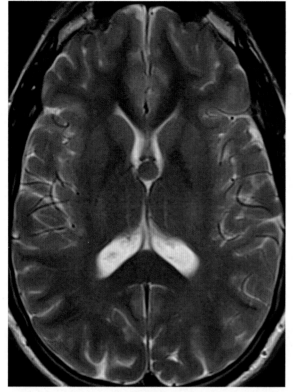

Fig. 42.3

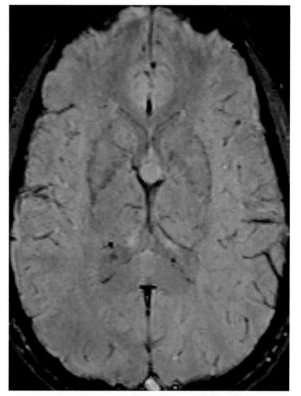

Fig. 42.4

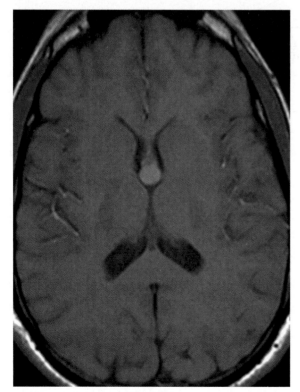

Fig. 42.5

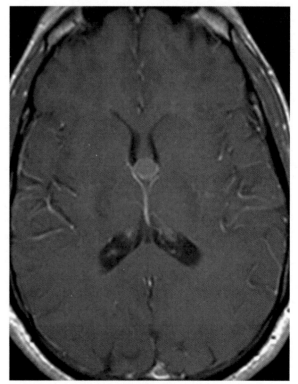

Fig. 42.6

Case 43

History:

Patient 1: 19-year-old male presents with a new-onset seizure (Figures ?).

Patient 2: 18-year-old male presents with headache and feelings of lightheadedness and slowed response (Figures?).

1. What is the most likely diagnosis for patient 1?
   A. Brain abscess
   B. Glioblastoma
   C. Tumefactive demyelination
   D. Pilocytic astrocytoma
   E. Hemangioblastoma
2. What is the differential diagnosis of a cystic mass with an eccentric mural nodule?
   A. Hemangioblastoma
   B. Pilocytic astrocytoma
   C. Ganglioglioma
   D. Pleomorphic xanthoastrocytoma
   E. All of the above

3. What is the common location of a pilocytic astrocytoma in a young adult?
   A. Optic nerve
   B. Parietal lobe
   C. Frontal lobe
   D. Cerebellum
4. What disorder is associated with pilocytic astrocytomas involving the visual pathway?
   A. Neurofibromatosis type 1 (NF1)
   B. Neurofibromatosis type 2 (NF2)
   C. Von Hippel–Lindau (VHL)
   D. Tuberous sclerosis (TS)

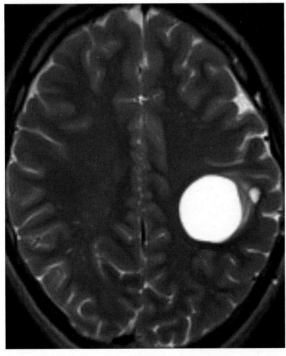

Fig. 43.1

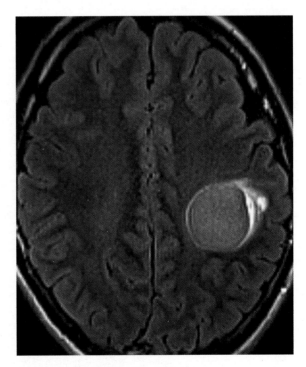

Fig. 43.2

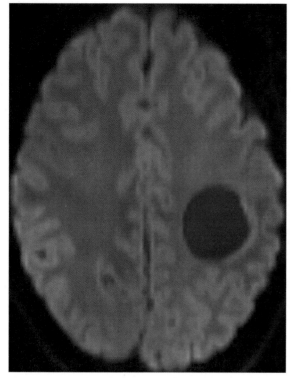

Fig. 43.3

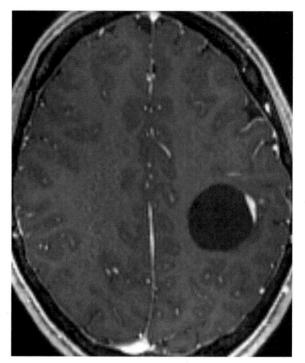

Fig. 43.4

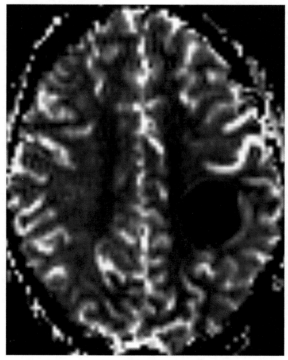

Fig. 43.5

Case 44

History: This 60-year-old female with type 2 diabetes mellitus presents with a swollen red eye and purulent drainage.

1. Which of the following is true regarding preseptal orbital cellulitis?
   A. Inflammation extends posterior to the orbital septum
   B. Managed with IV antibiotics
   C. The most common cause is a bug bite
   D. The most common cause in ethmoid sinusitis
2. Which of the following is/are true regarding postseptal orbital cellulitis?
   A. Inflammation extends posterior to the orbital septum
   B. Managed with IV antibiotics
   C. The most common cause is sinusitis
   D. All of the above
3. What is the diagnosis in this case?
   A. Preseptal orbital cellulitis
   B. Orbital pseudotumor
   C. Orbital cellulitis and abscess
   D. Orbital lymphoma
4. Which of the following is true regarding orbital compartment syndrome (OCS)?
   A. The most common cause is posttraumatic retrobulbar hemorrhage.
   B. Manifests as severe proptosis with tenting of the posterior globe and stretching of the optic nerve.
   C. It is a clinical diagnosis, and emergent canthotomy and orbital decompression are needed as just 60–100 minutes of elevated pressure can cause permanent vision loss.
   D. All of the above

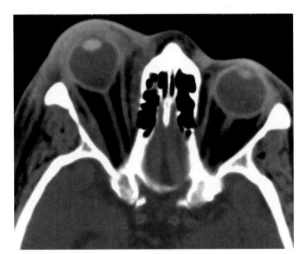

Fig. 44.1

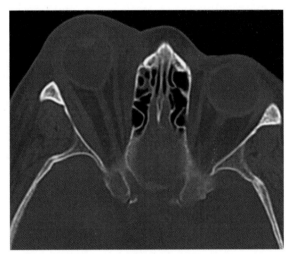

Fig. 44.2

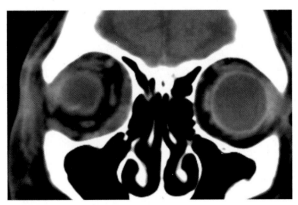

Fig. 44.3

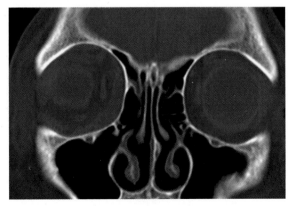

Fig. 44.4

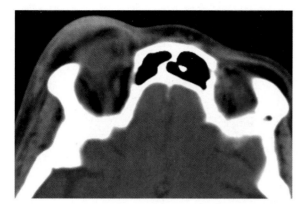

Fig. 44.5

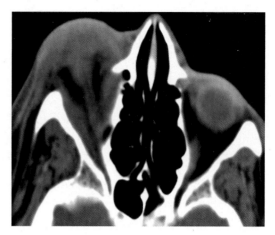

Fig. 44.6

Case 45

History: This is a 59-year-old male with COPD and intermittent headaches.

1. What is the most likely diagnosis?
   A. Superior sagittal sinus thrombosis
   B. Normal study
   C. Acute meningitis
   D. Subdural hemorrhage
2. Bilateral subacute subdural hematomas can be difficult to detect on CT particularly when they become isodense to the adjacent brain parenchyma. Which of the following imaging feature(s) can be helpful in its identification?
   A. CSF-filled sulci do not reach the inner table of the calvarium
   B. Mass effect including sulcal and ventricular effacement and midline shift
   C. Apparent thickening of the cortex
   D. All of the above

3. What are the MR imaging signal characteristics of subacute (weeks to months old) hematomas?
   A. Isointense on T1 and T2
   B. Hypointense on T1 and T2
   C. Hyperintense on T1 and T2
   D. Hypointense on T2 and FLAIR

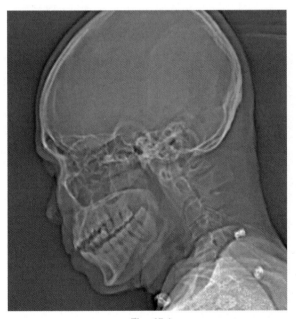

Fig. 45.1

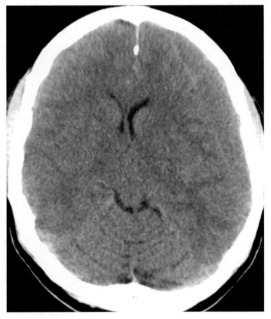

Fig. 45.2

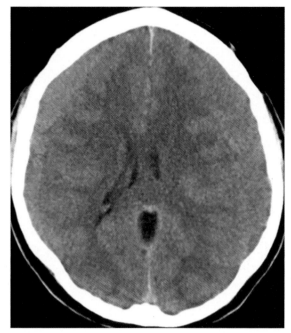

Fig. 45.3

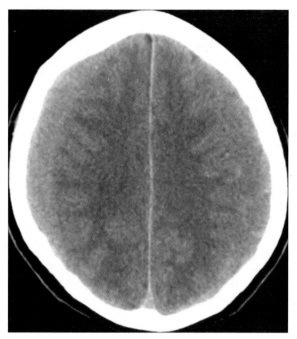

Fig. 45.4

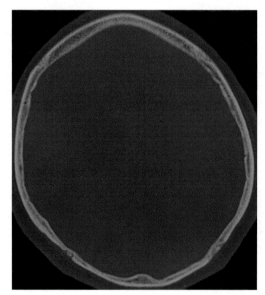

Fig. 45.5

Case 46

History: This 55-year-old right-handed female presents with high fever, repeated vomiting, and a strange sensation throughout her whole body.

1. What is the diagnosis?
   A. Status epilepticus
   B. Herpes simplex encephalitis
   C. Subacute left MCA infarction
   D. Limbic encephalitis
2. Which of the following imaging features is helpful in distinguishing herpes simplex encephalitis from middle cerebral artery infarction?
   A. Reduced diffusion in the acute phase
   B. Gyriform enhancement in the subacute phase
   C. Mass effect and cerebral swelling
   D. Sparing of the basal ganglia structures

3. Which herpes simplex virus is responsible for causing neonatal herpes simplex encephalitis?
   A. HSV-2
   B. HSV-1
   C. HSV 1 and 2
   D. Flavivirus
4. The arrow in Figure 46.5 points to which anatomical structure?
   A. Superior frontal gyrus
   B. Fusiform gyrus
   C. Inferior frontal gyrus
   D. Cingulate gyrus

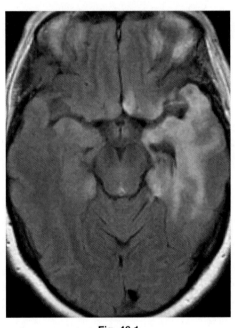

Fig. 46.1

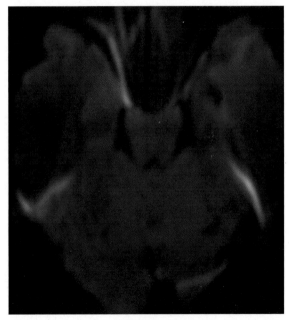

Fig. 46.2

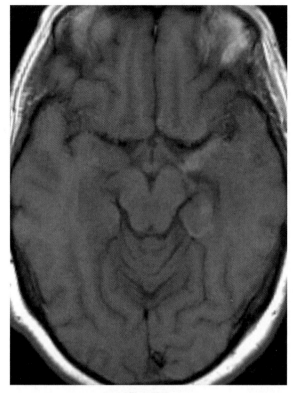

Fig. 46.3

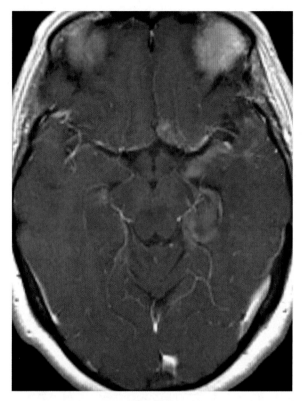

Fig. 46.4

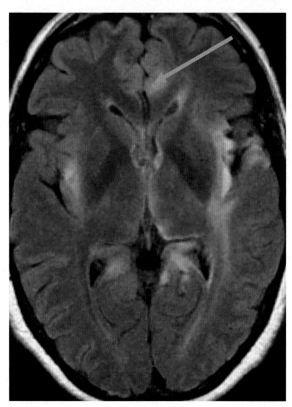

Fig. 46.5

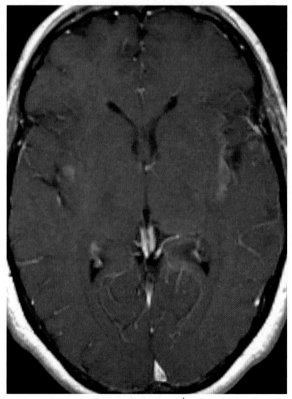

Fig. 46.6

Case 47

History: A 62-year-old man status post PEA arrest two days ago reportedly in myoclonic status epilepticus.

1. What is the diagnosis?
   A. Normal study
   B. Hypoglycemia
   C. Hypoxic ischemic encephalopathy
   D. Viral encephalitis
2. Which of the following radiographic signs is not associated with hypoxic-ischemic encephalopathy?
   A. White cerebellum sign
   B. Pseudosubarachnoid hemorrhage sign
   C. Reversal sign
   D. Hot nose sign
   E. Insular ribbon sign
3. Which of the following is true regarding brain death?
   A. Conventional angiography is considered the gold standard imaging test demonstrating no forward flow above the terminal internal carotid arteries.
   B. Nonvisualization of the intracranial vessels on a CT or MR angiography
   C. Increased external carotid artery perfusion to the nasal region, "hot nose sign," on radionuclide blood flow scans
   D. All of the above

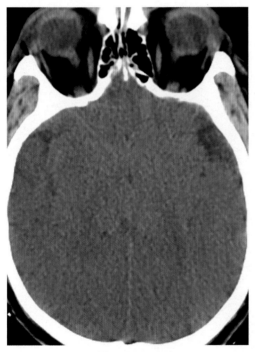

Fig. 47.1

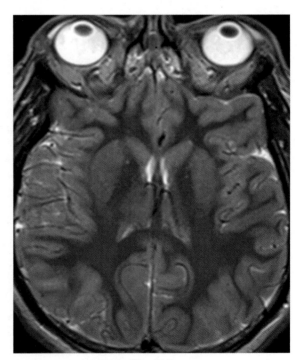

Fig. 47.2

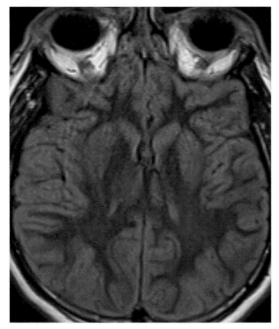

Fig. 47.3

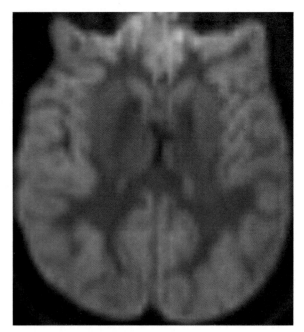

Fig. 47.4

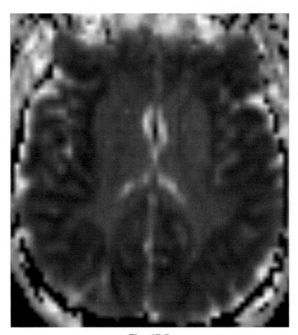

Fig. 47.5

Case 48

History: This 27-year-old female presents for the evaluation of seizures.

1. What is the diagnosis in this patient?
   A. Chiari I malformation
   B. Chiari II malformation
   C. Chiari III malformation
   D. Chiari IV malformation
2. Which of the following signs are classically described in these patients on ultrasonography?
   A. Apple sign
   B. Strawberry sign
   C. Banana sign
   D. Watermelon sign

3. Tethered cord syndrome is a clinico-radiological diagnosis with low-lying conus medullaris most commonly terminating below?
   A. Lower border of L1
   B. L1–L2 intervertebral disc space
   C. Lower border of L2
   D. Lower border of L3
4. Which of the following is a characteristic of Chiari III malformation?
   A. Lumbosacral myelomeningocele
   B. Occipital encephalocele
   C. Cerebellar hypoplasia
   D. Syringohydromyelia

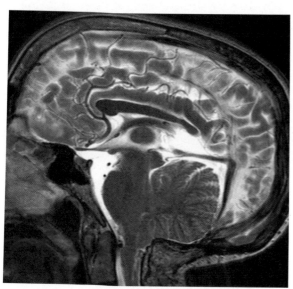

Fig. 48.1

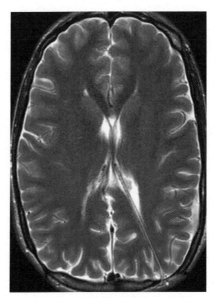

Fig. 48.2

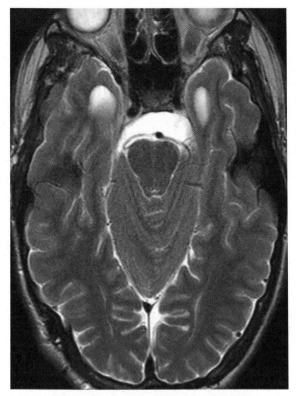

Fig. 48.3

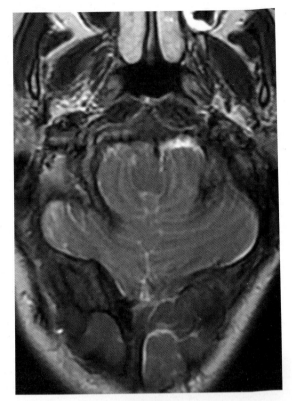

Fig. 48.4

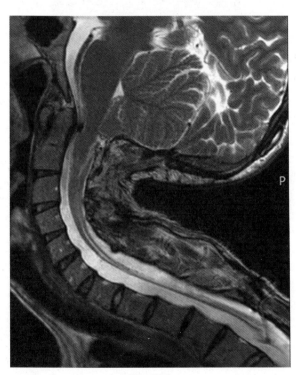

Fig. 48.5

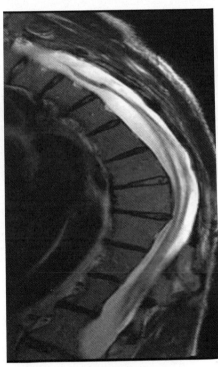

Fig. 48.6

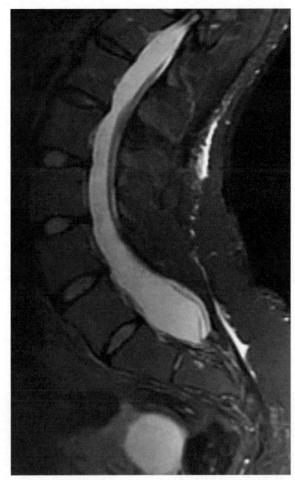

Fig. 48.7

Case 49

History: A 33-year-old patient with a new-onset seizure.

1. What is the most likely diagnosis?
   A. Primary glial neoplasm
   B. Metastatic disease
   C. Brain abscess
   D. Right MCA infarction
2. T2-FLAIR mismatch sign is predictive of which subgroup of infiltrating gliomas?
   A. IDH mutant, 1p/19q non-codeleted astrocytoma
   B. IDH mutant, 1p/19q codeleted oligodendroglioma
   C. IDH wild-type astrocytoma
   D. H3 K27M (diffuse midline glioma)
3. Which imaging biomarker is highly specific for the prediction of isocitrate dehydrogenase (IDH) mutant gliomas on MR spectroscopy?
   A. 2-hydroxyglutarate at 2.25 ppm
   B. Creatine at 3.0 ppm
   C. Acetate at 1.9 ppm
   D. Succinate at 2.4 ppm

4. cIMPACT (Consortium to Inform Molecular and Practical Approaches to CNS Tumor Taxonomy) recommends which of the following proposed changes to the upcoming WHO classification of CNS tumors.
   A. All glioblastomas will be designated as IDH wild-type tumors.
   B. All diffuse astrocytomas will be IDH mutant and graded based on histological and molecular phenotype as grade 2, grade 3, and grade 4.
   C. All gliomas will be graded using Arabic numerals (Roman numerals are no longer used).
   D. All of the above

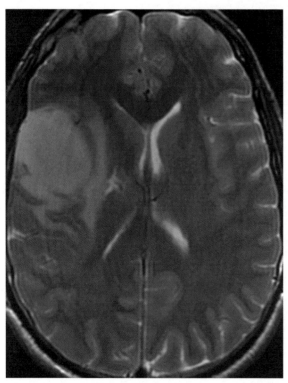

Fig. 49.1

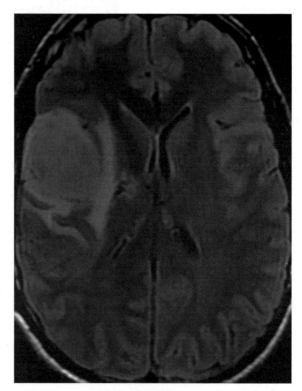

Fig. 49.2

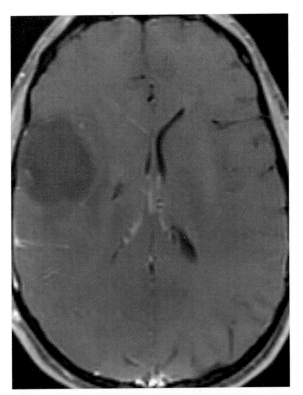

Fig. 49.3

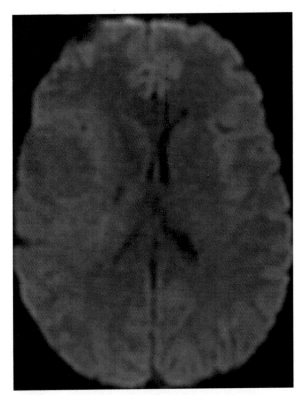

Fig. 49.4

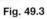

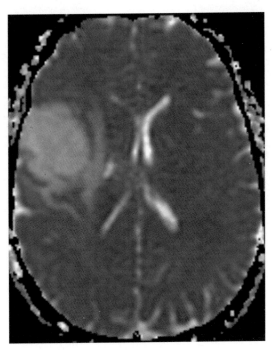

Fig. 49.5

Case 50

History: This 64-year-old female presents with headaches associated with intermittent blurry vision.

1. What is the likely cause of the patient's presenting symptoms?
   A. Hypertensive hemorrhage
   B. Ruptured aneurysm and intraventricular hemorrhage
   C. Reversible cerebral vasoconstriction syndrome (RCVS)
   D. Amyloid angiitis
2. What aneurysm may present with fourth ventricular hemorrhage and little or no hemorrhage in the basal cisterns?
   A. Posterior inferior cerebellar artery aneurysm
   B. Anterior inferior cerebellar artery aneurysm
   C. Posterior communicating artery aneurysm
   D. Anterior communicating artery aneurysm
3. Which of the following type(s) of hemorrhage is/are not commonly seen in patients with a closed-head injury?
   A. Intraventricular hemorrhage
   B. Subdural hemorrhage
   C. Thalamic hemorrhage
   D. Epidural hemorrhage
4. What does the arrow in Figure 50.6 point to?
   A. Right posterior inferior cerebellar artery aneurysm
   B. Right anterior inferior cerebellar artery aneurysm
   C. Left posterior inferior cerebellar artery
   D. Left anterior inferior cerebellar artery

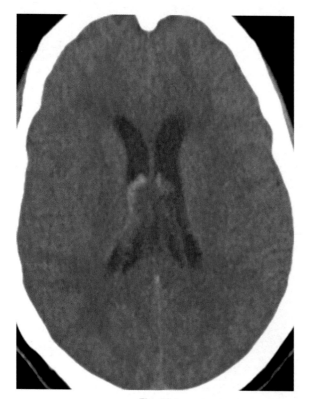

Fig. 50.1

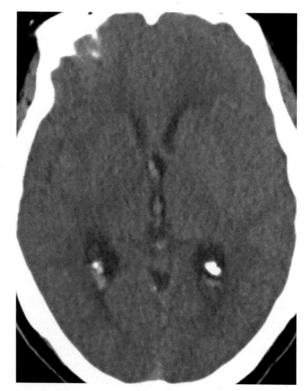

Fig. 50.2

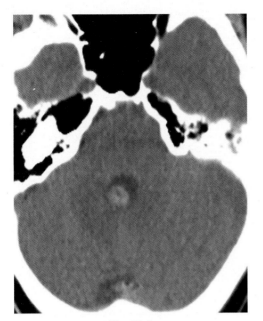

Fig. 50.3

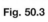

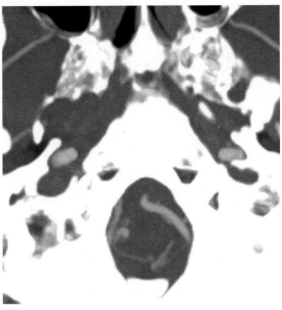

Fig. 50.4

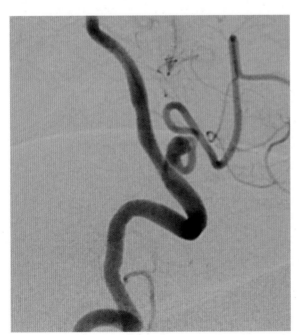

Fig. 50.5

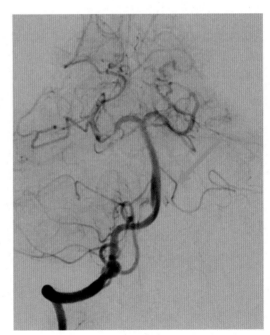

Fig. 50.6

Case 51

History: This 45-year-old male presents with eye pain.

1. What is the most common cause of nontraumatic proptosis?
   A. Thyroid-associated orbitopathy
   B. Cavernous venous malformation
   C. Idiopathic orbital inflammation
   D. Orbital venous varix

2. Which of the following is incorrect regarding idiopathic orbital inflammation (orbital pseudotumor)?
   A. Myositic pseudotumor is the most common subgroup
   B. Presence of periorbital edema is common
   C. Pain, proptosis, and decreased ocular motility are the typical presenting symptoms
   D. Poor response to corticosteroid therapy

3. What structure runs between the superior rectus muscle and the optic nerve?
   A. Superior ophthalmic vein
   B. Inferior ophthalmic vein
   C. Infraorbital nerve
   D. Inferior rectus muscle

4. What is the most common vascular lesion of the orbit in adults?
   A. Cavernous venous malformation
   B. Idiopathic orbital inflammation
   C. Orbital venous varix
   D. Carotid cavernous fistula

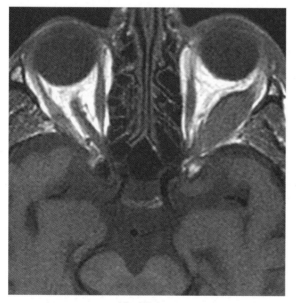

Fig. 51.1

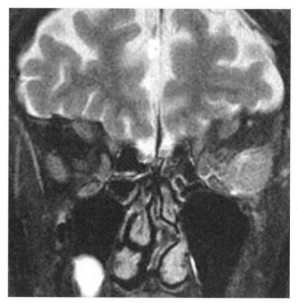

Fig. 51.2

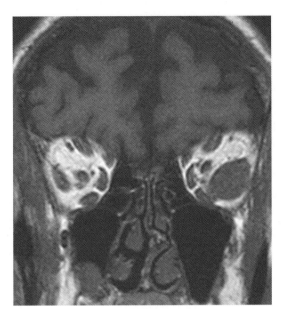

Fig. 51.3

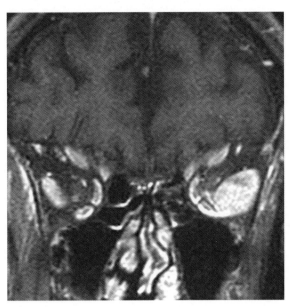

Fig. 51.4

Case 52

History: This is a 29-year-old female with vaginal bleeding, headaches, and skin pigmentation.

1. What is the most common extraskeletal manifestation of this disorder?
   A. Koplik's spots
   B. Erythema nodosum
   C. Café au lait spots
   D. Port-wine stain
2. Which of the following can be seen in patients with fibrous dysplasia?
   A. Elevated levels of serum alkaline phosphatase
   B. Elevated levels of urine hydroxyproline
   C. Increased tracer uptake on Tc99 bone scan
   D. All of the above

3. Which of the following imaging features is incorrect regarding craniofacial fibrous dysplasia?
   A. Expanded bones with a ground-glass attenuation on CT
   B. Relative preservation of the cort
   C. Heterogenous signal on T1 and T2 with no post-contrast enhancement on MRI
   D. Hot spot on a bone scan
4. What are the clinical manifestations of McCune–Albright syndrome?
   A. Precocious puberty
   B. Polyostotic fibrous dysplasia
   C. Cutaneous pigmentation "café au lait spots"
   D. All of the above

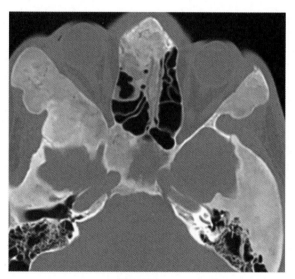

Fig. 52.1

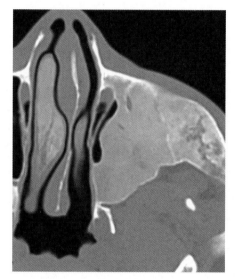

Fig. 52.2

Case 53

History: This 2-year-old child presents with leukocoria.

1. What are the causes of intraocular calcification in children?
   A. Retinoblastoma
   B. Persistent hyperplastic primary vitreous
   C. Toxocariasis
   D. Coats' disease
   E. Retrolental fibroplasia
   F. All of the above
2. What is the most common clinical presentation of retinoblastoma?
   A. Painful red eye
   B. Acute vision loss
   C. Red reflex
   D. Loss of red reflex
3. What is meant by the "third eye" in trilateral retinoblastoma?
   A. Pituitary gland
   B. Pineal gland
   C. Either of these
   D. None of these
4. In what percentage of cases are retinoblastomas bilateral?
   A. 15%–30%
   B. 30%–40%
   C. 50%–70%
   D. 70%–90%

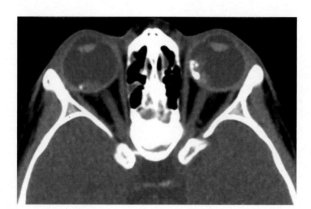

Fig. 53.1

Case 54

History: A 34-year-old participant in a research study.

1. What is the most likely diagnosis?
   A. Perivascular spaces
   B. Neurosarcoidosis
   C. Neurocysticercosis
   D. Toxoplasmosis
2. Which of the following statements is incorrect regarding tumefactive perivascular spaces?
   A. Can be large and mimic cystic tumors
   B. Can have surrounding edema with post-contrast enhancement
   C. Can cause mass effect and hydrocephalus
   D. Usually suppress on FLAIR images

3. Which of the following low-grade cystic neoplasms can mimic the appearance of dilated PVSs?
   A. Dysembryoplastic neuroepithelial tumors (DNETs)
   B. Multinodular and vacuolating neuronal tumors (MVNT)
   C. Both of these
   D. None of these
4. What CNS infection is associated with dilated Virchow–Robin spaces and pseudocysts within the basal ganglia?
   A. *Cytomegalovirus*
   B. *Cryptococcus*
   C. *Toxoplasma gondii*
   D. JC virus

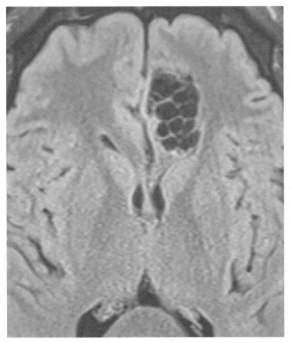

Fig. 54.1

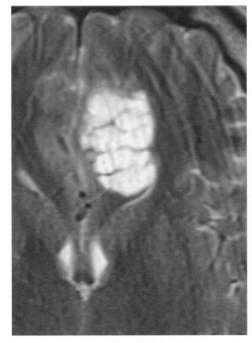

Fig. 54.2

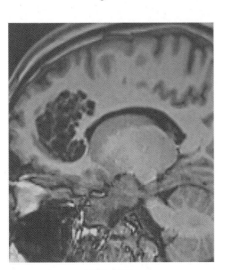

Fig. 54.3

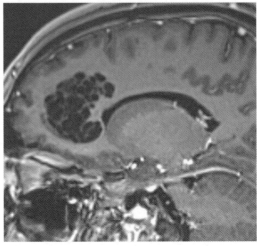

Fig. 54.4

Case 55

History: This 2-year-old nonverbal boy (per father) fell off the couch and hit the front of his head on the floor.

1. What is the diagnosis?
   - A. Colpocephaly
   - B. Porencephaly
   - C. Schizencephaly
   - D. Holoprosencephaly
2. What is the most common clinical presentation of isolated partial dysgenesis of the corpus callosum?
   - A. Seizures
   - B. Developmental delay
   - C. Asymptomatic
   - D. Nystagmus

3. Which part of the corpus callosum forms last?
   - A. Genu
   - B. Body
   - C. Splenium
   - D. Rostrum
4. What congenital anomalies are associated with this entity?
   - A. Chiari II malformation
   - B. Dandy–Walker spectrum
   - C. Heterotopias
   - D. Intracranial lipoma
   - E. All of the above

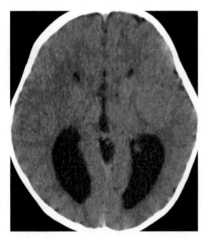

Fig. 55.1

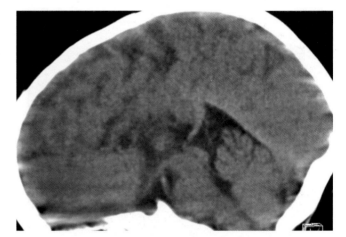

Fig. 55.2

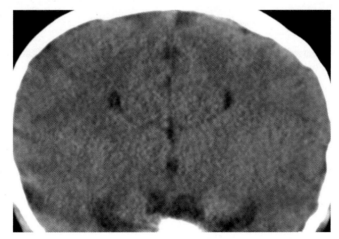

Fig. 55.3

Case 56

History: This is a 62-year-old female with metastatic non-small-cell lung cancer, MSSA bacteremia, and altered mental status.

1. What is the most likely diagnosis in this case?
   A. Calvarial hemangiomas
   B. Multiple myeloma
   C. Calvarial metastases
   D. Paget's disease
2. Which of the following primary cancers can present with sclerotic metastases?
   A. Prostate carcinoma
   B. Breast carcinoma
   C. Carcinoid
   D. Neuroblastoma
   E. Medulloblastoma
   F. All of the above

3. Which of the following primary cancers can present with lytic metastases?
   A. Thyroid cancer
   B. Renal cell cancer
   C. Melanoma
   D. Non-small-cell lung cancer
   E. All of the above
4. Which of the following is most sensitive for the detection of small focal skull metastases?
   A. Bone window CT scan
   B. FLAIR
   C. GRE
   D. DWI

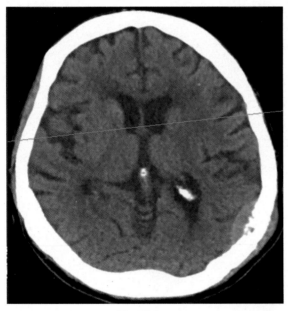

Fig. 56.1

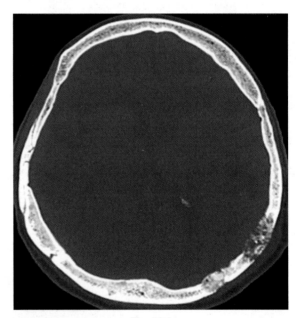

Fig. 56.2

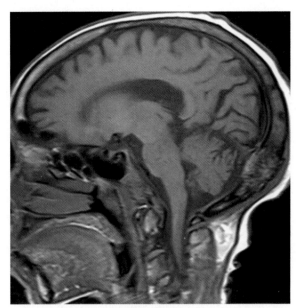

Fig. 56.3

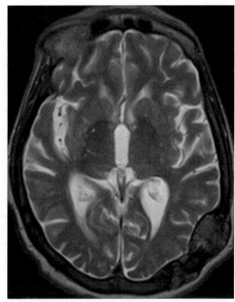

Fig. 56.4

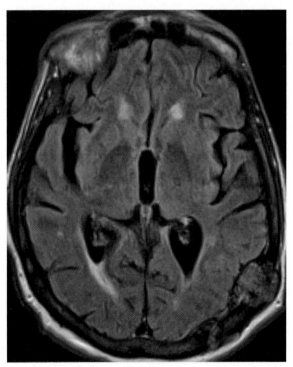

Fig. 56.5

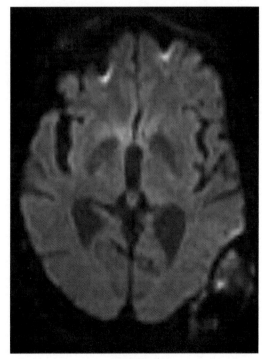

Fig. 56.6

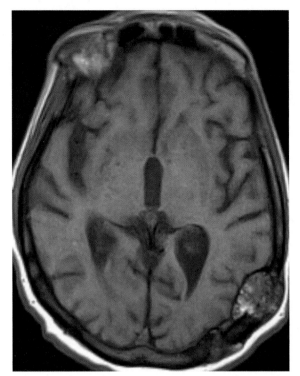

Fig. 56.7

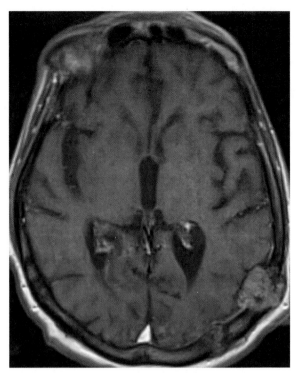

Fig. 56.8

Case 57

History: This 53-year-old female presents with headaches and intermittent left blurry vision.

1. What is the diagnosis?
   A. Primary CNS lymphoma
   B. Acute intracranial hemorrhage
   C. Giant aneurysm
   D. Ganglioglioma
2. What is the clinical presentation of these lesions when they involve the cavernous internal carotid artery?
   A. Worst headache of my life
   B. Seizures
   C. Painful ophthalmoplegia
   D. Optic neuritis

3. What is the definition of a giant aneurysm?
   A. Size more than 5 mm
   B. Size more than 15 mm
   C. Size more than 25 mm
   D. Size more than 4 cm
4. What are the common vessels of origin of these lesions?
   A. Middle cerebral artery
   B. Cavernous internal carotid artery
   C. Tip of the basilar artery
   D. All of the above

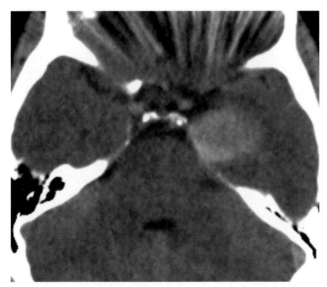

Fig. 57.1

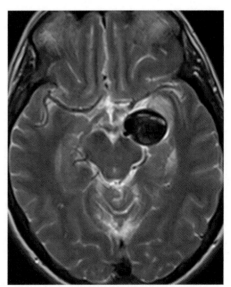

Fig. 57.2

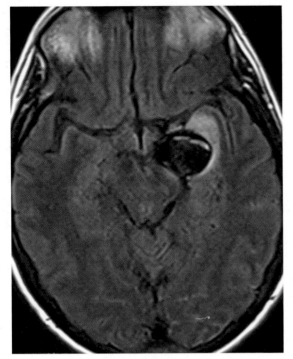

Fig. 57.3

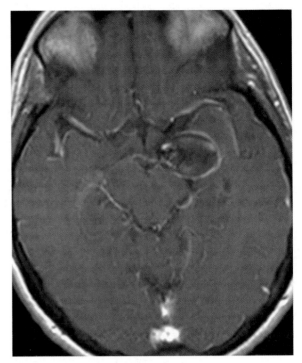

Fig. 57.4

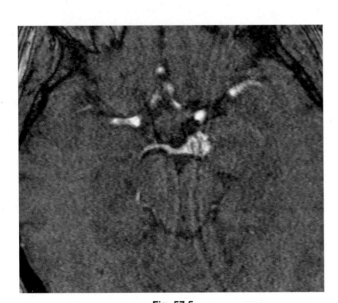

Fig. 57.5

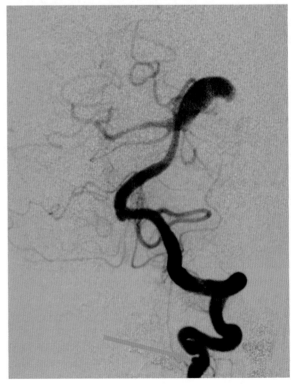

Fig. 57.6

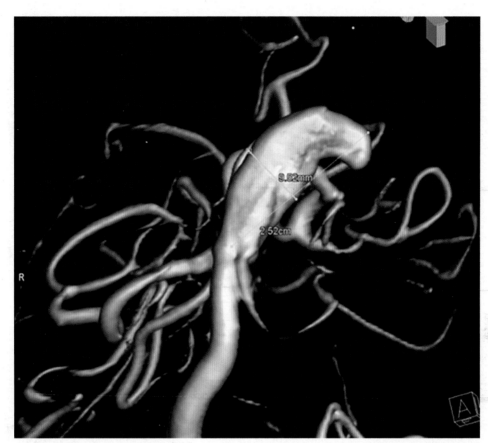

Fig. 57.7

Case 58

History: A 25-year-old female presents with gradual severe headache with radiation to the right neck and concern for aneurysm.

1. What is the first branch to arise from the supraclinoid internal carotid artery?
   A. Posterior communicating artery
   B. Ophthalmic artery
   C. Anterior choroidal artery
   D. Anterior communicating artery
2. What is the most common location for an intracranial infundibulum?
   A. Posterior communicating artery
   B. Ophthalmic artery
   C. Anterior choroidal artery
   D. Anterior communicating artery

3. Which of the following features are helpful in differentiating a posterior communicating artery infundibulum from an aneurysm?
   A. Size: 3 mm or smaller
   B. Shape: triangular or funnel-shaped
   C. Posterior communicating artery arising from its apex
   D. All of the above
4. What percentage of patients with nontraumatic subarachnoid hemorrhage will have unrevealing (negative) angiograms?
   A. 5%
   B. 15%
   C. 25%
   D. 50%

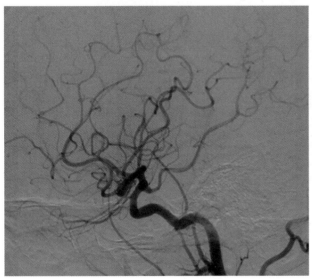

Fig. 58.1

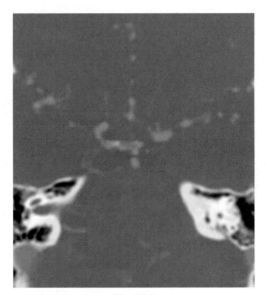

Fig. 58.2

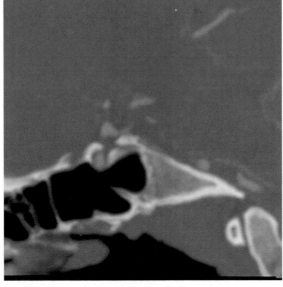

Fig. 58.3

Case 59

History: A 23-year-old male involved in a motorcycle accident presents with cognitive difficulties.

1. What is the most likely diagnosis?
   A. Acute Disseminated Encephalomyelitis (ADEM)
   B. Multiple sclerosis (MS)
   C. Susac's syndrome
   D. Diffuse axonal injury DAI
2. Which of the following conditions is unlikely to result in multiple small foci of susceptibility on SWI?
   A. Acute Disseminated Encephalomyelitis (ADEM)
   B. Multiple sclerosis (MS)
   C. Cerebral amyloid angiopathy (CAA)
   D. Diffuse axonal injury (DAI)
   E. Both A and B
   F. Both C and D
3. Which of the following anatomic locations are classically involved in diffuse axonal injury?
   A. Gray–white matter junction
   B. Corpus callosum
   C. Brainstem
   D. All of the above
4. Which of the following is incorrect regarding DAI?
   A. Results in severe cognitive difficulties
   B. Diagnosis is easily established on CT
   C. SWI is more sensitive than GRE to detect DAI
   D. Stage 3 DAI involves the brainstem in addition to the lobar white matter and corpus callosum

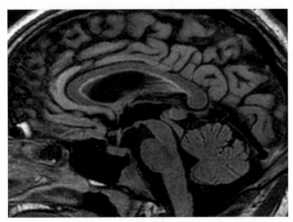

Fig. 59.1

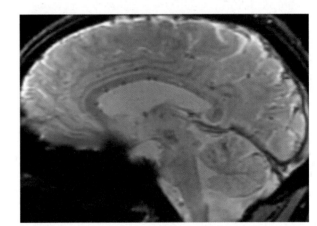

Fig. 59.2

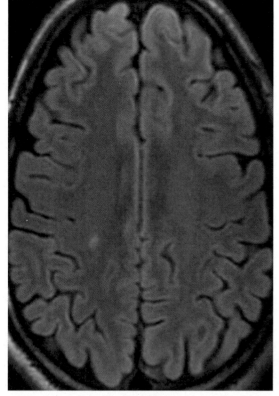

Fig. 59.3

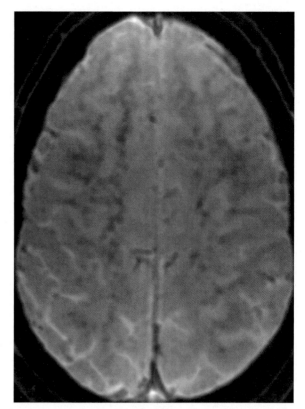

Fig. 59.4

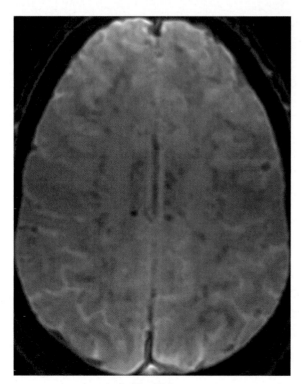

Fig. 59.5

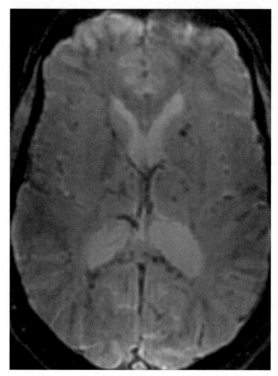

Fig. 59.6

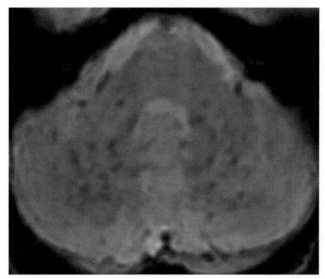

Fig. 59.7

Case 60

History: This 84-year-old man presents with mild cognitive impairment.

1. Which of the following conditions can present with multiple small foci of susceptibility on SWI?
   A. Hypertensive angiopathy
   B. Familial multiple cavernous malformation syndrome
   C. Cerebral amyloid angiopathy
   D. Diffuse axonal injury
   E. Neurocysticercosis
   F. All of the above
2. Which of the following is incorrect regarding hypertensive angiopathy?
   A. Cerebellar hemispheres and pons are common locations
   B. Basal ganglia and thalami are common locations
   C. Microhemorrhages are usually seen peripherally in a lobar distribution
   D. Hypertensive hemorrhages are typically not associated with superficial siderosis
3. Which of the following features are commonly seen in cerebral amyloid angiopathy?
   A. Lobar hemorrhage
   B. Microhemorrhages
   C. Subarachnoid hemorrhage
   D. Superficial siderosis
   E. All of the above
4. Scattered lobar microhemorrhages in the brain increase the likelihood of which neurodegenerative disease?
   A. Pick's disease
   B. Alzheimer's disease
   C. Lewy body disease
   D. Parkinson's disease

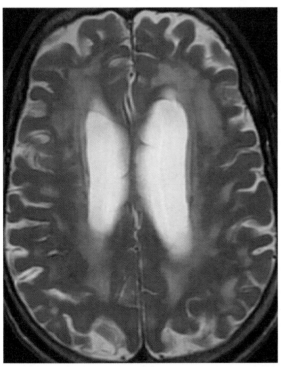

Fig. 60.1

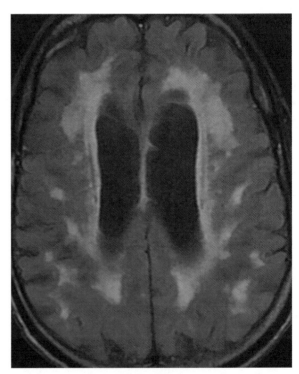

Fig. 60.2

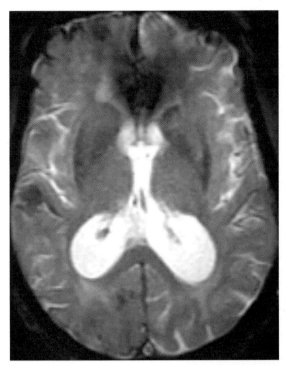

Fig. 60.3

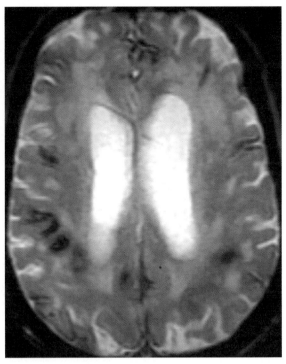

Fig. 60.4

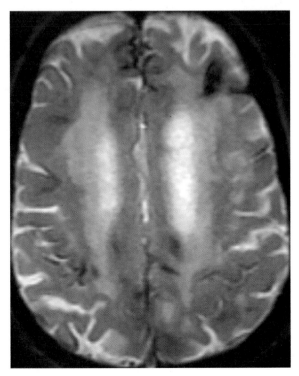

Fig. 60.5

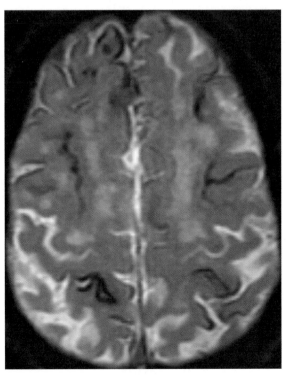

Fig. 60.6

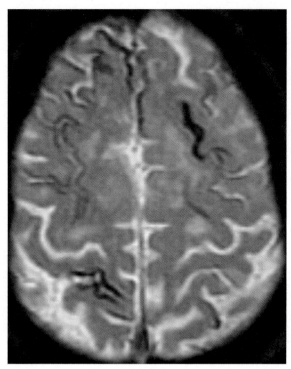

Fig. 60.7

Case 61

History: A 45-year-old patient with seizures from age 5.

1. The arrow in Figure 61.1 points to what anatomic structure?
   A. Anterior commissure
   B. Massa intermedia
   C. Mammillary body
   D. Optic nerve
2. What is the patient's diagnosis?
   A. Normal study
   B. Multiple sclerosis
   C. Mesial temporal sclerosis
   D. Wernicke's encephalopathy
3. The arrow in Figure 61.4 points to what anatomic structure?
   A. Posterior commissure
   B. Septum pellucidum
   C. Tail of the caudate nucleus
   D. Fornix
4. Which of the following is incorrect regarding imaging in mesial temporal sclerosis (MTS)?
   A. Atrophy of the ipsilateral fornix and mammillary body
   B. Atrophy of the cingulate gyrus
   C. Enlargement of the ipsilateral temporal horn is the least specific finding.
   D. Intravenous gadolinium is necessary to establish the diagnosis.

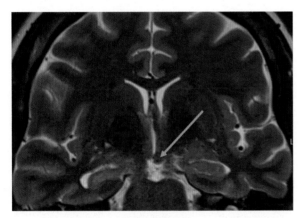

Fig. 61.1

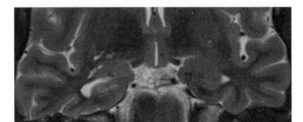

Fig. 61.2

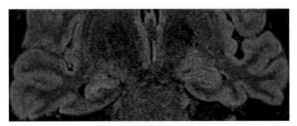

Fig. 61.3

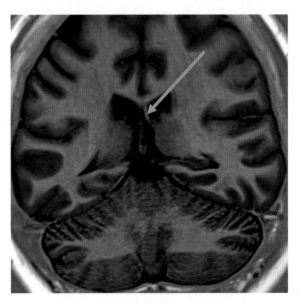

Fig. 61.4

Case 62

History: A 29-year-old with a history of medulloblastoma, status-post gross total resection and chemoradiation 26 years ago.

1. What is the most likely diagnosis?
   A. Radiation necrosis
   B. Recurrent medulloblastoma
   C. Mineral deposition
   D. Cortical laminar necrosis
2. Which of the following can be seen in survivors of childhood brain tumors treated with radiotherapy?
   A. Cavernomas
   B. Microbleeds
   C. Large-vessel vasculopathy
   D. Lacunar infarcts
   E. Mineralizing microangiopathy
   F. All of the above

3. What neurocutaneous syndrome is associated with high signal intensity foci in the brain on unenhanced T1W images?
   A. Neurofibromatosis type 1 (NF1)
   B. Neurofibromatosis type 2 (NF2)
   C. Sturge–Weber syndrome
   D. Tuberous sclerosis
4. Which of the following acauses of T1 hyperintensity in the basal ganglia?
   A. Hyperglycemia
   B. Wilson disease
   C. Hepatic encephalopathy
   D. Administration of linear gadolinium chelates
   E. All of the above

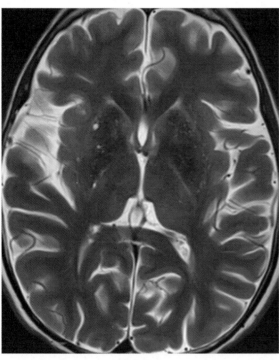

Fig. 62.1

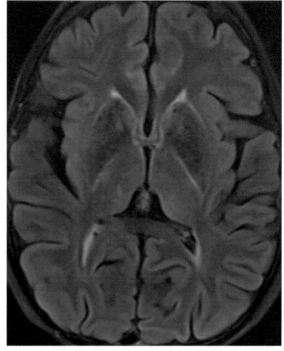

Fig. 62.2

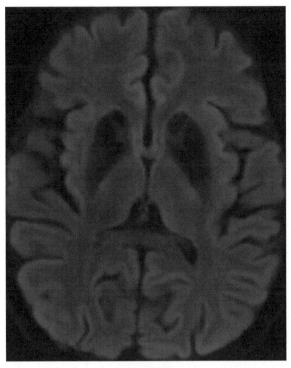

Fig. 62.3

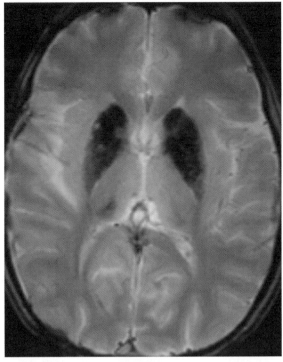

Fig. 62.4

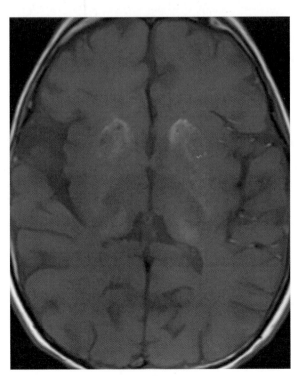

Fig. 62.5

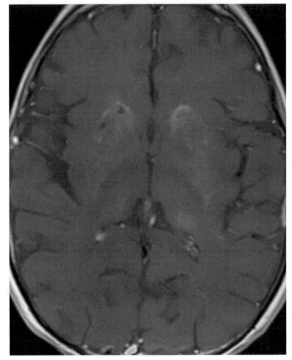

Fig. 62.6

Case 63

History: This 54-year-old male presents with HIV and altered mental status.

1. What is the most likely diagnosis?
   A. Acute pyogenic meningitis
   B. Tuberculous meningitis
   C. Cryptococcal meningitis
   D. Carcinomatous meningitis
2. Which of the following disease processes can affect the basilar meninges?
   A. Leptomeningeal carcinomatosis
   B. Fungal meningitis
   C. Neurosarcoidosis
   D. All of the above
3. Which of the following is correct regarding imaging in tuberculous meningitis?
   A. Hydrocephalus associated with TB meningitis is typically communicating.
   B. Intracranial tuberculosis has two related pathologic correlates—TB meningitis and tuberculoma—which coexist in 100% of cases.
   C. Tuberculous pachymeningitis is the most common form of CNS tuberculosis.
   D. Anti-tuberculosis treatment is ineffective.
4. Which primary CNS neoplasm can present with predominant nodular meningeal enhancement particularly around the basal cisterns, mimicking chronic meningitis?
   A. Diffuse leptomeningeal glioneuronal tumor
   B. Hemangiopericytoma/solitary fibrous tumor
   C. Pleomorphic xanthoastrocytoma
   D. Multinodular and vacuolating neuronal tumor

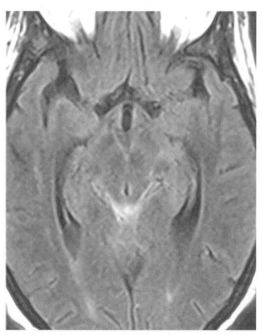

Fig. 63.1

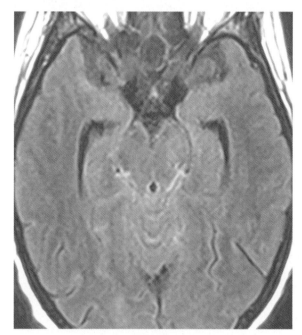

Fig. 63.2

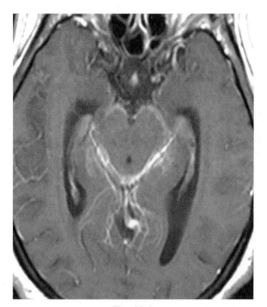

Fig. 63.3

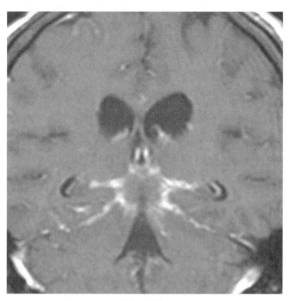

Fig. 63.4

Case 64

History: This 72-year-old female became confused while grocery shopping.

1. What is the most likely diagnosis?
   A. Atypical meningioma
   B. Metastatic disease
   C. Lymphoma
   D. Multiple myeloma
2. What metastases may be associated with minimal or no edema such that they are frequently missed on T2W imaging and necessitate the administration of intravenous contrast for their detection?
   A. Cortex
   B. White matter
   C. Basal ganglia
   D. Thalamus
3. What is the most common neoplasm associated with dural metastases?
   A. Breast cancer
   B. Prostate cancer
   C. Lung cancer
   D. Melanoma
   E. Glioblastoma
4. Dural metastases in children are most commonly associated with which primary extracranial tumor?
   A. Nephroblastoma
   B. Neuroblastoma
   C. Wilms tumor
   D. Hepatoblastoma

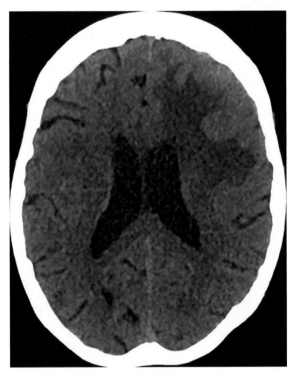

Fig. 64.1

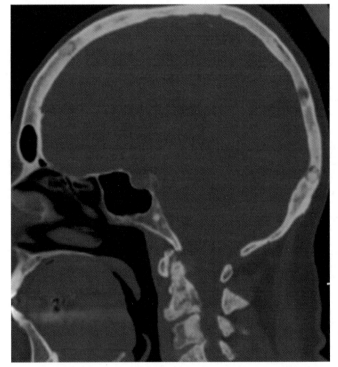

Fig. 64.2

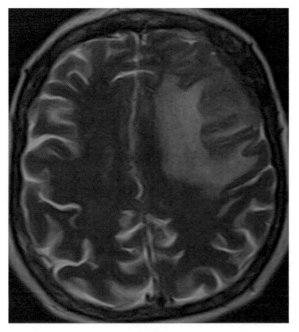

Fig. 64.3

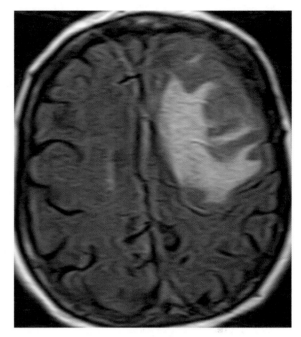

Fig. 64.4

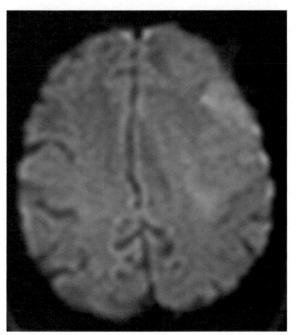

Fig. 64.5

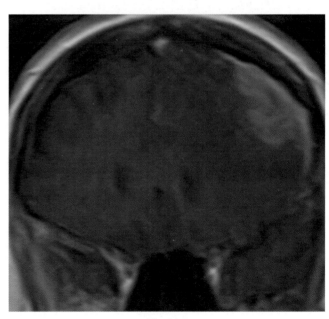

Fig. 64.6

Case 65

History: An 18-year-old female participant in a research study.

1. What is the diagnosis?
   A. Normal study
   B. Pituitary apoplexy
   C. Craniopharyngioma
   D. Rathke's cleft cyst
2. What is the most common clinical presentation of a Rathke's cleft cyst?
   A. Asymptomatic
   B. Precocious puberty
   C. Nipple discharge
   D. Amenorrhea and infertility

3. Most Rathke's cleft cysts are localized in what part of the pituitary gland?
   A. Pars tuberalis
   B. Pars intermedia
   C. Pars nervosa
   D. Pituitary infundibulum
4. Eccentric nonenhancing intracystic nodule is considered a distinguishing feature of a Rathke's cleft cyst and is seen in what percent of patients?
   A. 25%
   B. 50%
   C. 75%
   D. 100%

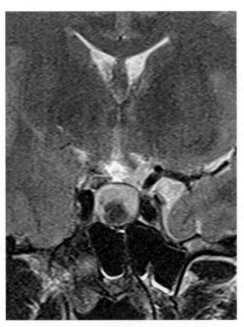

Fig. 65.1

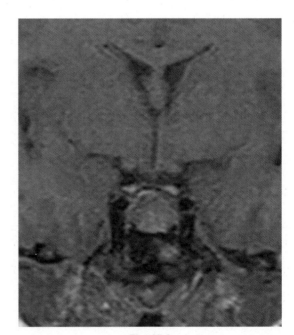

Fig. 65.2

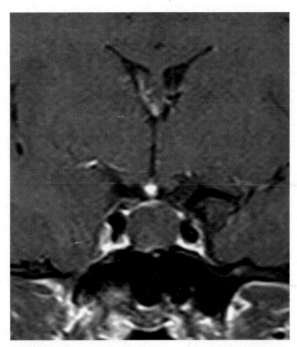

Fig. 65.3

Case 66

History: This 34-year-old patient presents with right eye pain and vision loss for 2 months.

1. What is the most likely diagnosis?
   A. Optic sheath meningioma
   B. Optic nerve glioma
   C. Optic atrophy
   D. Optic neuritis
2. Which clinical sign is seen in patients with optic neuritis?
   A. Argyll Robertson pupil
   B. Marcus Gunn pupil
   C. Holmes-Adie pupil
   D. Pinpoint pupil

3. Enhancement of the optic nerve on fat-suppressed T1W images is a sensitive marker for disease activity and can be seen in what percent of patients with acute optic neuritis?
   A. 25%
   B. 50%
   C. 75%
   D. 95%

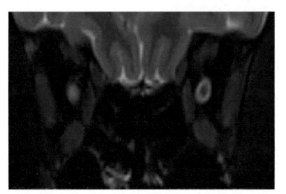

Fig. 66.1

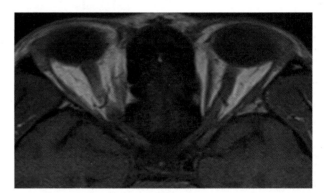

Fig. 66.2

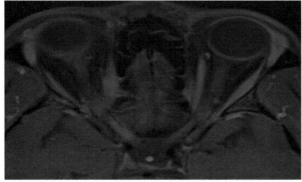

Fig. 66.3

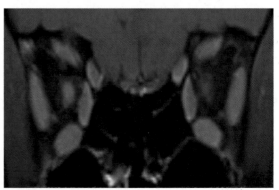

Fig. 66.4

Case 67

History: This is a 41-year-old male with HIV infection and new-onset seizure.

1. According to the American Academy of Neurology (AAN) guidelines, what is the next best step for the management of ring-enhancing lesions in the immunocompromised host?
   A. Go directly to brain biopsy
   B. Treat empirically for toxoplasmosis
   C. Treat empirically for pyogenic abscess
   D. Treat empirically with steroids
2. Which of the following would be the least likely cause of ring-enhancing brain lesions in an immunocompetent patient?
   A. Metastases
   B. Pyogenic abscess
   C. Toxoplasmosis
   D. Multiple sclerosis

3. Which radiotracer scan is useful in differentiating toxoplasmosis from primary CNS lymphoma in an immunocompromised patient?
   A. Thallium-201 scintigraphy
   B. I-131-MIBG scan
   C. Gallium-67 scintigraphy
   D. Indium-111-labeled WBC scintigraphy
4. In infants infected in utero with toxoplasmosis, what are the typical neuroimaging findings?
   A. Eccentric target sign
   B. Concentric target sign
   C. Multiple calcifications in the basal ganglia
   D. Subependymal cysts

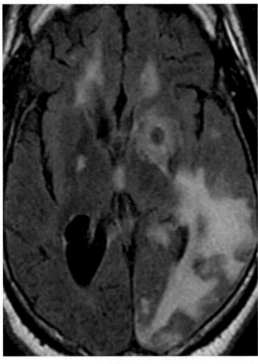

Fig. 67.1

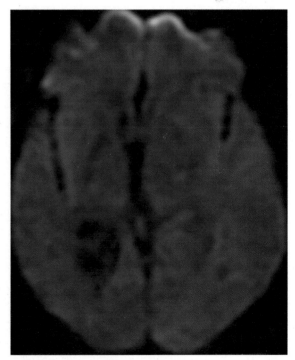

Fig. 67.2

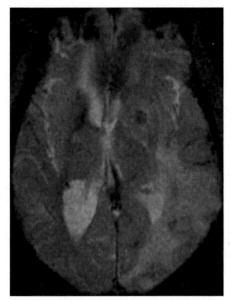

Fig. 67.3

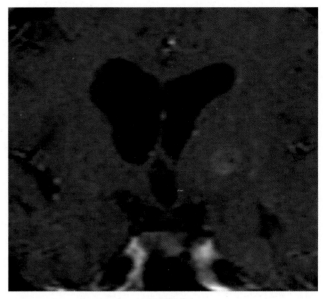

Fig. 67.4

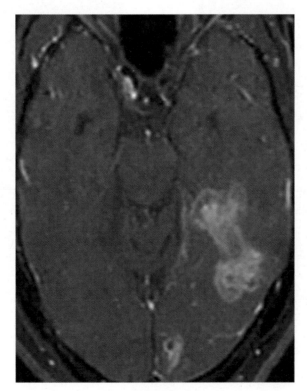

Fig. 67.5

Case 68

History: A 55-year-old patient with seizures reportedly for the past 10 years. The patient is Burmese speaking.

1. What is the most likely diagnosis?
   A. Septic emboli
   B. Pyogenic abscesses
   C. Cysticercosis
   D. Metastatic disease
2. Which of the following is the most common parasitic infection affecting the CNS in humans?
   A. Cysticercosis
   B. Toxoplasmosis
   C. Echinococcosis
   D. Schistosomiasis
3. What is the most common clinical presentation of patients with this entity?
   A. Headache
   B. Seizures
   C. Dizziness and giddiness
   D. Vertigo and vomiting
4. What is the most common location of intraventricular neurocysticercosis?
   A. Foramen on Monro
   B. Third ventricle
   C. Fourth ventricle
   D. Aqueduct of Sylvius

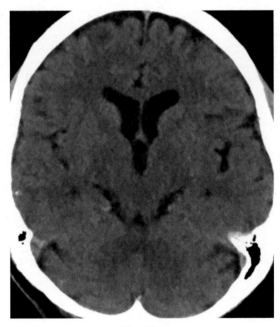

Fig. 68.1

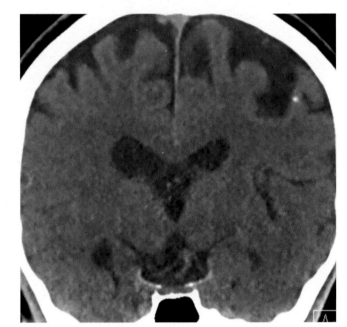

Fig. 68.2

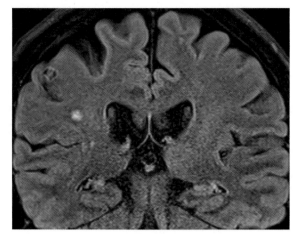

Fig. 68.3

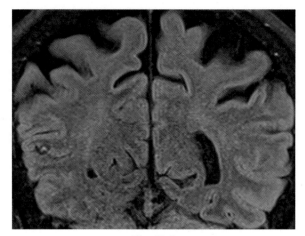

Fig. 68.4

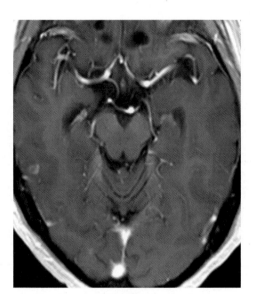

Fig. 68.5

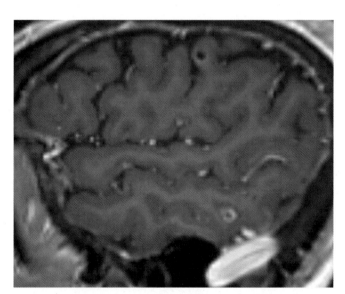

Fig. 68.6

Case 69

History: A 70-year-old female status-post fall within a moving bus.

1. What is the name of this characteristic radiographic appearance?
   A. Osteoporosis circumscripta
   B. Hyperostosis frontalis interna
   C. Fibrous dysplasia
   D. Osteogenesis imperfecta
2. Which of the following helps in distinguishing Paget's disease from fibrous dysplasia?
   A. Paget's disease is typically seen in children and young adults.
   B. Paget's disease usually affects the outer table of the skull.
   C. Extensive involvement of the facial bones is uncommon in Paget's disease.
   D. Pagetoid lesions demonstrate increased tracer uptake on Tc99 bone scan.

3. Which of the following are the potential complications of Paget's disease?
   A. Pathological fractures
   B. Hearing loss
   C. Cranial nerve palsies
   D. High-output cardiac failure
   E. Osteosarcoma
   F. Basilar invagination
   G. All of the above

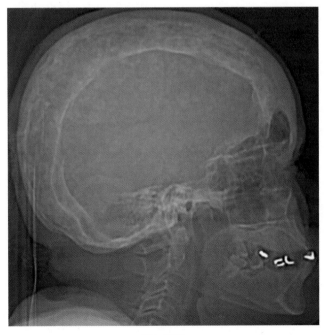

Fig. 69.1

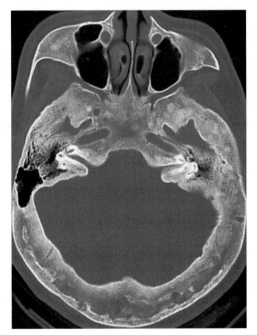

Fig. 69.2

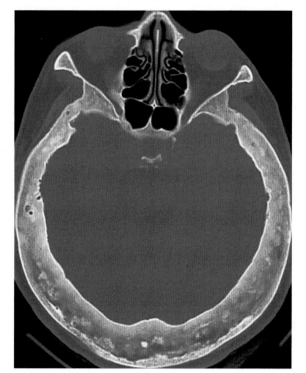

Fig. 69.3

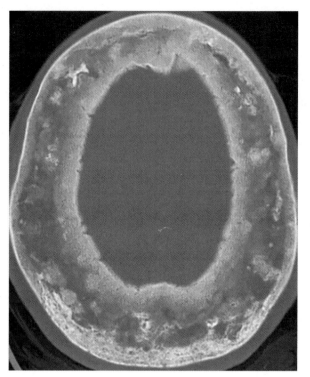

Fig. 69.4

Case 70

History: This 26-year-old attempted suicide.

1. What basal ganglionic structures are involved in these cases?
   A. Caudate nucleus
   B. Globus pallidus
   C. Putamen
   D. Globus pallidus and putamen
2. What is the most common cause of accidental poisoning in the United States?
   A. Cyanide
   B. Cocaine
   C. Carbon monoxide
   D. Heroin
3. Which of the following conditions can present with abnormalities in bilateral globus pallidi?
   A. Pantothenate kinase-associated neurodegeneration (PKAN)
   B. Hepatic encephalopathy
   C. Kernicterus (bilirubin encephalopathy)
   D. All of the above

4. After the globus pallidus, the second most commonly affected site is cerebral white matter which can show delayed leukoencephalopathy in the subacute phase of carbon monoxide poisoning. Which of the following is correct regarding toxic leukoencephalopathy?
   A. Extensive bilaterally symmetric restricted diffusion involving the centrum semiovale
   B. Can be caused by other chemotherapeutic agents such as methotrexate and opioids (heroin).
   C. Reversible and believed to be due to intramyelinic edema
   D. All of the above

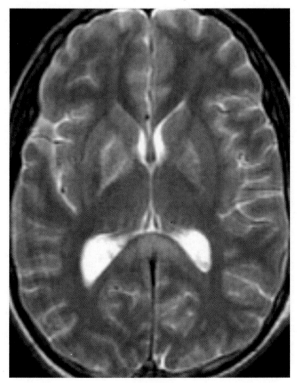

Fig. 70.1

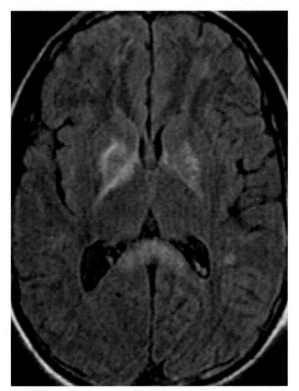

Fig. 70.2

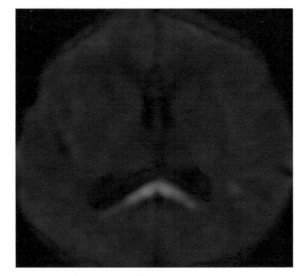

Fig. 70.3

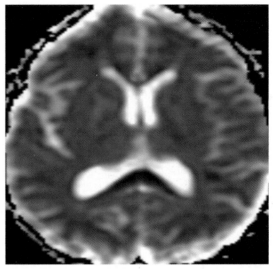

Fig. 70.4

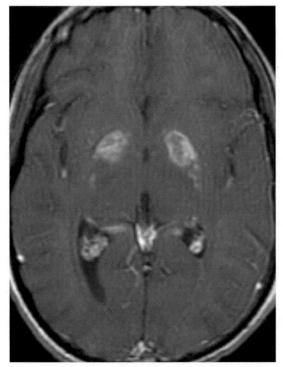

Fig. 70.5

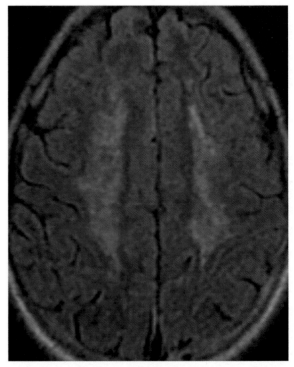

Fig. 70.6

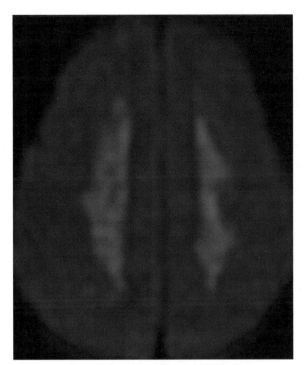

Fig. 70.7

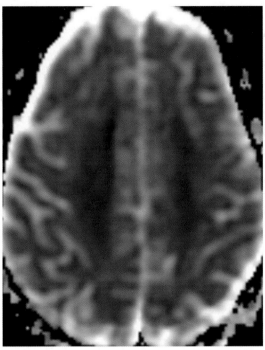

Fig. 70.8

Case 71

History: A 6-day-old male (born at 40 weeks 3-day gestation) with seizure.

1. What does the arrow in Figure 71.4 and Figure 71.6 represent?
   A. Acute infarction
   B. Seizure-related changes
   C. Hypoxic ischemic encephalopathy
   D. Acute Wallerian degeneration
2. Which of the following statements is incorrect regarding Wallerian degeneration (WD)?
   A. WD is defined as a progressive anterograde disintegration of axons and accompanying demyelination after an injury to the proximal axon or cell body.
   B. WD occurs after axonal injury in both the central and peripheral nervous systems.
   C. Diffusion abnormality can be seen in the distal descending white matter tract ipsilateral to the infarction.
   D. WD is not seen in the spinal cord.

3. What will be the salient finding of this entity in its chronic stage?
   A. Ipsilateral hypertrophy of the corticospinal tract
   B. Ipsilateral atrophy of the corticospinal tract
   C. Ipsilateral hypertrophy of the pontocerebellar tract
   D. Ipsilateral hypertrophy of the inferior olivary nucleus
4. Which of the following neural tracts can demonstrate WD?
   A. Corticopontocerebellar tract
   B. Dentate-rubro-olivary pathway
   C. Posterior column of the spinal cord
   D. Corpus callosum
   E. Limbic circuit
   F. All of the above

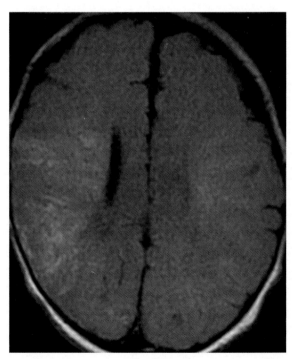

Fig. 71.1

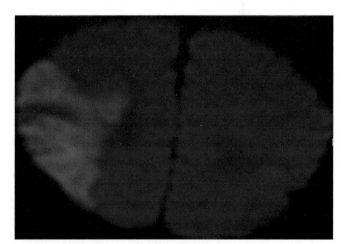

Fig. 71.2

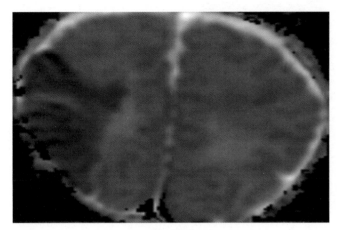

Fig. 71.3

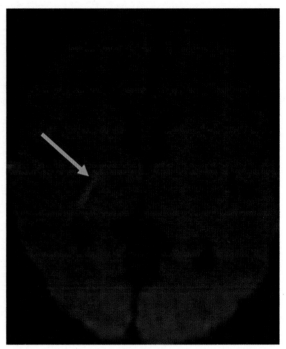

Fig. 71.4

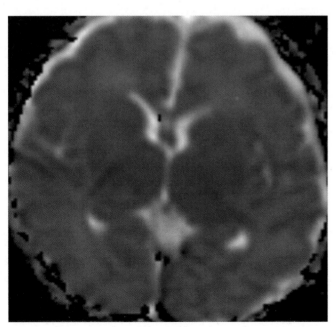

Fig. 71.5

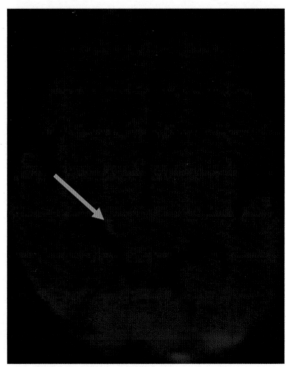

Fig. 71.6

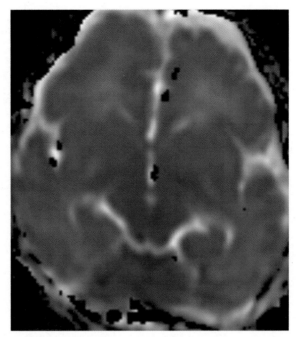

Fig. 71.7

Case 72

History:
Patient 1: A 38-year-old female with proptosis (Figure 72.1).
Patient 2: A 42-year-old female with proptosis (Figure 72.2).

1. What is the most common cause of proptosis in adults?
   A. Orbital cellulitis
   B. Orbital lymphoma
   C. Thyroid orbitopathy
   D. Orbital metastasis
   E. Orbital venous malformation
   F. Orbital pseudotumor
2. Isolated involvement of which extraocular muscle is extremely rare in thyroid-associated orbitopathy?
   A. Superior rectus
   B. Inferior rectus
   C. Medial rectus
   D. Lateral rectus

3. Which of the following are vascular causes of enlargement of the extraocular muscles?
   A. Carotid–cavernous fistula
   B. Superior ophthalmic vein thrombosis
   C. Cavernous sinus thrombosis
   D. All of the above
4. Which of the following is incorrect regarding thyroid-associated orbitopathy?
   A. The tendinous insertions of the extraocular muscles are characteristically spared, also known as the "Coca-Cola bottle sign."
   B. It is more frequently seen in women than men.
   C. Patients classically present with rapid-onset of unilateral, painful proptosis and diplopia.
   D. It is self-limiting with spontaneous improvement within 2–5 years.

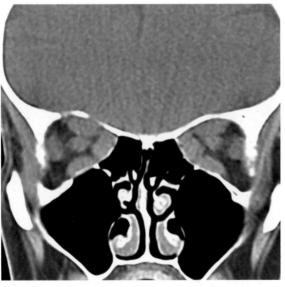

Fig. 72.1

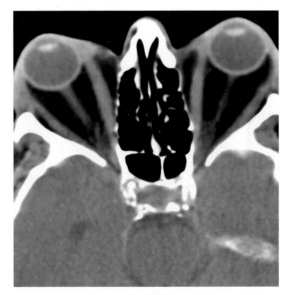

Fig. 72.2

Case 73

History: This 44-year-old man with a remote history of sinus surgery, presents complaining of left frontal headache, left eye swelling, and blurry vision.

1. What is the most likely diagnosis?
   A. Sinonasal undifferentiated carcinoma (SNUC)
   B. Orbital dermoid cyst
   C. Mucocele
   D. Meningioma
2. Which paranasal sinus is most prone to develop mucoceles?
   A. Frontal sinus
   B. Ethmoid sinus
   C. Maxillary sinus
   D. Sphenoid sinus
3. What determines the signal characteristics of these lesions on MR imaging?
   A. Viral load
   B. Patient's immune status
   C. Protein concentration, water content, viscosity, and cross-linking of glycoproteins
   D. Intrinsic hemorrhage

4. Which of the following is true regarding a "pseudo-pneumatized sinus"?
   A. Involved sinus demonstrates variable signal intensity on T1W image
   B. Involved sinus demonstrates low signal intensity on T2W image mimicking air
   C. In patients in whom invasive fungal infection is suspected, the recommendation is to start with an unenhanced CT, and then get an MRI to evaluate the orbit, cavernous sinus, and intracranial compartment.
   D. All of the above

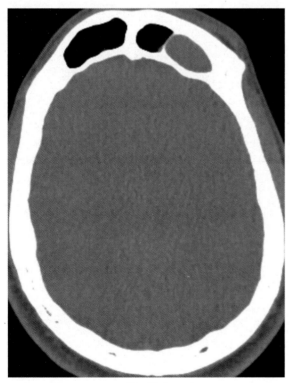

Fig. 73.1

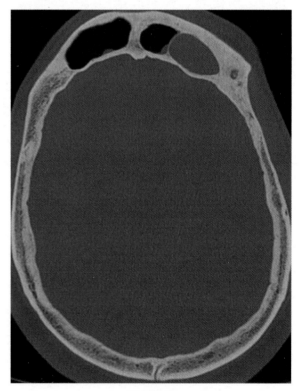

Fig. 73.2

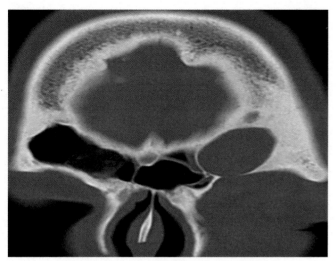

Fig. 73.3

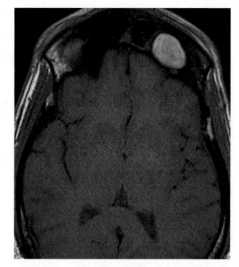

Fig. 73.4

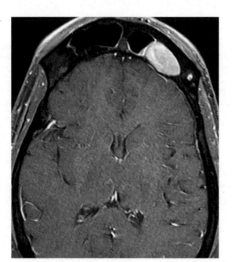

Fig. 73.5

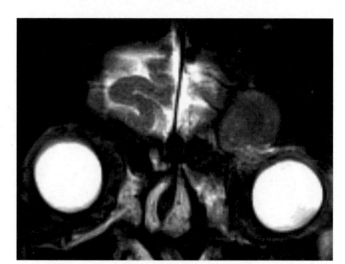

Fig. 73.6

Case 74

History: This is a 22-month-old male with developmental delay and seizure.

1. What is the diagnosis?
   A. Craniopharyngioma
   B. Medulloblastoma
   C. Meningioma
   D. Vein of Galen malformation
2. What are the classic clinical presentations for this entity in the neonatal period?
   A. Developmental delay
   B. Seizures
   C. Heart failure
   D. Asymptomatic

3. What anatomic structure is denoted by the arrow in Figure 74.4?
   A. Internal cerebral vein
   B. Vein of Galen
   C. Falcine sinus
   D. Straight sinus
4. What is the preferred management strategy for Vein of Galen malformations (VOGM)?
   A. Surgery
   B. Radiosurgery
   C. Endovascular therapy
   D. Ventricular shunting

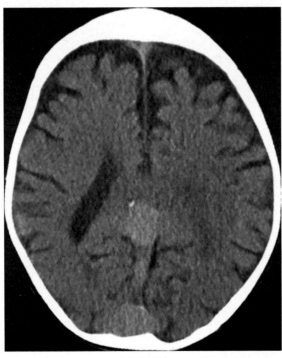

Fig. 74.1

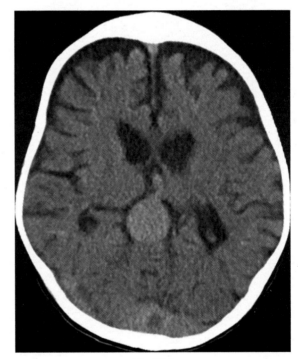

Fig. 74.2

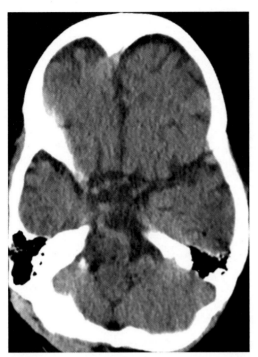

Fig. 74.3

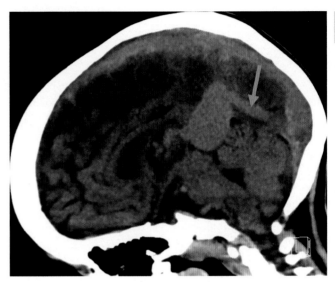

Fig. 74.4

Case 75

History: A 2-month-old male with a lump on the right forehead.

1. What is your recommendation based on these skull radiographs (Figures 75.1–75.3)?
   A. MRI to evaluate for a soft tissue neoplasm
   B. CT scan for possible craniosynostosis
   C. No further imaging is necessary
   D. Skeletal survey for evaluation of child abuse
2. Which is the most common form of craniosynostosis?
   A. Trigonocephaly
   B. Dolichocephaly
   C. Plagiocephaly
   D. Brachycephaly
3. What is the most common suture to close prematurely?
   A. Sagittal suture
   B. Metopic suture
   C. Lambdoid suture
   D. Coronal suture
4. Trigonocephaly and hypotelorism are characteristic of premature closure of which suture?
   A. Sagittal suture
   B. Metopic suture
   C. Lambdoid suture
   D. Coronal suture

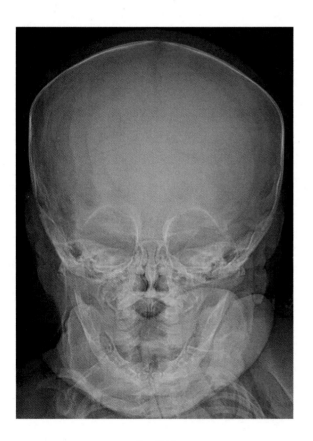

Fig. 75.1

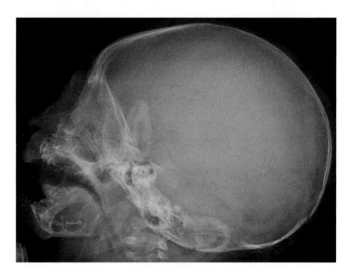

Fig. 75.2

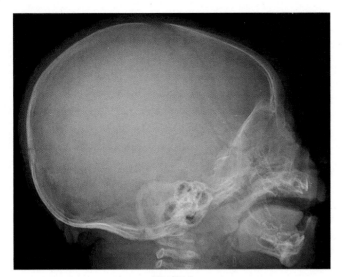

Fig. 75.3

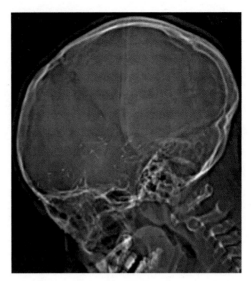

Fig. 75.4

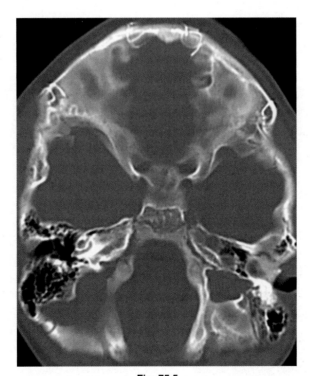

Fig. 75.5

Case 76

History: This 46-year-old male presents with increasing confusion for the past three months, accompanied by weakness and dizziness. The patient denies visual symptoms.

1. What is the diagnosis in this case?
   A. Craniopharyngioma
   B. Pituitary macroadenoma
   C. Meningioma
   D. Vein of Galen malformation
2. Which of the following is incorrect regarding a craniopharyngioma?
   A. Craniopharyngiomas are WHO grade I tumors that arise in the sellar/suprasellar region.
   B. The adamantinomatous subtype is more common than the papillary subtype.
   C. There is a bimodal age of presentation, with the first peak between 5 and 15 years, and a second smaller peak in adults older than 40 years.
   D. Thin peripheral or stippled calcification is seen in ~90% of papillary craniopharyngiomas on CT.
3. Adamantinomatous craniopharyngiomas are 3–9 times more common than the papillary subtype and are typically characterized on imaging as which of the following?
   A. Cystic with peripheral calcification
   B. Solid with peripheral calcification
   C. Cystic with no calcification
   D. Solid with no calcification

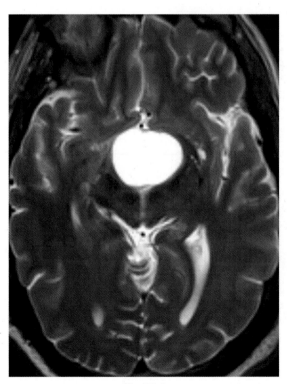

Fig. 76.1

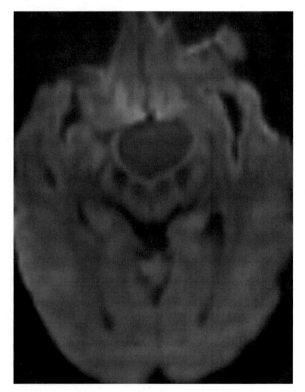

Fig. 76.2

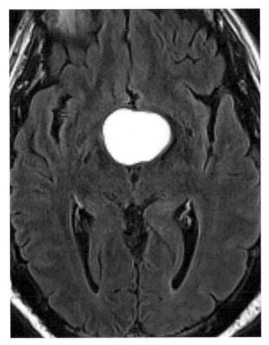

Fig. 76.3

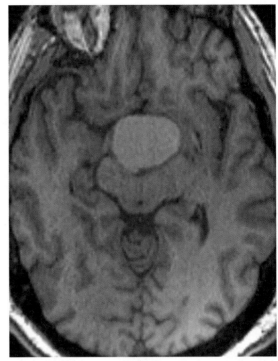

Fig. 76.4

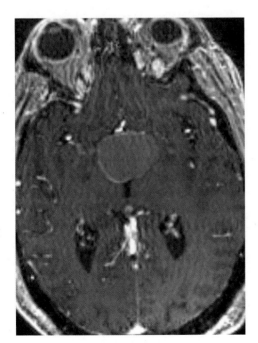

Fig. 76.5

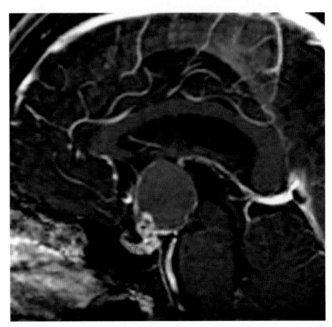

Fig. 76.6

Case 77

History: A 5-month-old infant with an abnormal skull shape.

1. What is the most likely clinical presentation in this 5-month-old infant?
   A. Asymptomatic
   B. Vomiting
   C. Seizures
   D. Developmental delay
2. What is the diagnosis?
   A. Normal study
   B. Hydrocephalus
   C. Heterotopia
   D. Schizencephaly

3. What heritable pattern has been described in some cases of this entity?
   A. X-linked inheritance
   B. Autosomal dominant
   C. Autosomal recessive
   D. Mitochondrial inheritance
4. What percentage of subependymal tubers in tuberous sclerosis are calcified?
   A. 10%
   B. 25%
   C. 50%
   D. 90%

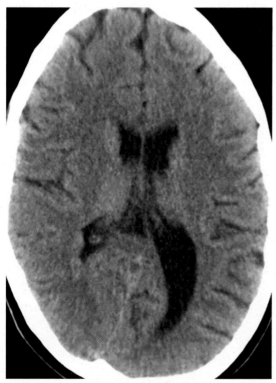

Fig. 77.1

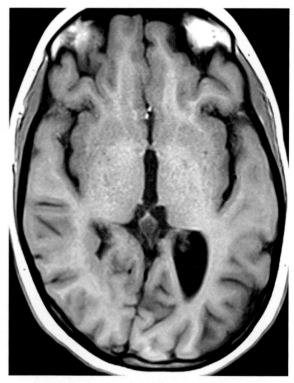

Fig. 77.2

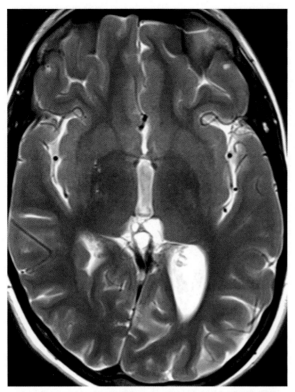

Fig. 77.3

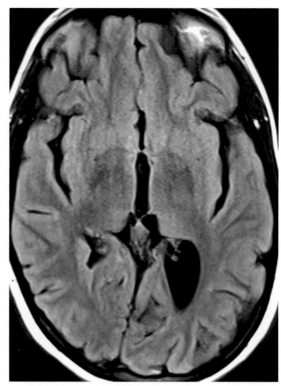

Fig. 77.4

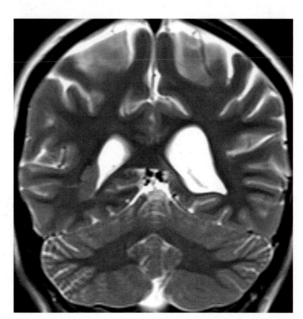

Fig. 77.5

Case 78

History: This 46-year-old male presents with right eye vision loss.

1. What is the diagnosis?
   A. Optic neuritis
   B. Optic atrophy
   C. Optic nerve glioma
   D. Optic nerve meningioma
2. Which of the following is incorrect regarding optic nerve meningiomas?
   A. The majority are direct extensions from intracranial meningiomas.
   B. The most common presenting symptom is painful and progressive vision loss.
   C. On sagittal oblique images, the enhancing tumor surrounding the nonenhancing optic nerve results in the so-called "tram-track sign"
   D. Conservative management is preferred in patients with preserved vision.

3. What does the arrow in Figure 78.2 represent?
   A. Pneumosinus dilatans
   B. Pneumatocele
   C. Concha bullosa
   D. Onodi cell

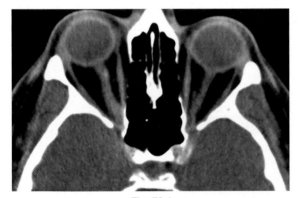

Fig. 78.1

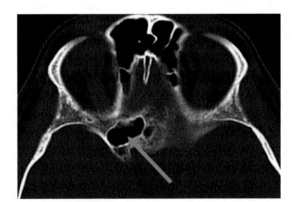

Fig. 78.2

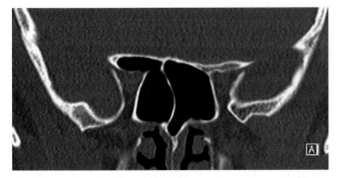

Fig. 78.3

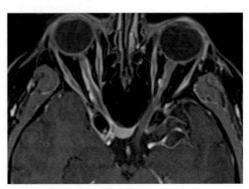

Fig. 78.4

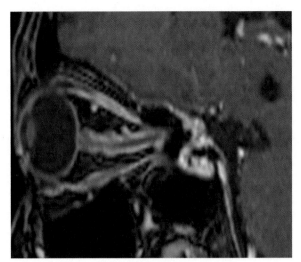

Fig. 78.5

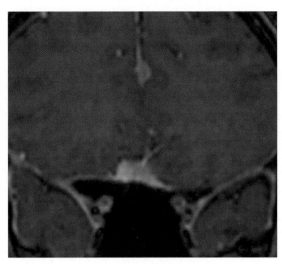

Fig. 78.6

Case 79

History: This 42-year-old female presents with headache, left-sided neck pain, and seizure activity lasting approximately 2 minutes.

1. What is the diagnosis?
   A. Low-grade astrocytoma
   B. Atypical PRES
   C. Acute ischemic infarction
   D. Cerebral venous thrombosis
2. Which of the following is considered a risk factor for cerebral venous sinus thrombosis?
   A. Oral contraceptive pill
   B. Pregnancy
   C. Protein S deficiency
   D. Malignancy
   E. All the above
3. Giant arachnoid (Pacchionian) granulations are projections of the arachnoid membrane into the dural sinuses and can mimic dural venous sinus thrombosis. Which of the following is correct regarding these arachnoid granulations?
   A. Hyperintense on T1
   B. Blooming artifact on GRE
   C. Isointense to CSF on T2 with no enhancement
   D. Isointense to CSF on T1 with contrast enhancement
4. The arrow in Figure 79.6 points to what anatomical structure?
   A. Vein of Trolard
   B. Basal vein of Rosenthal
   C. Vein of Labbe
   D. Superficial middle cerebral vein

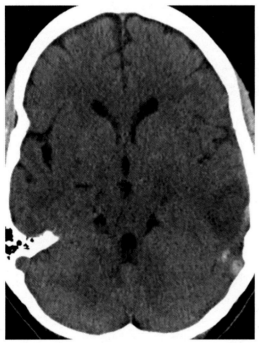

Fig. 79.1

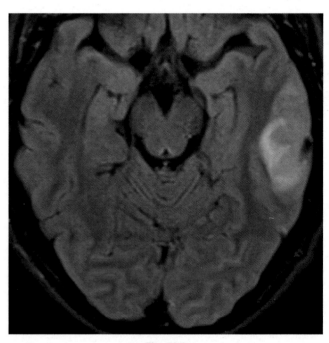

Fig. 79.2

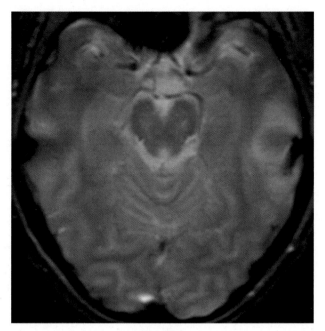

Fig. 79.3

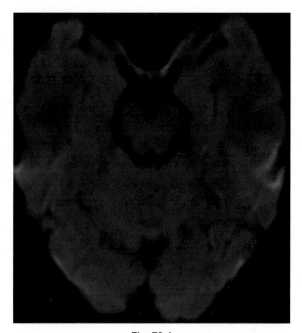

Fig. 79.4

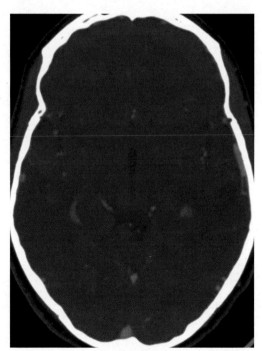

Fig. 79.5

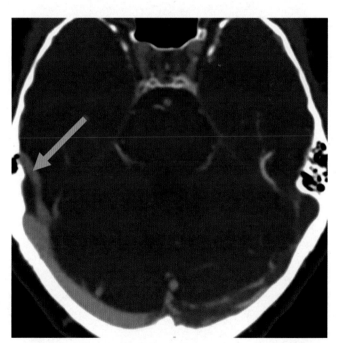

Fig. 79.6

Case 80

History: A 51-year-old female with oral cavity adenoid cystic carcinoma, status-post left hemimandibulectomy, left neck dissection, and fibular free flap reconstruction now complaining of neck pain, burning in the facial region, and trismus.

1. What is the diagnosis?
   A. Fatty replacement of the left occipital condyle from prior radiation therapy
   B. Metastases to the left occipital condyle
   C. Metastases to the right occipital condyle
   D. Degenerative changes along the right craniocervical junction
2. The arrow in Figure 80.6 points to which skull base foramina?
   A. Pars nervosa of the jugular foramen
   B. Pars vascularis of the jugular foramen
   C. Hypoglossal canal
   D. Carotid canal

3. Extension of skull base disease into the hypoglossal canal may result in what cranial nerve palsy?
   A. IX CN
   B. X CN
   C. XI CN
   D. XII CN
4. Which of the following is correct regarding occipital condyle fractures?
   A. Mostly occur in the setting of high-speed motor vehicle collision
   B. Mechanism of injury is usually axial loading with associated ipsilateral flexion
   C. History and clinical examination are usually unreliable
   D. Treatment is generally conservative
   E. All of the above

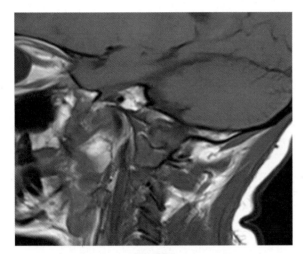

Fig. 80.1

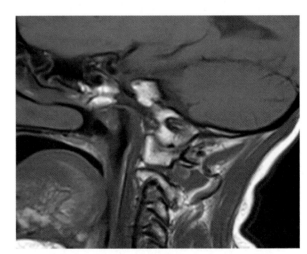

Fig. 80.2

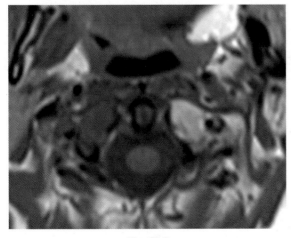

Fig. 80.3

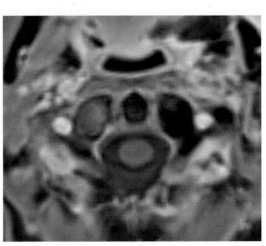

Fig. 80.4

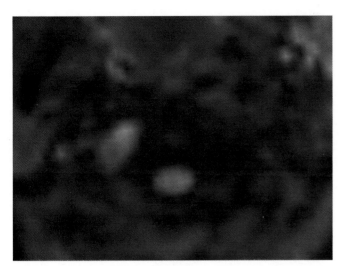

Fig. 80.5

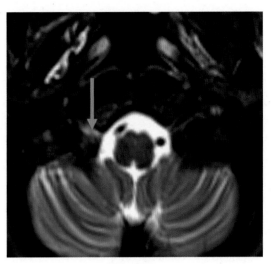

Fig. 80.6

Case 81

History: A 26-year-old male with left-sided weakness.

1. What disorders have been associated with these angiographic findings?
   A. Atherosclerosis
   B. Radiation-induced vasculopathy
   C. Neurofibromatosis type-1 (NF1)
   D. Varicella zoster vasculitis
   E. Antiphospholipid syndrome
   F. Sickle cell disease
   G. All of the above
2. Which of the following is true regarding Moyamoya disease?
   A. An idiopathic condition with characteristic intracranial vascular findings
   B. Usually secondary to radiation
   C. Usually secondary to neurofibromatosis type-1 (NF1)
   D. Usually secondary to sickle cell disease
   E. Usually secondary to systemic lupus erythematosus (SLE)

3. What is the characteristic clinical presentation in children with this disorder?
   A. Transient ischemic attacks or strokes
   B. Intracranial hemorrhage
   C. Seizures
   D. Chorea and hemiballismus
4. What is the most common clinical presentation in adults with this disorder?
   A. Transient ischemic attacks or strokes
   B. Intracranial hemorrhage
   C. Seizures
   D. Chorea and hemiballismus

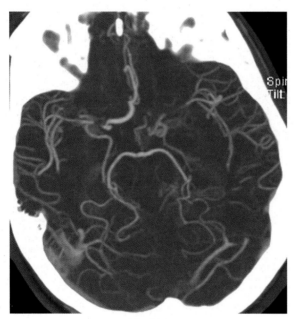

Fig. 81.1

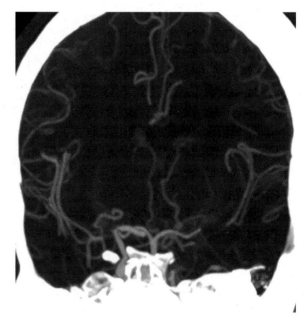

Fig. 81.2

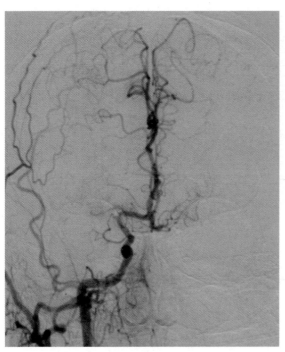

Fig. 81.3

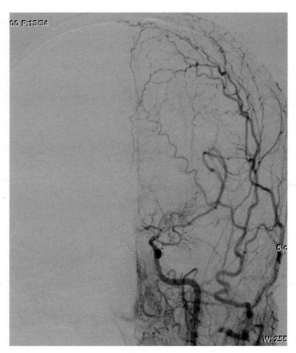

Fig. 81.4

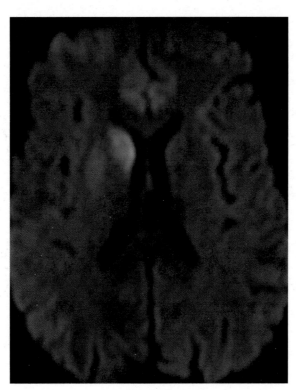

Fig. 81.5

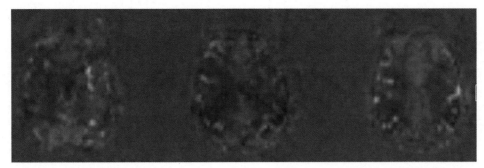

Fig. 81.6

Case 82

History: This 50-year-old female presents with occipital headaches, worse with coughing.

1. What is the most likely diagnosis?
   A. Chiari 1 malformation
   B. Idiopathic intracranial hypertension
   C. Idiopathic pachymeningitis
   D. Spontaneous intracranial hypotension
2. What do the arrows in Figures 82.5 and 82.6 represent?
   A. Normal spinal nerves
   B. Disc herniations
   C. Arachnoid cysts
   D. CSF leak

3. Which of the following can present with diffuse dural enhancement?
   A. Metastatic disease
   B. Neurosarcoidosis
   C. Spontaneous intracranial hypotension
   D. Idiopathic pachymeningitis
   E. All of the above

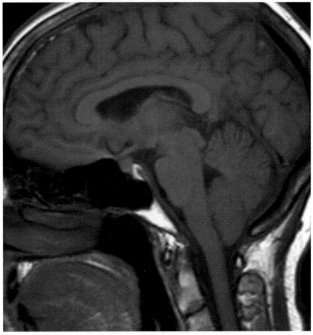

Fig. 82.1

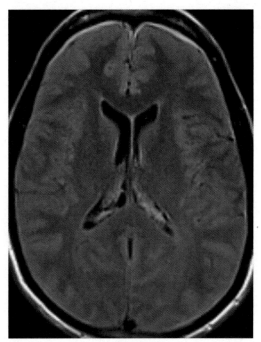

Fig. 82.2

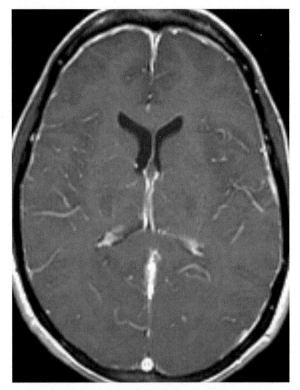

Fig. 82.3

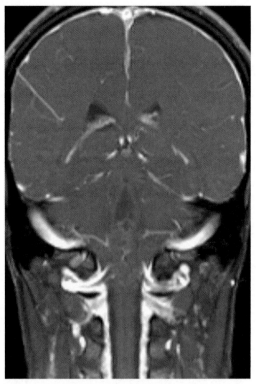

Fig. 82.4

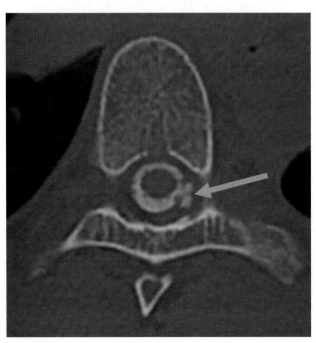

Fig. 82.5

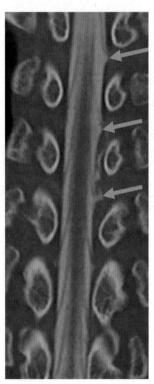

Fig. 82.6

Case 83

History: A 43-year-old female with a history of migraines and cryptogenic lymphadenopathy presented with a sudden severe headache.

1. What would you recommend next based on the findings on this unenhanced head CT (Figure 83.1)?
   A. CTA of the head to rule out an aneurysm
   B. Vessel wall imaging MRI to exclude vasculitis
   C. Conventional angiography to exclude dissection
   D. MRI of the cervical spine to exclude spinal dural AVF
2. CTA of the circle was performed (Figure 83.2) which was unrevealing. What percentage of cases with perimesencephalic subarachnoid hemorrhage (pmSAH) will have a normal cerebral angiogram?
   A. 15%
   B. 25%
   C. 75%
   D. 95%
3. Which of the following is believed to be the most likely cause of this entity?
   A. Ruptured saccular aneurysm
   B. Venous bleed
   C. Underlying occult dural AVF
   D. Vertebrobasilar dolichoectasia
4. What do the arrows in Figures 83.3 and 83.4 point to?
   A. Vertebral artery
   B. Superior cerebellar artery
   C. Anterior inferior cerebellar artery (AICA)
   D. Posterior inferior cerebellar artery (PICA)

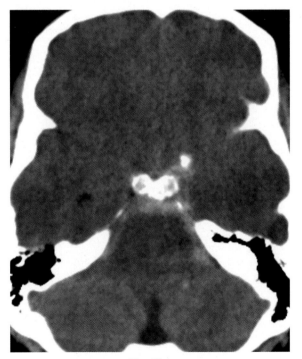

Fig. 83.1

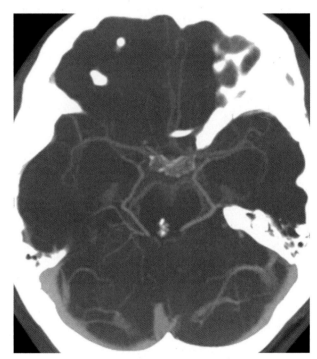

Fig. 83.2

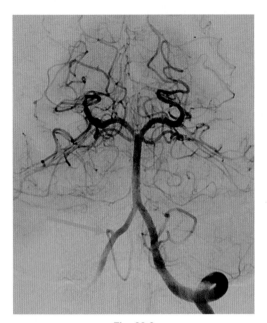

Fig. 83.3

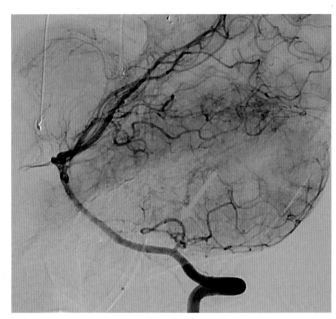

Fig. 83.4

Case 84

History: This is a 56-year-old man with headaches and anisocoria (left pupil 2 mm—sluggish, right pupil 3 mm—normally reactive).

1. What is the most likely diagnosis?
   A. Normal study
   B. Left IJV thrombosis
   C. Left ICA dissection
   D. Left vertebral artery dissection
2. Which of the following can be potential risk factors for internal carotid artery dissection?
   A. Hypertension
   B. Trauma
   C. Fibromuscular dysplasia
   D. Ehlers–Danlos syndrome
   E. Marfan syndrome
   F. All of the above
3. Which of the following is incorrect regarding Horner's syndrome (HS) in internal carotid artery dissection?
   A. In ICA dissections, HS is preganglionic due to the involvement of the pericarotid sympathetic plexus that is compressed by the intramural hematoma.
   B. HS is present in 40% to 50% of patients and may be transient.
   C. Miosis in HS is a decrease in pupil size due to paralysis of the iris dilator muscles.
   D. HS can sometimes be the only manifestation of ICA dissection.
4. Intracranial arterial dissections typically present with which of the following?
   A. Subarachnoid hemorrhage
   B. Subdural hemorrhage
   C. Epidural hemorrhage
   D. Intraventricular hemorrhage

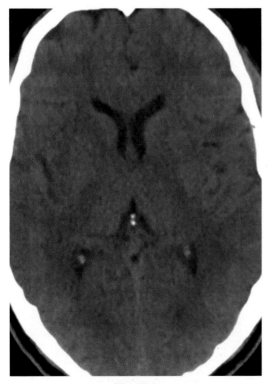

Fig. 84.1

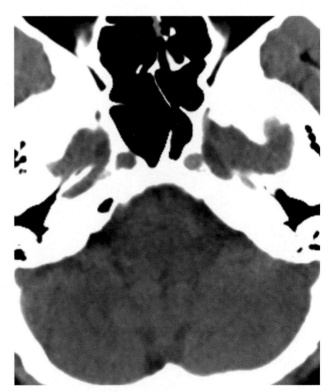

Fig. 84.2

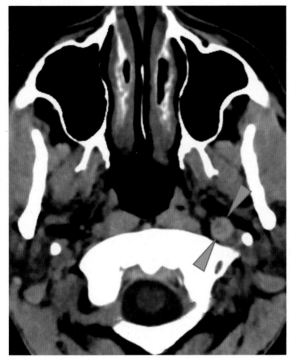

Fig. 84.3

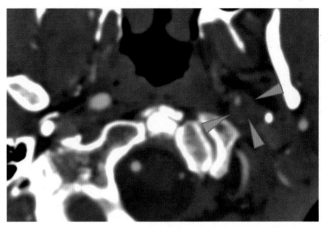

Fig. 84.4

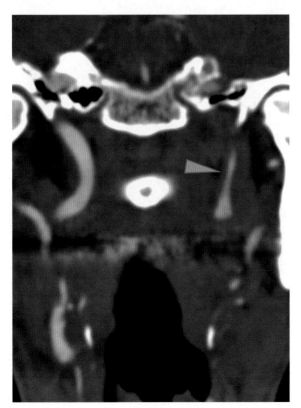

Fig. 84.5

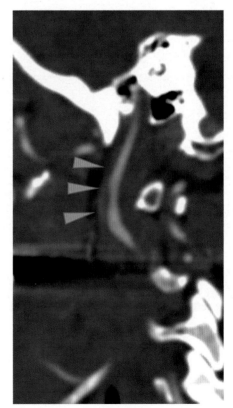

Fig. 84.6

Case 85

History: This 69-year-old female with a history of NASH cirrhosis, hypothyroidism, diabetes complicated by renal failure, septic shock, and worsening liver failure presents with progressive encephalopathy.

1. What is the most common fungal infection of the central nervous system?
   A. *Cryptococcus neoformans*
   B. *Candida*
   C. *Aspergillus*
   D. *Mucor*
2. What fungal infections may occur in both immunocompetent and immunocompromised patients?
   A. *Cryptococcus*
   B. *Coccidioides*
   C. *Histoplasma*
   D. All of the above

3. What is the most common imaging finding of CNS cryptococcal infection in immunocompromised patients?
   A. Spread along the perivascular spaces in the basal ganglia
   B. Hydrocephalus
   C. CNS vasculitis and cerebral infarcts
   D. Scattered cerebral abscesses
4. Why is there a lower incidence of both hydrocephalus and enhancement of parenchymal lesions in immunocompromised patients with CNS infections compared with immunocompetent patients with the same infections?
   A. This likely reflects the inability of these patients to mount significant inflammatory and cell-mediated immune responses.
   B. Decreased permeability of blood–brain barrier
   C. Both of the above
   D. None of the above

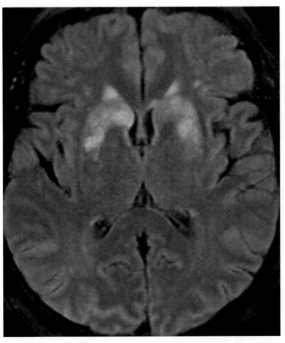

Fig. 85.1

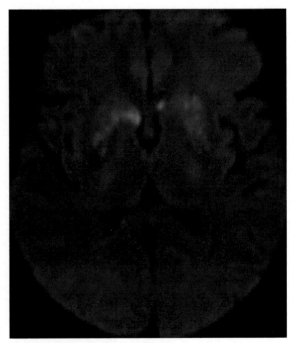

Fig. 85.2

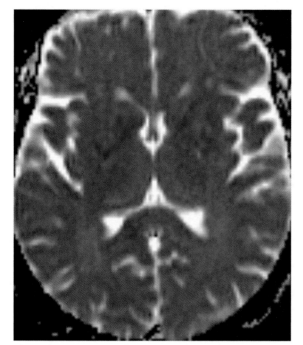

Fig. 85.3

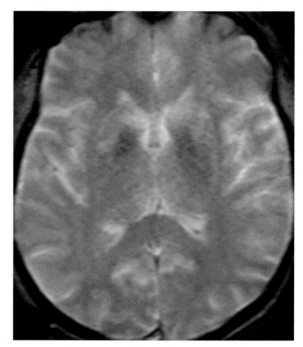

Fig. 85.4

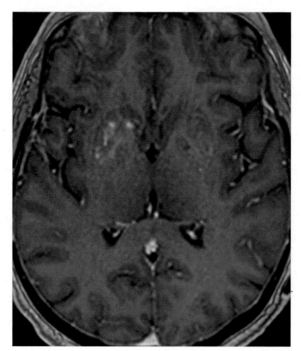

Fig. 85.5

Case 86

History: A 43-year-old woman with headaches. Stage IV breast cancer, on therapeutic anticoagulation.

1. What is the most likely diagnosis?
   A. Neurofibromatosis type-2 (NF-2)
   B. Optic neuritis
   C. Bacterial meningitis
   D. Leptomeningeal carcinomatosis
2. Which of the following primary malignancies is most commonly associated with leptomeningeal carcinomatosis?
   A. Ovarian carcinoma
   B. Breast carcinoma
   C. Gastric carcinoma
   D. Pancreatic carcinoma
   E. Renal cell carcinoma
   F. Prostate carcinoma

3. Which of the following can present with subarachnoid space (sulcal) hyperintensity on the FLAIR sequence?
   A. Susceptibility artifact
   B. Subarachnoid hemorrhage
   C. Meningitis
   D. Leptomeningeal carcinomatosis
   E. Moyamoya disease
   F. Supplemental oxygenation
   G. CSF flow artifact
   H. Motion artifact
   I. All of the above
4. Blockage of the basal cisterns and arachnoid villi may result in what condition?
   A. Leptomeningeal carcinomatosis
   B. Dizziness
   C. Sensorineural hearing loss
   D. Hydrocephalus

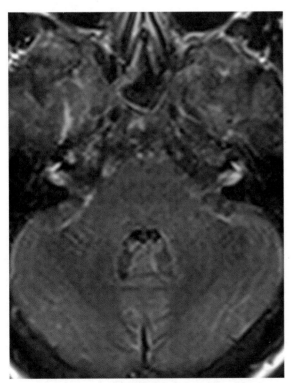

Fig. 86.1

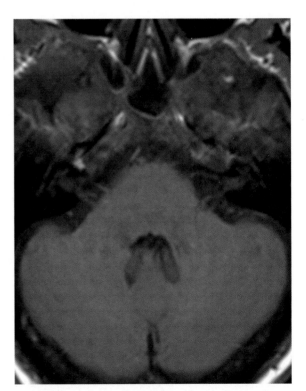

Fig. 86.2

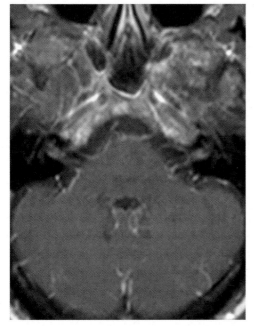

Fig. 86.3

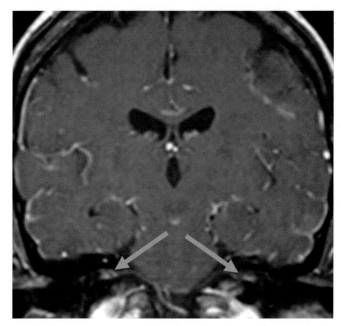

Fig. 86.4

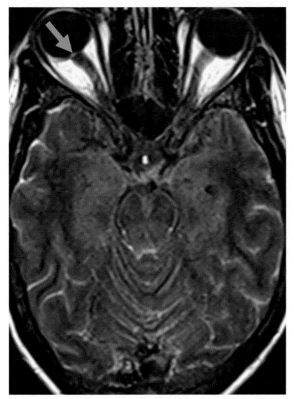

Fig. 86.5

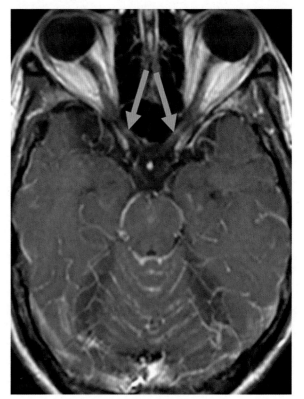

Fig. 86.6

Case 87

History: This 26-year-old female presents with right ear pain and tinnitus, episodic vertiginous dizziness and imbalance. Denies hearing difficulties.

1. What is the most likely diagnosis?
   A. Giant ICA aneurysm
   B. Cholesteatoma
   C. Chondrosarcoma
   D. Cholesterol granuloma
2. Which of the following is responsible for the high T1 signal in a cholesterol granuloma on MRI?
   A. Cholesterol crystals and blood breakdown products
   B. Bone fragments and keratinizing squamous epithelium, admixed with inflammatory cells, granulation tissue, and newly formed vessels
   C. Gelatinous mucoid material
   D. Epidermal appendages, such as hair follicles, sweat glands, and fatty sebum

3. What is the most likely etiology of this lesion?
   A. Changes in tympanic pressure resulting in repeated hemorrhages
   B. Cerumen impaction
   C. Prior trauma and CSF leak
   D. Petrous apex effusion
4. What is the recommended treatment for a symptomatic cholesterol granuloma?
   A. Surgical drainage
   B. Radiation therapy
   C. Observation
   D. Cochlear implantation

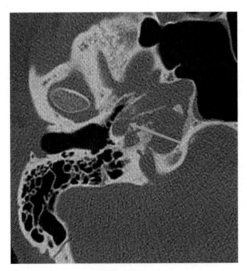

Fig. 87.1

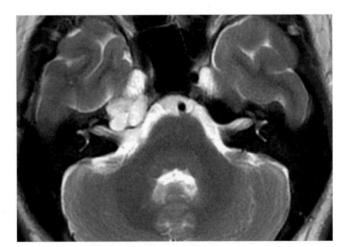

Fig. 87.2

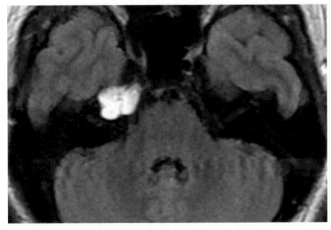

Fig. 87.3

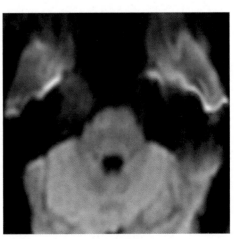

Fig. 87.4

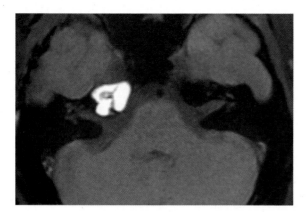

Fig. 87.5

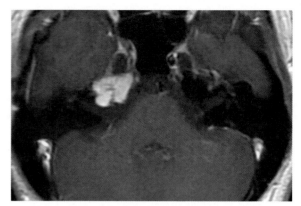

Fig. 87.6

Case 88

History: A 37-year-old male presented with vomiting, dizziness, and vertigo.

1. What is the most likely diagnosis?
   A. Ependymoma
   B. Medulloblastoma
   C. Choroid plexus papilloma
   D. Subependymoma
2. Which molecular subgroup of medulloblastoma arises laterally within the cerebellar hemispheres?
   A. Wingless (WNT)
   B. Sonic hedgehog (SHH)
   C. Group 3
   D. Group 4

3. Which of the following entities has been removed from the most recent 2016 update to the WHO classification of CNS tumors?
   A. Primitive neuroectodermal tumor (PNET)
   B. Dysembryoplastic neuroepithelial tumor (DNET)
   C. Multinodular and vacuolating neuronal tumors (MVNT)
   D. Embryonal tumors with multilayered rosettes (ETMR)
4. What percentage of patients with medulloblastomas present with subarachnoid seeding at the time of diagnosis?
   A. 10%
   B. 30%
   C. 50%
   D. 90%

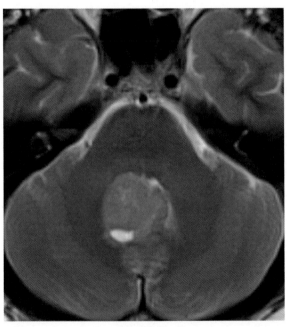

Fig. 88.1

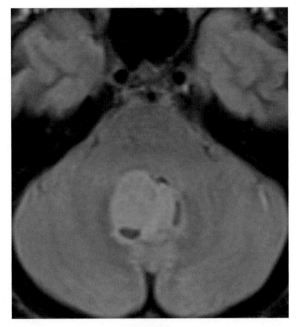

Fig. 88.2

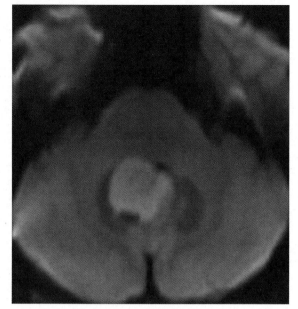

Fig. 88.3

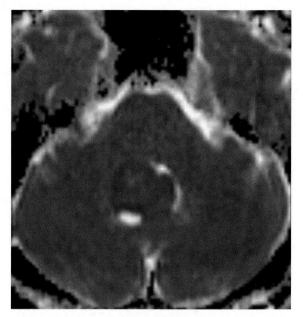

Fig. 88.4

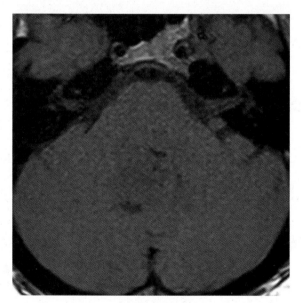

Fig. 88.5

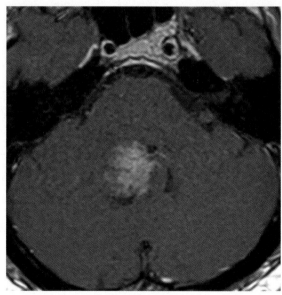

Fig. 88.6

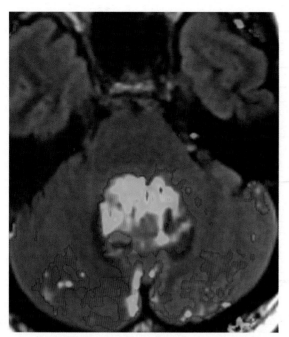

Fig. 88.7

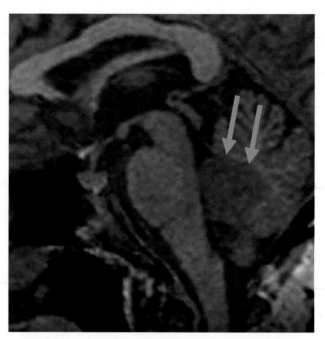

Fig. 88.8

Case 89

History: This 43-year-old man presents with a "mass" seen on an outside hospital head CT.

1. What is the diagnosis?
   A. Calcified granuloma
   B. Cavernous malformation
   C. Capillary telangiectasia
   D. Cavernous malformation and developmental venous anomaly
2. Which vascular malformation is most commonly associated with a developmental venous anomaly (DVA)?
   A. Arteriovenous malformation
   B. Cavernous malformation
   C. Capillary telangiectasias
   D. Mycotic aneurysms
3. Which of the following is the most common cerebral vascular malformation?
   A. Cavernous malformation
   B. Capillary telangiectasia
   C. Developmental venous anomaly
   D. Cavernous malformation and developmental venous anomaly
4. Which type of cavernous malformation is depicted in the present case?
   A. Type I
   B. Type II
   C. Type III
   D. Type IV

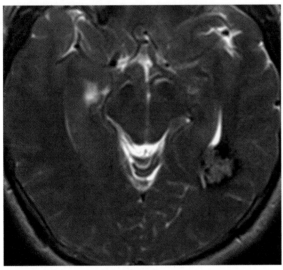

Fig. 89.1

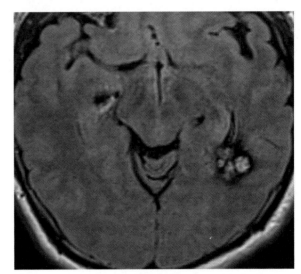

Fig. 89.2

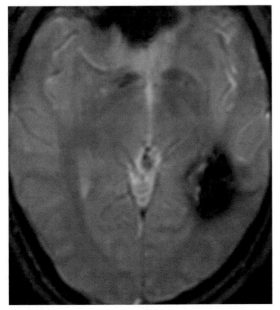

Fig. 89.3

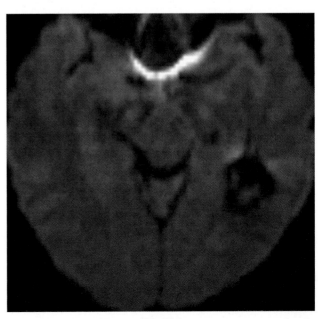

Fig. 89.4

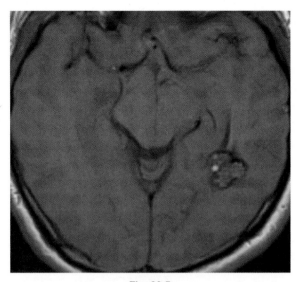

Fig. 89.5

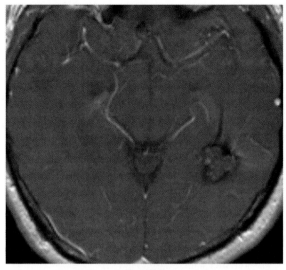

Fig. 89.6

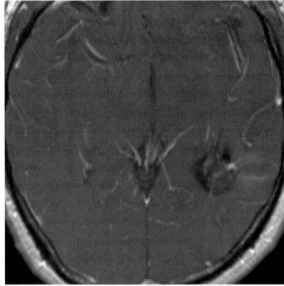

Fig. 89.7

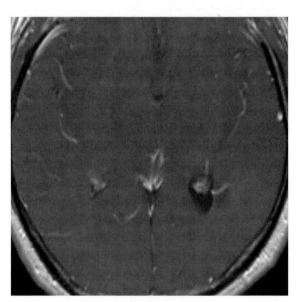

Fig. 89.8

Case 90

History: A 55-year-old vegan female presents with progressive difficulties with memory, language, cognition, and behavior. She also has type II diabetes on metformin, hyperlipidemia on rosuvastatin, and prior hospital admission for hypertensive crisis.

1. What is the diagnosis?
   A. Chronic hypoxic-ischemic encephalopathy from prior hypertensive urgency
   B. Hypoglycemia
   C. Central nervous system vasculitis
   D. Creutzfeldt–Jakob disease (CJD)
2. Which of the following radiological signs is associated with Creutzfeldt–Jakob disease (CJD)?
   A. Hockey stick sign
   B. Pulvinar sign
   C. Cortical ribbon sign
   D. All of the above
3. The definitive diagnosis of Creutzfeldt–Jakob disease (CJD) is established by which of the following?
   A. Characteristic findings on brain MRI
   B. CSF 14-3-3 protein
   C. CSF and/or olfactory mucosa real-time quaking-induced conversion (RT-QuIC) assay
   D. Brain biopsy
4. Which MRI sequence is depicted by Figures 90.4 and 90.8?
   A. b-1000
   B. b-0
   C. Apparent diffusion coefficient (ADC)
   D. Exponential apparent diffusion coefficient (e-ADC)

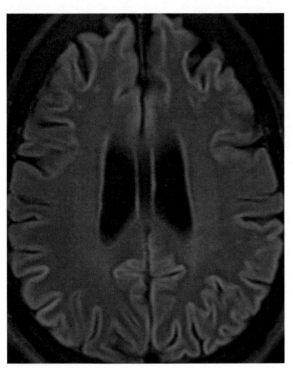

Fig. 90.1

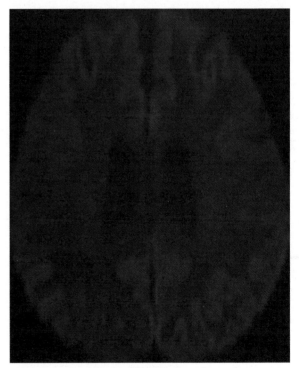

Fig. 90.2

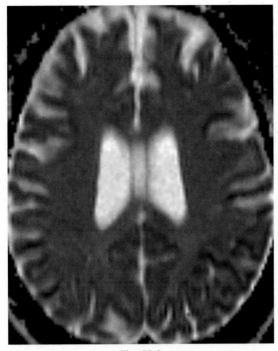

Fig. 90.3

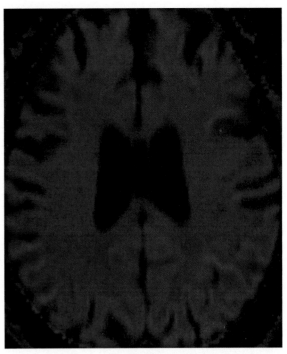

Fig. 90.4

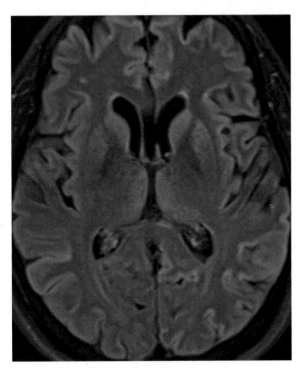

Fig. 90.5

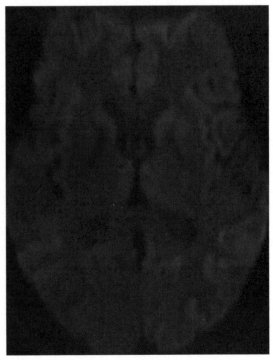

Fig. 90.6

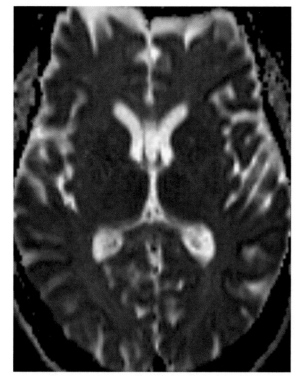

Fig. 90.7

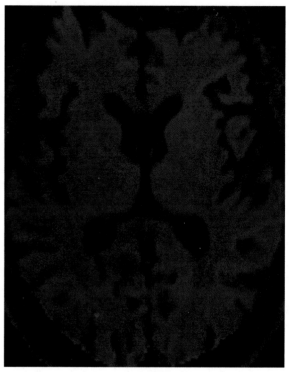

Fig. 90.8

Case 91

History: A 27-year-old with a known inherited disorder presented with throbbing pulsatile occipital headache, ataxic gait, nystagmus, imbalance, and hearing loss.

1. What is the likely inherited disorder in this patient?
   A. Neurofibromatosis type-1 (NF1)
   B. Neurofibromatosis type-2 (NF2)
   C. Neurofibromatosis type-3 (NF3)
   D. Von Hippel–Lindau disease (VHL)
2. Neurofibromatosis type-2 is associated with increased incidence of which of the following conditions?
   A. Intracranial schwannomas
   B. Intracranial as well as spinal meningiomas
   C. Ependymomas
   D. All of the above

3. Alterations in which protein are associated with neurofibromatosis type-2?
   A. Neurofibromin
   B. Merlin
   C. Hamartin
   D. Tuberin
4. What primary glial neoplasm is this disorder associated with?
   A. Ependymoma
   B. Glioblastoma
   C. Astrocytoma
   D. Oligodendroglioma

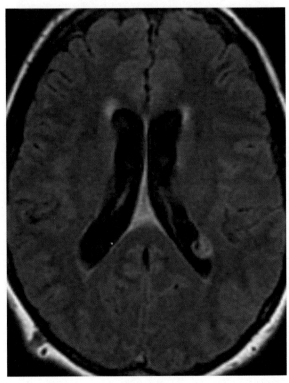

Fig. 91.1

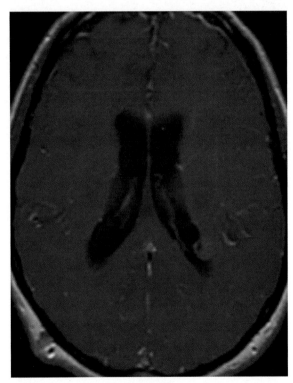

Fig. 91.2

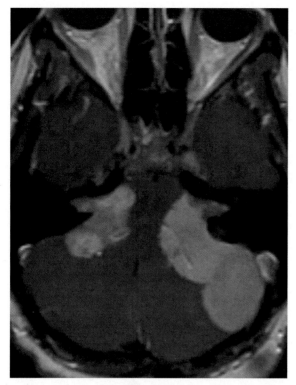

Fig. 91.3

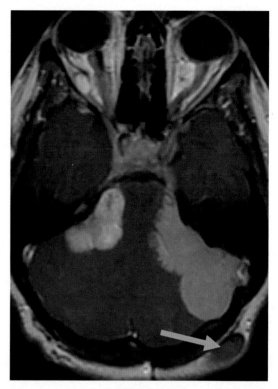

Fig. 91.4

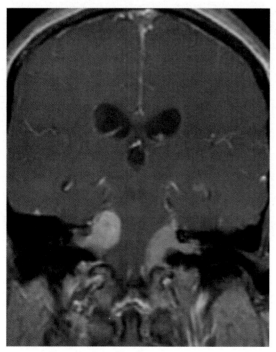

Fig. 91.5

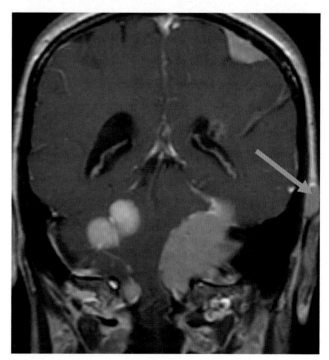

Fig. 91.6

Case 92

History: This is a 45-year-old male with HIV-AIDS and a CD4 count of 52 cells/μL.

1. What is the most likely diagnosis in this immunocompromised patient?
   A. Progressive multifocal leukoencephalopathy (PML)
   B. Lymphoma
   C. Toxoplasmosis
   D. HIV encephalitis
2. Which of the following infectious agents is responsible for progressive multifocal leukoencephalopathy (PML)?
   A. Human immunodeficiency virus (HIV)
   B. Epstein-Barr virus (EBV)
   C. Herpes simplex virus (HSV)
   D. John Cunningham virus (JCV)

3. Which of the following is incorrect regarding imaging in patients with progressive multifocal leukoencephalopathy (PML)?
   A. Asymmetric white matter lesions with sparing of the subcortical U-fibers
   B. Usually, there is little or no mass effect.
   C. Enhancement can be seen in PML-immune reconstitution inflammatory syndrome (IRIS).
   D. On MR spectroscopy, there is reduced NAA, presence of lipids/lactate, and increased choline.
4. Progressive multifocal leukoencephalopathy is a known complication in patients with multiple sclerosis with positive JC virus serology treated with which agent?
   A. Corticosteroids
   B. Interferon beta
   C. Fingolimod
   D. Natalizumab

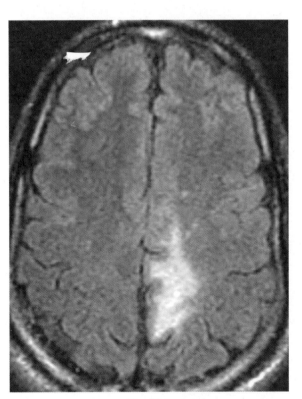

Fig. 92.1

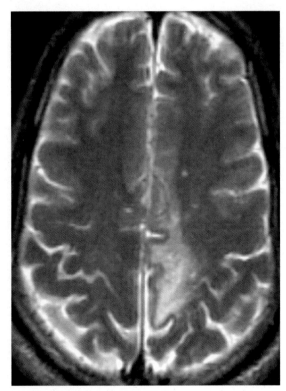

Fig. 92.2

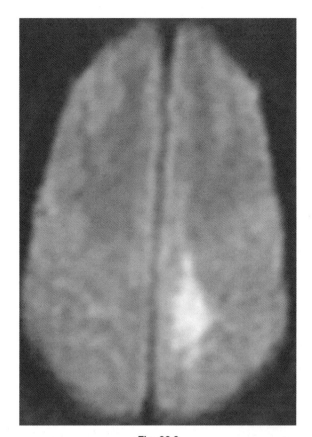

Fig. 92.3

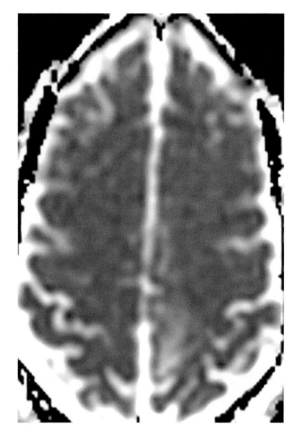

Fig. 92.4

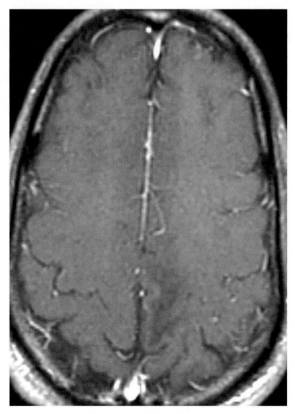

Fig. 92.5

Case 93

History: This 27-year-old female history of primary hypothyroidism (diagnosed 3 years ago) presents with right neck pain, right eyelid droop, and right leg and arm paresthesias.

1. What is the most likely diagnosis?
   A. Prolactinoma
   B. Pituitary apoplexy
   C. Pituitary hyperplasia
   D. Lymphocytic hypophysitis
2. The arrow in Figure 93.3 is pointing to what anatomical structure?
   A. Optic nerve
   B. Cavernous internal carotid artery
   C. Oculomotor nerve
   D. Trigeminal ganglion

3. A focal T1 hyperintense region is usually observed at the posterior aspect of the sella turcica, immediately anterior to the dorsum sellae. What is the etiology of this "posterior pituitary bright spot" on T1-weighted images?
   A. Storage of vasopressin
   B. Flow artifacts from adjacent arteries
   C. Volume averaging with fatty marrow in the dorsum sella
   D. Magnetic susceptibility effects
4. Which of the following can mimic a "posterior pituitary bright spot"?
   A. Pituitary apoplexy
   B. Rathke cleft cysts
   C. Manganese accumulation in the anterior pituitary in patients with liver disease
   D. Hyperactive hormone secretion in the anterior pituitary in newborns
   E. All of the above

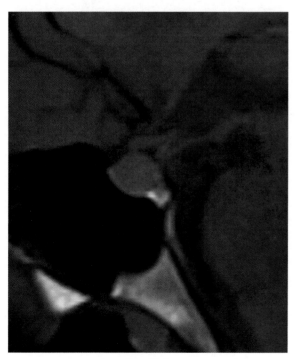

Fig. 93.1

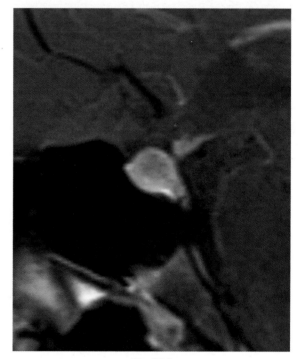

Fig. 93.2

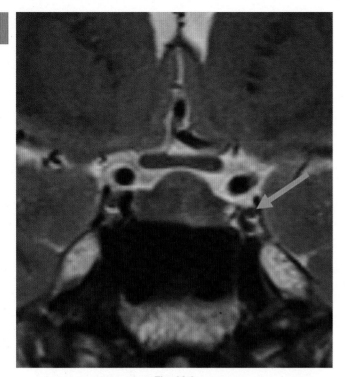

Fig. 93.3

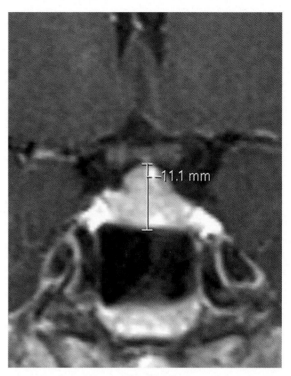

Fig. 93.4

Case 94

History: A 43-year-old female with a sore throat, pain and swelling in the right submandibular region, and fatigue.

1. What is the most common vascular lesion of the orbit in adults?
   A. Optic nerve meningioma
   B. Lymphoma
   C. Venous varix
   D. Metastases
   E. Cavernous hemangioma
2. What is the most common presenting symptom of an orbital cavernous hemangioma?
   A. Pain
   B. Proptosis
   C. Diplopia
   D. Vision loss
3. Which of the following is incorrect regarding imaging of orbital cavernous hemangiomas?
   A. Well-circumscribed intraconal masses with sparing of the orbital apex
   B. Usually managed conservatively, with surgical excision reserved for those causing severe proptosis or optic nerve compression
   C. Cavernous malformations demonstrate progressive accumulation of the contrast material on late-phase dynamic images and delayed images
   D. On MRI, multiple fluid-fluid levels within the lesion are characteristic
4. The arrow in Figure 94.6 is pointing to what anatomical structure?
   A. Levator palpebrae superioris
   B. Superior rectus
   C. Superior oblique
   D. Medial rectus

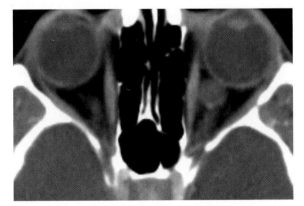

Fig. 94.1

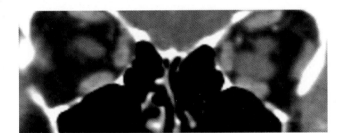

Fig. 94.2

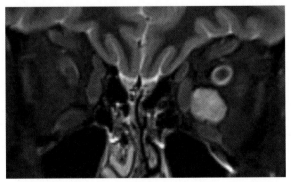

Fig. 94.3

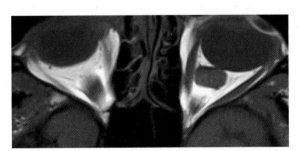

Fig. 94.4

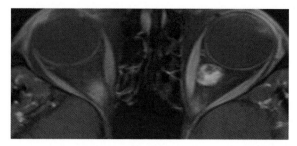

Fig. 94.5

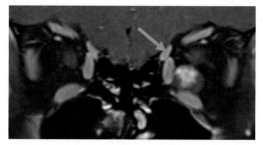

Fig. 94.6

Case 95

History: This 86-year-old male presents with confusion and delirium.

1. What is the most likely diagnosis?
   A. Orbital dermoid
   B. Orbital lymphoma
   C. Orbital venous varix
   D. Orbital metastases
   E. Orbital cavernous hemangioma
2. What is the most common presenting symptom of an orbital dermoid?
   A. Painful swelling
   B. Painless subcutaneous lump
   C. Diplopia
   D. Vision loss
3. What is the etiology of an orbital dermoid cyst?
   A. Congenital
   B. Posttraumatic
   C. Iatrogenic
   D. Postinfectious
4. What does the arrow in Figure 95.4 represent?
   A. Zygomaticotemporal suture
   B. Zygomaticomaxillary suture
   C. Zygomaticofrontal suture
   D. Zygomaticosphenoid suture

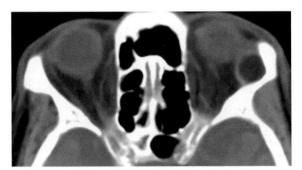

Fig. 95.1

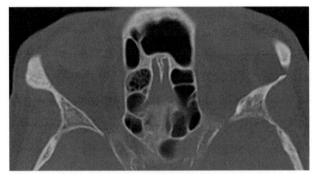

Fig. 95.2

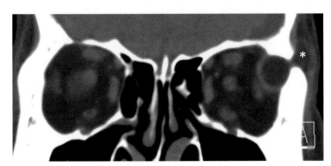

Fig. 95.3

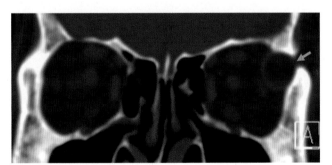

Fig. 95.4

Case 96

History: This is a 27-year-old male with a headache.

1. What substances are hyperintense on unenhanced T1-weighted imaging?
   A. Fat
   B. Methemoglobin
   C. Manganese
   D. Melanin
   E. All of the above
2. What is the diagnosis in this case?
   A. Metastatic melanoma
   B. Ruptured dermoid cyst
   C. Fat embolism
   D. Epidermoid cyst
3. On MR imaging, what artifact is indicative of the presence of fat?
   A. Chemical shift artifact
   B. Moiré fringes
   C. Aliasing artifact
   D. Susceptibility artifact
4. Which of the following is true regarding chemical shift artifact?
   A. Seen as white and dark bands flanking an object along a frequency-encoding direction
   B. Seen because the protons of fat resonate at a higher frequency than those of water
   C. Chemical shift artifact is only seen in the brain
   D. Chemical shift artifact decreases with magnetic field strength

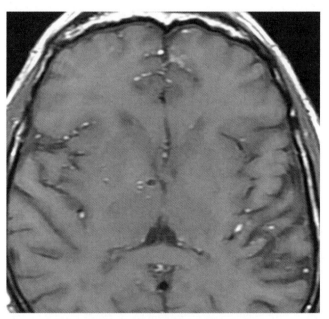

Fig. 96.1

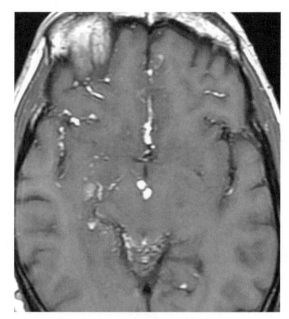

Fig. 96.2

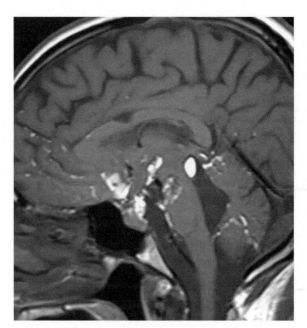

Fig. 96.3

Case 97

History: A 45-year-old female with migraine headaches and a family history of stroke presented with throbbing in the ear.

1. What is the diagnosis?
   A. Takayasu's arteritis
   B. Atherosclerosis
   C. Loeys–Dietz syndrome
   D. Fibromuscular dysplasia with a dissecting pseudoaneurysm
2. Which layer of the vessel wall is most commonly affected in fibromuscular dysplasia (FMD)?
   A. Tunica adventitia
   B. Tunica media
   C. Tunica intima
   D. Endothelial layer

3. Which vessel is most commonly involved in fibromuscular dysplasia (FMD)?
   A. Internal carotid artery
   B. Abdominal aorta
   C. Left subclavian artery
   D. Renal artery
4. Which of the following is true regarding "arterial tortuosity syndrome"?
   A. Rare connective tissue disorder characterized by tortuosity of the large and medium-sized arteries, caused by mutations in SLC2A10
   B. Stenoses, tortuosity, and aneurysm formation are widespread occurrences
   C. Complications include aortic root aneurysms, neonatal intracranial hemorrhage as well as ischemic stroke
   D. Vascular dissections are not known
   E. All of the above

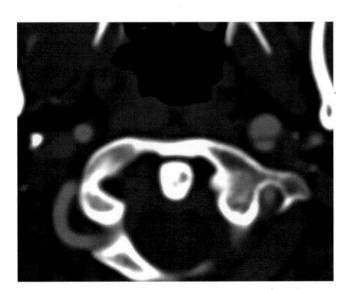

Fig. 97.1

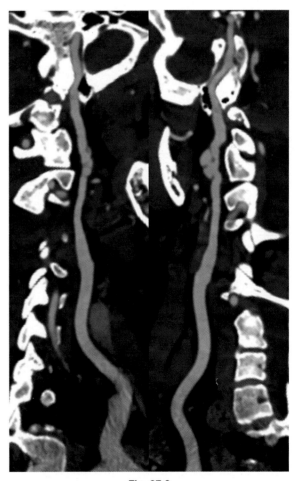

Fig. 97.2

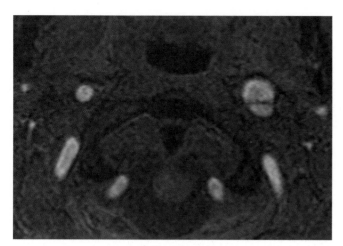

Fig. 97.3

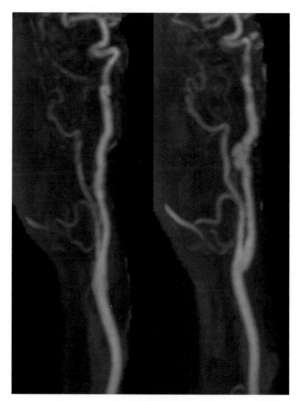

Fig. 97.4

Case 98

History: This is a 65-year-old female with word-finding difficulty and difficulty performing tasks. No headaches, weakness, or sensory changes.

1. Which of the following primary glial neoplasms are associated with hemorrhage?
   A. Pilocytic astrocytoma
   B. Glioblastoma
   C. Oligodendroglioma
   D. All of the above

2. What is the diagnosis in this case?
   A. Glioblastoma
   B. Oligodendroglioma
   C. Primary CNS lymphoma
   D. Toxoplasmosis

3. What is the added value of MRI perfusion in the evaluation of brain tumors?
   A. Glioma grading and prognostication
   B. Distinguishing a primary glioma from lymphoma and brain metastases
   C. Distinguishing high-grade gliomas from tumefactive demyelinating lesions, and infection
   D. Differentiation of true progression from pseudoprogression
   E. All of the above

4. Diffusion tensor imaging (DTI) and fiber tractography (FT) are commonly used MRI techniques for the presurgical mapping of brain tumors. Which white matter tract is depicted by the color blue in Figure 98.8?
   A. Corticospinal tract (CST)
   B. Inferior fronto-occipital fasciculus (IFOF)
   C. Arcuate fasciculus (AF)
   D. Optic radiation (OR)

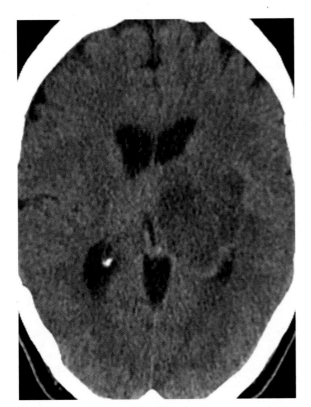

Fig. 98.1

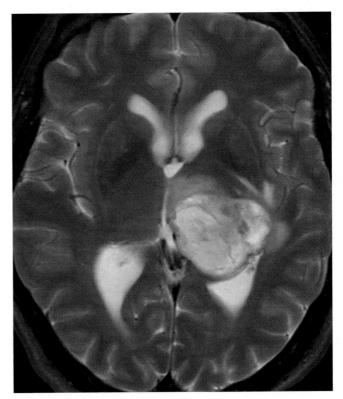

Fig. 98.2

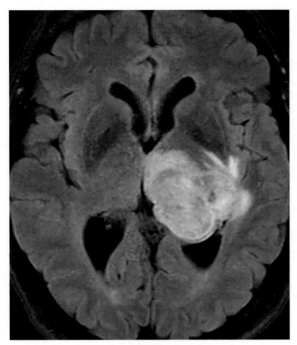

Fig. 98.3

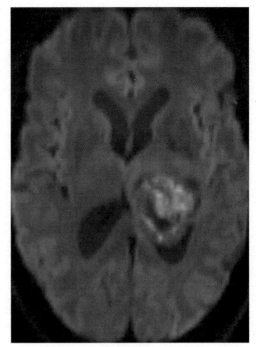

Fig. 98.4

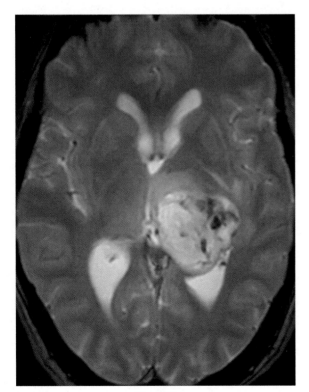

Fig. 98.5

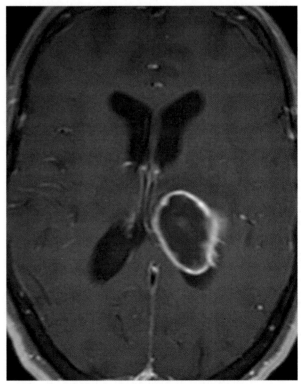

Fig. 98.6

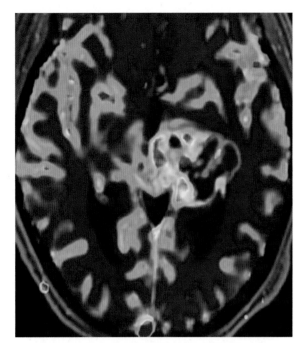

Fig. 98.7

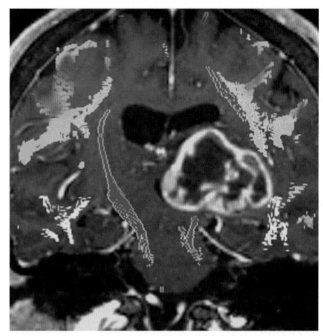

Fig. 98.8

Case 99

History: This 17-year-old boy presents with oculomotor apraxia, gait ataxia, learning disabilities, and complex behavioral health phenotype.

1. What is the diagnosis?
   A. Dandy–Walker malformation
   B. Joubert's syndrome
   C. Lhermitte–Duclos disease
   D. Mega cisterna magna
2. Which radiology sign describes the morphology of the fourth ventricle in Joubert's syndrome?
   A. Morning glory sign
   B. Bat wing sign
   C. Hummingbird sign
   D. Owl-eyes sign
3. Molar tooth appearance of the midbrain was initially described in patients with Joubert's syndrome, but it is now recognized in a number of other conditions. It results from a lack of normal decussation of which of the following?
   A. Superior cerebellar peduncles
   B. Middle cerebellar peduncles
   C. Inferior cerebellar peduncles
   D. Cerebral peduncles
4. Which of the following is correct regarding rhombencephalosynapsis?
   A. Absence of vermis and fusion of the dentate nuclei and superior cerebellar peduncles
   B. Cerebellar hyperplasia
   C. Vermian hypoplasia with elongated and horizontally oriented superior cerebellar peduncles
   D. Vermian hypoplasia with flattened ventral pons, vaulted pontine tegmentum, and partial absence of the middle cerebellar peduncles

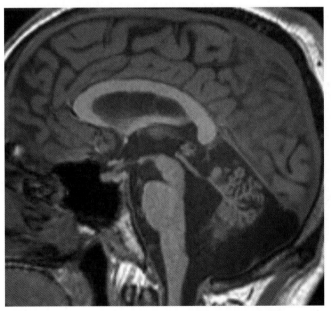

Fig. 99.1

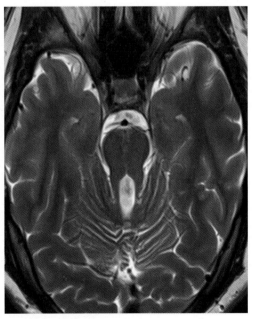

Fig. 99.2

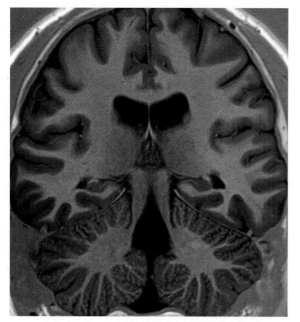

Fig. 99.3

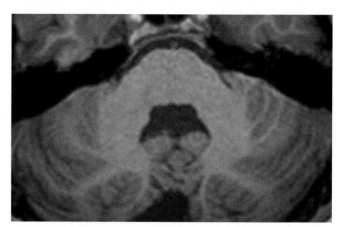

Fig. 99.4

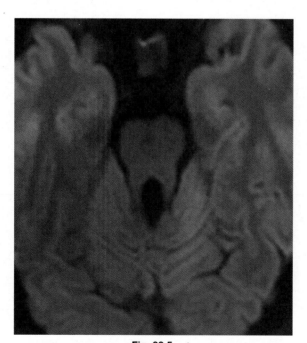

Fig. 99.5

Case 100

History: An 18-month-old boy with early difficulties with latching, head circumference in the 85th percentile, and nystagmus.

1. Which of the following conditions can present with enlargement of the head?
    A. Congenital hydrocephalus
    B. Mucopolysaccharidoses
    C. Alexander disease
    D. Canavan disease
    E. All of the above
2. What is the diagnosis in this case?
    A. Adrenoleukodystrophy
    B. Pelizaeus–Merzbacher disease
    C. Alexander disease
    D. Canavan disease

3. What enzyme deficiency is responsible for Canavan disease?
    A. Arylsulfatase A
    B. *N*-acetylaspartoacylase
    C. Galactocerebrosidase
    D. Beta-galactosidase
4. Which leukodystrophy typically spares the subcortical U-fibers and has a characteristic parieto-occipital periventricular white matter distribution?
    A. Adrenoleukodystrophy
    B. Pelizaeus–Merzbacher disease
    C. Alexander disease
    D. Canavan disease

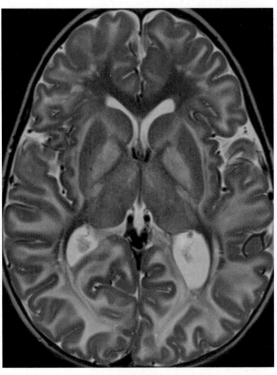

Fig. 100.1

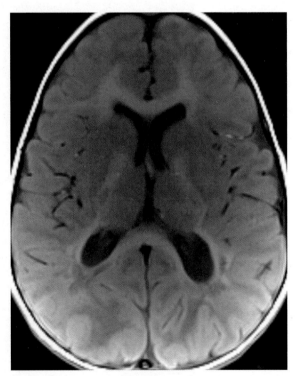

Fig. 100.2

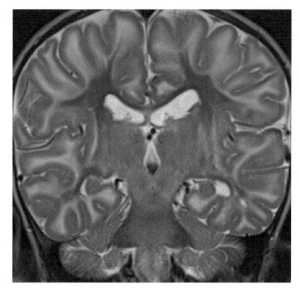

Fig. 100.3

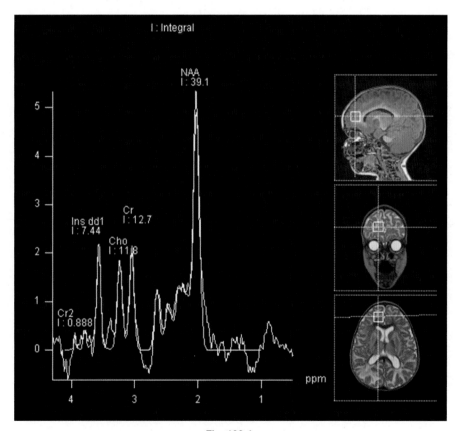

Fig. 100.4

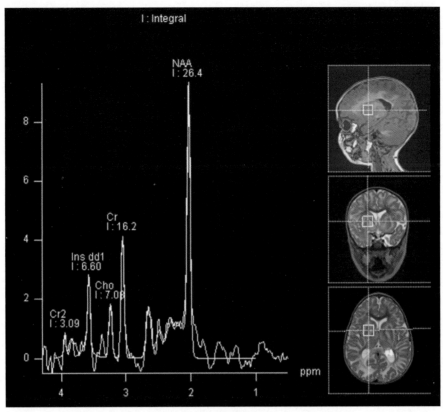

Fig. 100.5

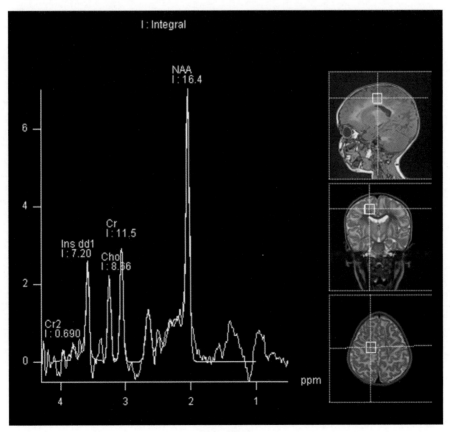

Fig. 100.6

Case 101

History:
Case 1: A 25-year-old female with headaches.
Case 2: A 67-year-old male with a history of sciatica and slowly progressive deterioration of gait.
Case 3: A 61-year-old male with nonspecific GI symptoms, low energy, abdominal bloating, and fatigue.

1. What is the common diagnosis in all three of these patients?
   A. Bone marrow reconversion
   B. Osseous metastases
   C. Chiari 1 malformation
   D. Spontaneous intracranial hypotension
2. What is the cause of hypointense marrow on T1W imaging in chronic anemia?
   A. Replacement of fat cells normally found in red marrow (yellow-to-red marrow reconversion)
   B. Prominent sclerosis in the bone marrow
   C. Replacement of hematopoietic cells with fat cells
   D. Decreased vascularity

3. Which of the following disorders are associated with extra-medullary hematopoiesis?
   A. Sickle cell disease
   B. Thalassemia
   C. Hereditary spherocytosis
   D. Leukemia
   E. Myelofibrosis
   F. All of the above
4. What is the most common site of extramedullary hematopoiesis in the body?
   A. Bone marrow
   B. Adrenal gland
   C. Lungs
   D. Liver

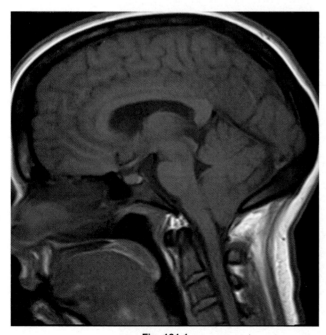

Fig. 101.1

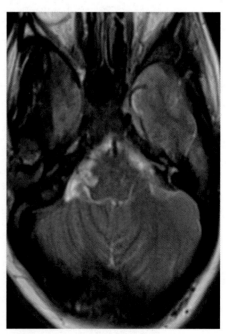

Fig. 101.2

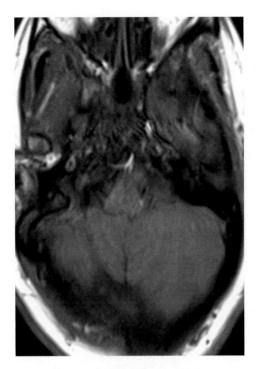

Fig. 101.3

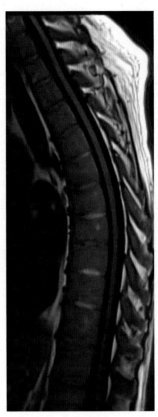

Fig. 101.4

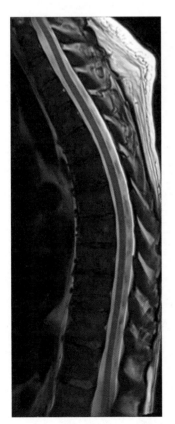

Fig. 101.5

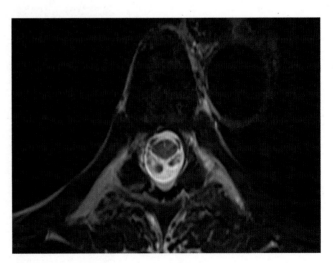

Fig. 101.6

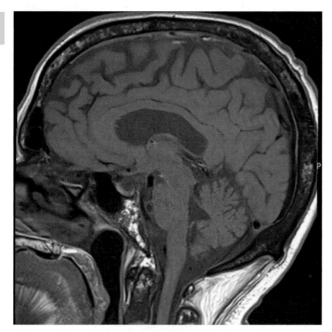

Fig. 101.7

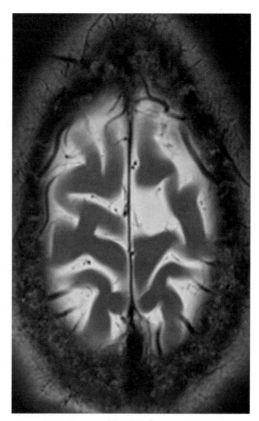

Fig. 101.8

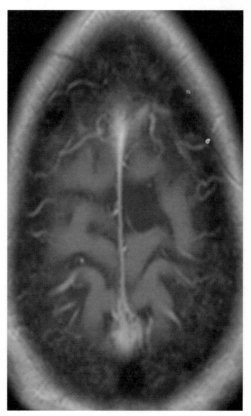

Fig. 101.9

Case 102

History: This is a 34-year-old female with a week of waxing and waning mental status, confusion, and drowsiness.

1. What would be the most appropriate next imaging test based on the initial head CT (Figure 102.1)?
   A. Contrast-enhanced head CT
   B. CT angiography
   C. MR venography
   D. PET scan
2. MRI and MR venography were performed (Figures 102.2–102.7). What is the final diagnosis based on these images?
   A. Hemorrhagic metastases
   B. Hemorrhagic venous infarction
   C. Hemorrhagic MCA territory infarction
   D. Hemorrhagic PRES

3. Which of the following is correct regarding hemorrhagic venous infarction?
   A. Parenchymal hemorrhage is observed in 5%–15% of cases.
   B. 2D time-of-flight MRV has better sensitivity to slow flow and is insensitive to short T1 tissue than 3D phase-contrast MRV.
   C. Both contrast-enhanced MRV and 3D contrast-enhanced gradient-recalled-echo T1W MRI are excellent methods for the diagnosis of cerebral venous thrombosis (CVT).
   D. Complete recanalization of thrombosed sinuses is necessary for clinical recovery.

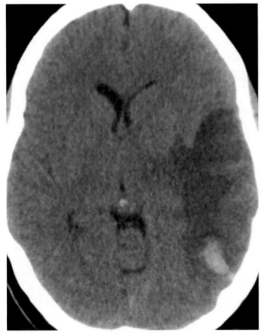

Fig. 102.1

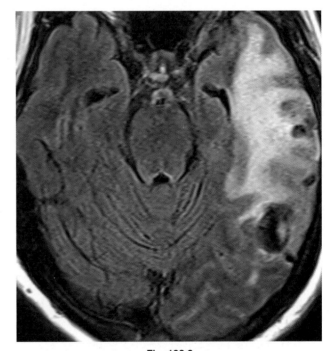

Fig. 102.2

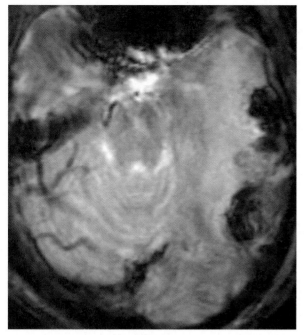

Fig. 102.3

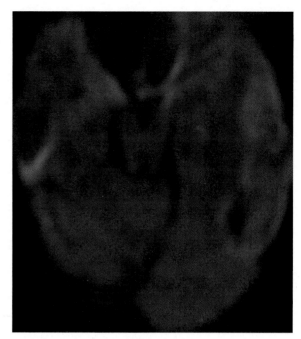

Fig. 102.4

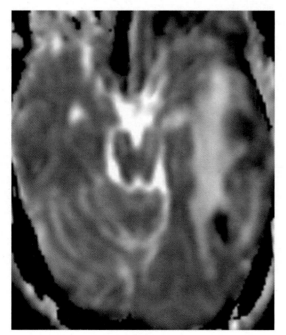

Fig. 102.5

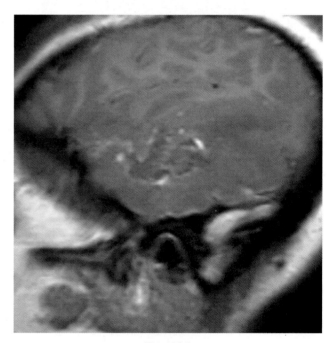

Fig. 102.6

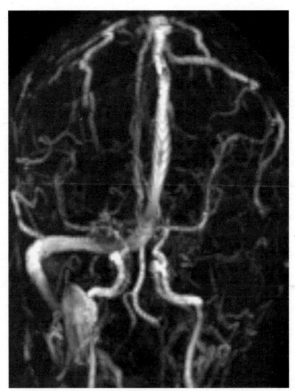

Fig. 102.7

Case 103

History: This 53-year-old female presents with headache, confusion, nausea, and vomiting. The patient has been coughing for a week with a recent diagnosis of bronchitis.

1. What is the most likely etiology of subarachnoid hemorrhage in this patient?
   A. Ruptured PICA aneurysm
   B. Ruptured vertebral artery aneurysm
   C. Ruptured posterior fossa AVM
   D. Right vertebral artery dissection and pseudoaneurysm
2. Which of the following is correct regarding intracranial vertebral artery dissections?
   A. Intracranial dissections are more common than extracranial dissections of the vertebral artery.
   B. Vertebral artery dissections are mostly located in the V2 or V3 segments.
   C. Conventional angiography is limited in assessing intracranial dissections.
   D. Anticoagulation and antiplatelet therapy are not contraindicated in patients with intracranial hemorrhage.

3. What is the likely etiology of acute infarcts seen on follow-up head CT (Figure 103.3)?
   A. Vasospasm following subarachnoid hemorrhage
   B. Primary CNS vasculitis
   C. Reversible cerebral vasoconstriction syndrome
   D. Cardioembolic stroke
4. What are common complications of intracranial vascular dissections?
   A. Thromboembolic stroke
   B. Pseudoaneurysm formation
   C. Subarachnoid hemorrhage
   D. All of the above

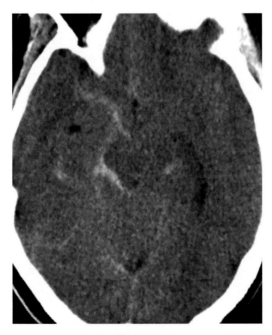

Fig. 103.1

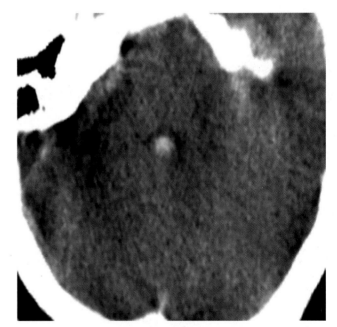

Fig. 103.2

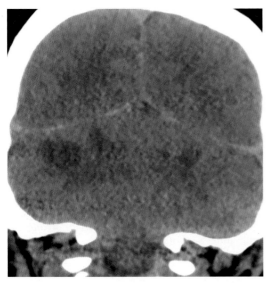

Fig. 103.3

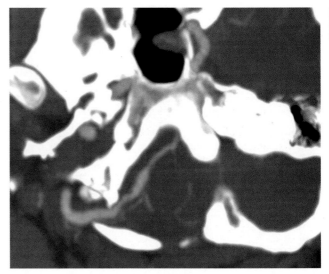

Fig. 103.4

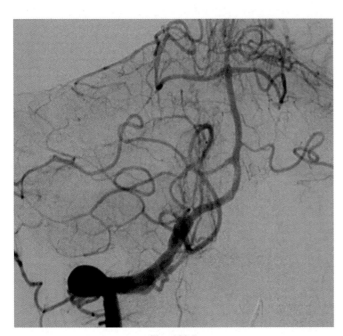

Fig. 103.5

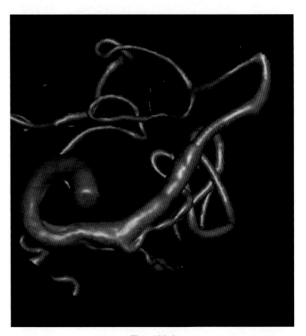

Fig. 103.6

Case 104

History: This is a 22-year-old male with visual disturbance, hematologic abnormalities, endocrine disturbance, and hypernatremia.

1. What is the diagnosis?
   A. Germinoma
   B. Craniopharyngioma
   C. Hamartoma
   D. Glioma
2. In what percentage of cases with suprasellar (hypothalamic) germinomas is a synchronous lesion seen in the pineal region?
   A. 10%
   B. 30%
   C. 50%
   D. 70%

3. Which of the following is correct regarding CNS germinomas?
   A. These tumors are derived from germ cells and are typically seen in the midline.
   B. Suprasellar location is most common and is seen in 80%–90% of cases.
   C. Pineal germinoma is the second most common and is seen in 15%–30% of cases.
   D. Posterior pituitary bright spot is generally preserved in suprasellar germinomas.
4. Which category of pineal tumors has a strong male sex predilection?
   A. Pineoblastoma
   B. Pineocytoma
   C. Germinoma
   D. Pineal parenchymal tumor with intermediate differentiation

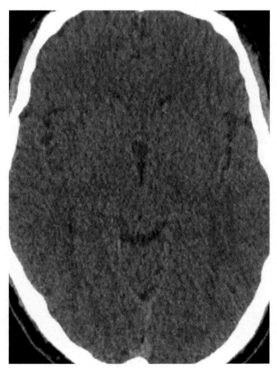

Fig. 104.1

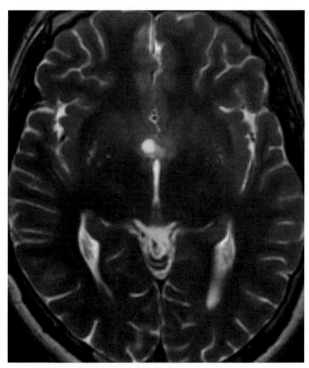

Fig. 104.2

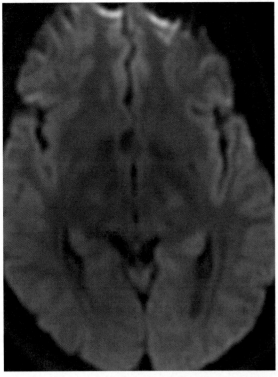

Fig. 104.3

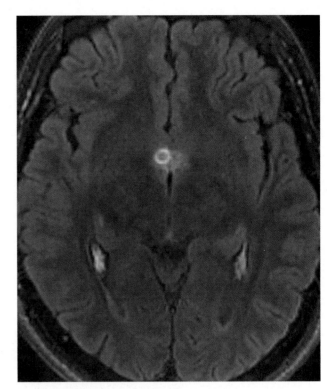

Fig. 104.4

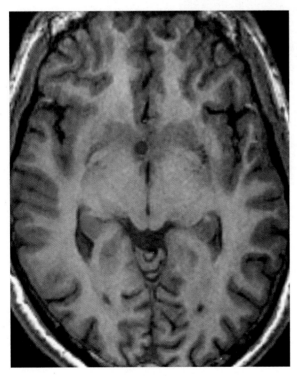

Fig. 104.5

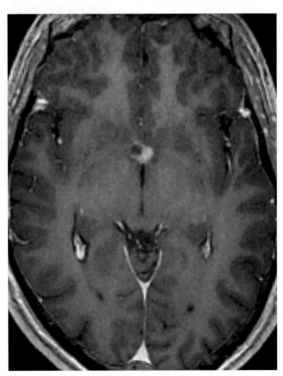

Fig. 104.6

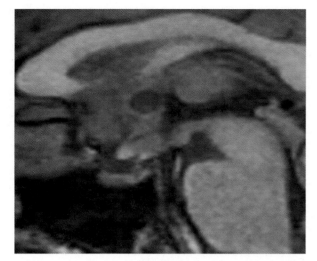

Fig. 104.7

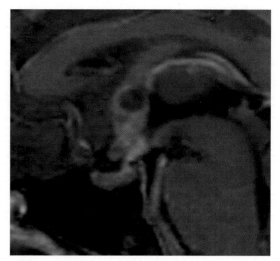

Fig. 104.8

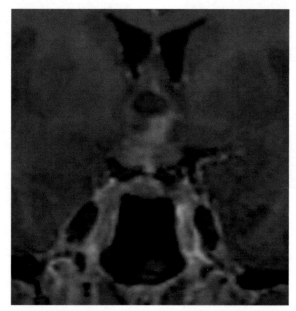

Fig. 104.9

Case 105

History: A 50-year-old male presents with fever and right eyelid drooping.

1. What is the most common orbital malignancy?
   A. Orbital lymphoma
   B. Orbital metastases
   C. Orbital sarcoma
   D. Orbital melanoma
2. Which of the following infections has been found to be associated with orbital lymphoma?
   A. *Chlamydia psittaci*
   B. *Borrelia burgdorferi*
   C. *Treponema pallidum*
   D. Herpes simplex
3. What is the most common site of primary orbital lymphoma?
   A. Superior lateral quadrant
   B. Retrobulbar compartment
   C. Inferior quadrants
   D. Optic nerve
4. What characteristic imaging finding, when present, is highly suggestive of metastatic breast carcinoma?
   A. Proptosis
   B. Double vision
   C. Vision loss
   D. Enophthalmos

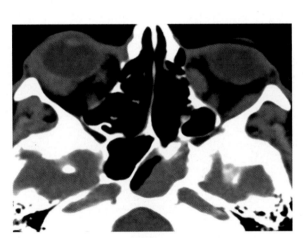

Fig. 105.1

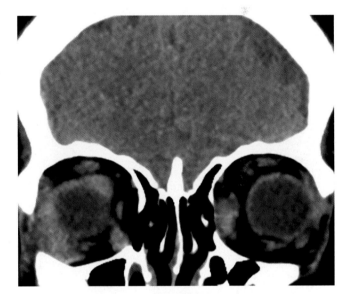

Fig. 105.2

209

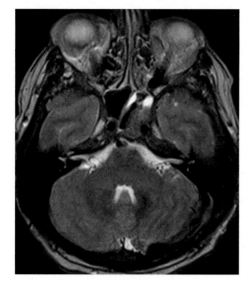

Fig. 105.3

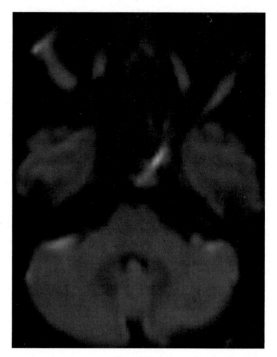

Fig. 105.4

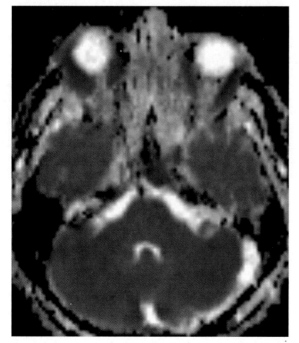

Fig. 105.5

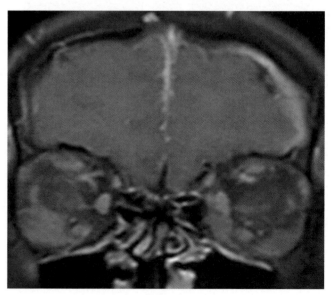

Fig. 105.6

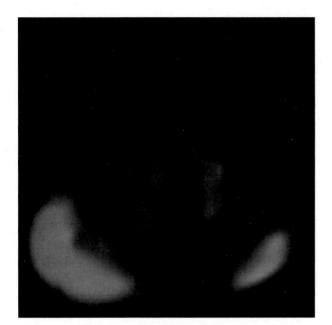

Fig. 105.7

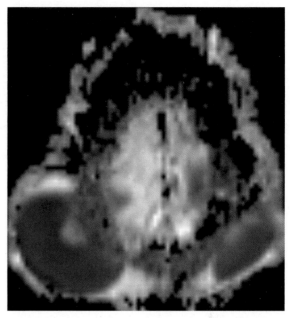

Fig. 105.8

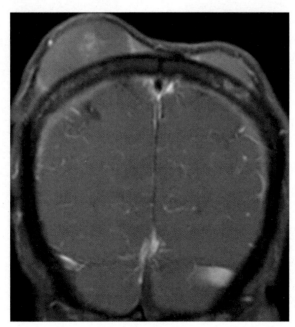

Fig. 105.9

Case 106

History: This 32-year-old male presents with myasthenia gravis and seizures. Long-standing headaches, especially in the mornings, which last for 1–2 hours before resolving. No visual problems.

1. What is the level of ventricular obstruction in this case?
   A. Foramen of Monro
   B. Third ventricle
   C. Aqueduct of Sylvius
   D. Foramen of Magendie
2. What is the diagnosis in this case?
   A. Normal pressure hydrocephalus
   B. Pineal cyst
   C. Aqueductal web
   D. Colloid cyst
3. What is the most common cause of congenital hydrocephalus?
   A. Intracranial hemorrhage
   B. Chiari malformation
   C. Aqueductal stenosis
   D. Vein of Galen malformation
4. What is the inheritance pattern in congenital aqueductal stenosis?
   A. Autosomal dominant
   B. Autosomal recessive
   C. X-linked recessive
   D. Complex inheritance

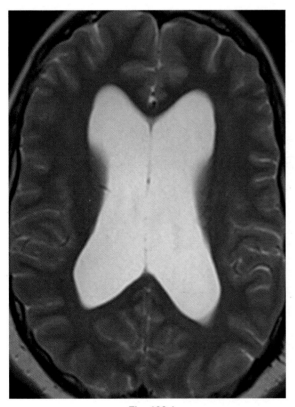

Fig. 106.1

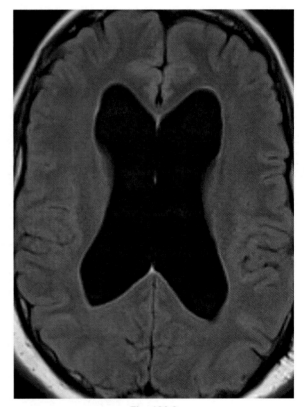

Fig. 106.2

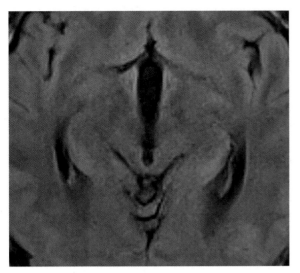

Fig. 106.3

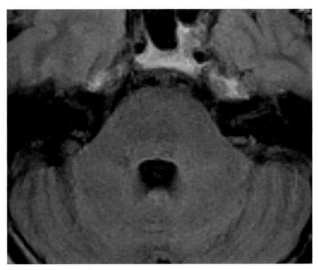

Fig. 106.4

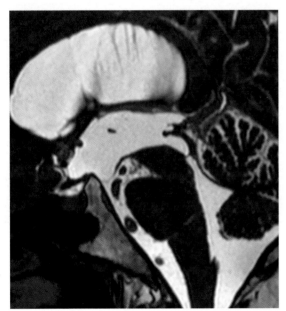

Fig. 106.5

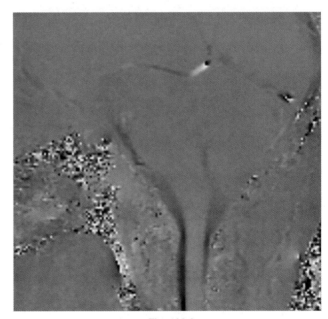

Fig. 106.6

Case 107

History: This is a 42-year-old female with left eye pain and numbness.

1. What is the anatomic location of the mass in this case?
   A. Pituitary gland
   B. Cavernous sinus
   C. Medial temporal lobe
   D. Sphenoid sinus
2. What cranial nerves course through this anatomic space?
   A. III
   B. IV
   C. V1
   D. V2
   E. VI
   F. All of the above

3. What is the most common tumor to involve the cavernous sinus?
   A. Meningioma
   B. Nerve sheath tumors
   C. Nasopharyngeal carcinoma
   D. Metastases
4. Given the presence of narrowing of the left cavernous internal carotid artery, what is the best diagnosis?
   A. Meningioma
   B. Nerve sheath tumor
   C. Nasopharyngeal carcinoma
   D. Metastasis

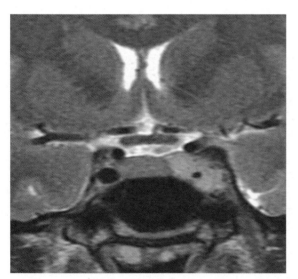

Fig. 107.1

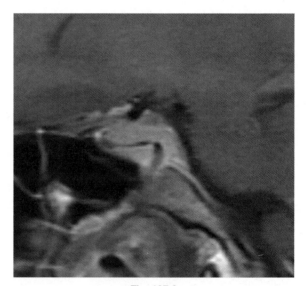

Fig. 107.2

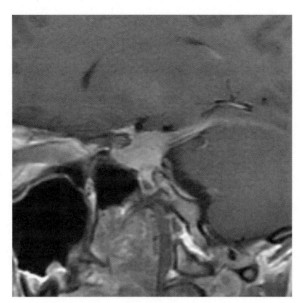

Fig. 107.3

Case 108

History: A 60-year-old female status-post fall hitting her head on a cabinet.

1. What is the diagnosis?
   A. Acute cerebellar infarct
   B. Medulloblastoma
   C. Metastases
   D. Dysplastic cerebellar gangliocytoma
2. Dysplastic gangliocytoma of the cerebellum (Lhermitte–Duclos disease) is associated with which uncommon neurocutaneous syndrome?
   A. Joubert syndrome
   B. Neurofibromatosis type 1 (NF1)
   C. Neurofibromatosis type 2 (NF2)
   D. Cowden syndrome

3. The recent WHO classification of CNS tumors recognizes dysplastic cerebellar gangliocytoma as a
   A. WHO grade 1 tumor
   B. WHO grade 2 tumor
   C. WHO grade 3 tumor
   D. WHO grade 4 tumor
4. Which of the following is true regarding imaging of dysplastic cerebellar gangliocytoma?
   A. Enhancement is typically seen with intravenous gadolinium administration
   B. FDG-PET shows increased tracer uptake
   C. Elevated choline levels on MR spectroscopy
   D. Hypointensity on T2 with loss of cerebellar striations

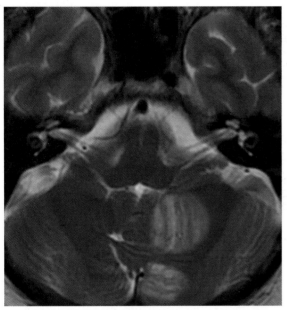

Fig. 108.1

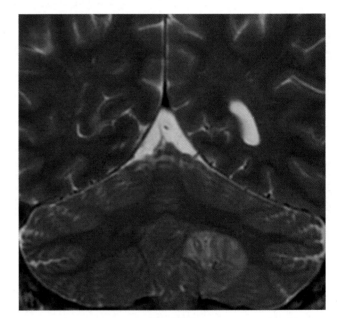

Fig. 108.2

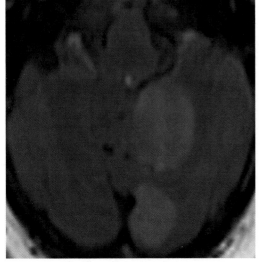

Fig. 108.3

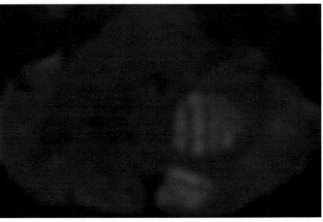

Fig. 108.4

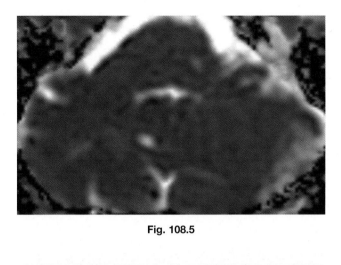

Fig. 108.5

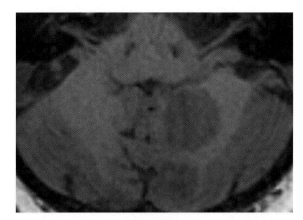

Fig. 108.6

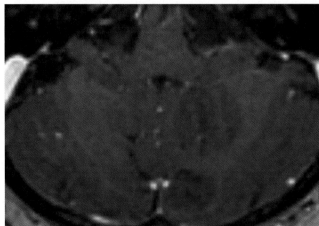

Fig. 108.7

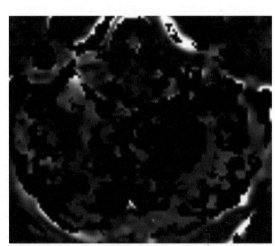

Fig. 108.8

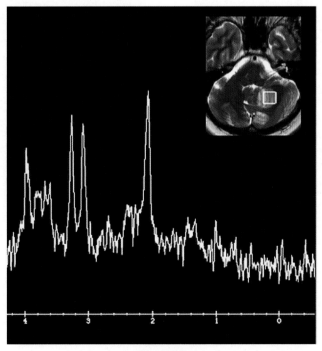

Fig. 108.9

Case 109

History: This 38-year-old female presents with bipolar disorder, chronic headache, decreased memory, weight loss, and not eating. Confusion and weakness with 3 falls over the past 2 days. No vision change.

1. Which of the following conditions can present with basilar meningitis?
   A. Tuberculosis
   B. Cryptococcus
   C. Sarcoidosis
   D. Carcinomatous meningitis
   E. All of the above
2. Which of the following statements regarding neurosarcoidosis is incorrect?
   A. Vast majority of patients have systemic sarcoidosis.
   B. Leptomeningeal involvement is rare.
   C. Involvement of the pituitary stalk is common.
   D. Involvement of the perivascular spaces can also be seen.

3. What primary CNS neoplasms have a predilection for subarachnoid seeding?
   A. Tectal glioma
   B. Diffuse midline glioma
   C. Hemangioblastoma
   D. Pineocytoma

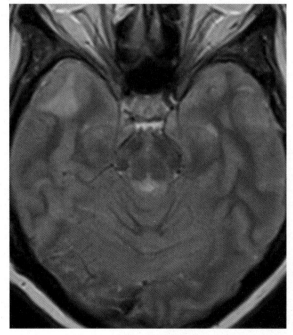

Fig. 109.1

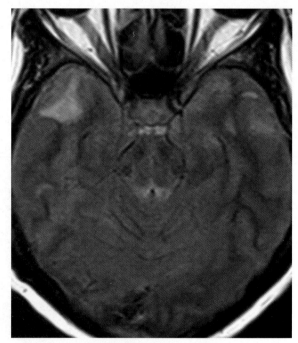

Fig. 109.2

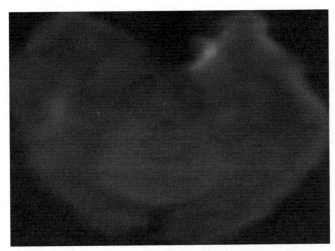

Fig. 109.3

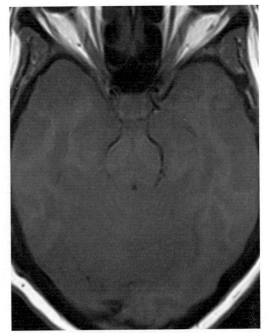

Fig. 109.4

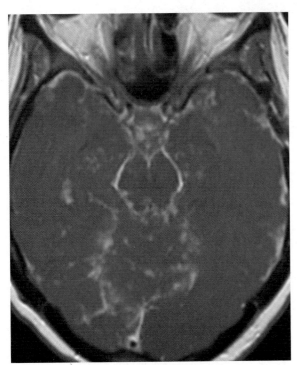

Fig. 109.5

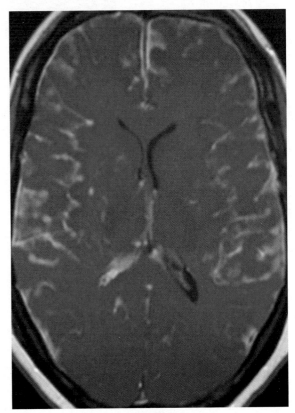

Fig. 109.6

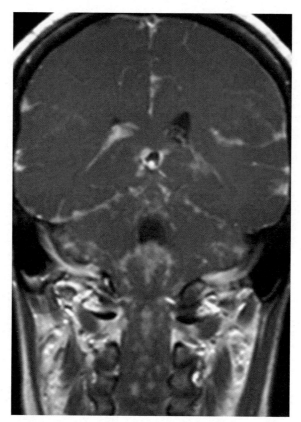

Fig. 109.7

Case 110

History: A 26-year-old with headaches.

1. What is the diagnosis?
   A. Germinoma
   B. Craniopharyngioma
   C. Epidermoid cyst
   D. Arachnoid cyst
2. What is the most common location of intracranial epidermoid cysts?
   A. Cerebellopontine angle cistern
   B. Suprasellar cistern
   C. Middle cranial fossa
   D. Calvarial

3. Which MRI sequence is most helpful in distinguishing epidermoid from arachnoid cysts?
   A. FLAIR
   B. ADC
   C. GRE
   D. Contrast-enhanced T1
4. Apparent diffusion coefficient (ADC) is a measure of the magnitude of diffusion of water molecules within a tissue. What is the unit of ADC value of a tissue?
   A. mm^2/s
   B. cm^2/s
   C. mm/s
   D. mm/s^2

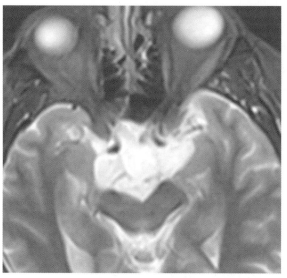

Fig. 110.1

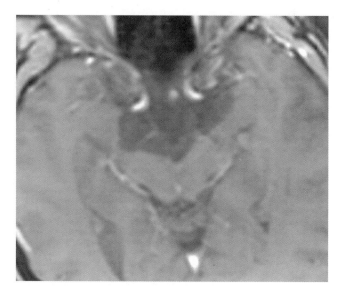

Fig. 110.2

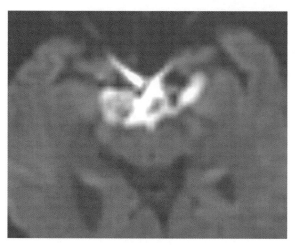

Fig. 110.3

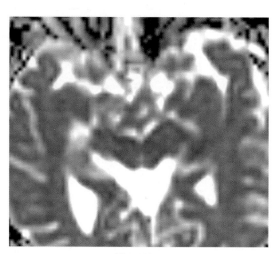

Fig. 110.4

Case 111

History: A 64-year-old male presents with remote cocaine abuse, psychiatric comorbidities, tinnitus, and seizures.

1. What is the likely cause of this patient's seizures?
   A. Left mesial temporal sclerosis
   B. Left otitis media
   C. Left temporal bone fracture
   D. Left temporal encephalocele
2. What is/are the common causes of acquired encephaloceles in adults?
   A. Trauma
   B. Cholesteatoma formation
   C. Iatrogenic
   D. Idiopathic intracranial hypertension
   E. All of the above
3. What is the recommended treatment for this patient?
   A. Observation
   B. Antiepileptic medication
   C. Surgical resection and repair
   D. Stereotactic electroencephalogaphy with placement of penetrating depth electrodes
4. What is the most common presentation of an encephalocele in the postoperative setting?
   A. Seizures
   B. CSF leak
   C. Headache
   D. Dizziness

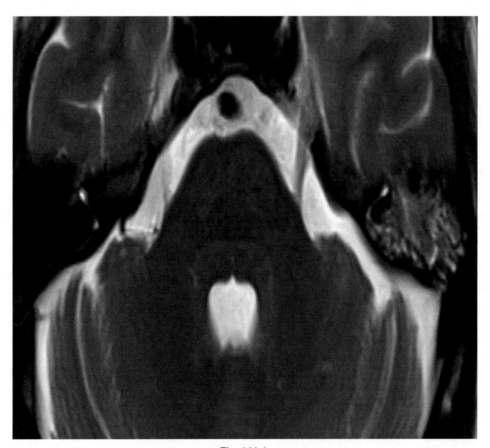

Fig. 111.1

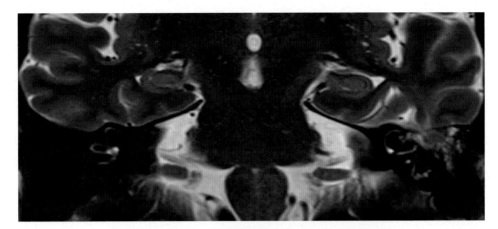

Fig. 111.2

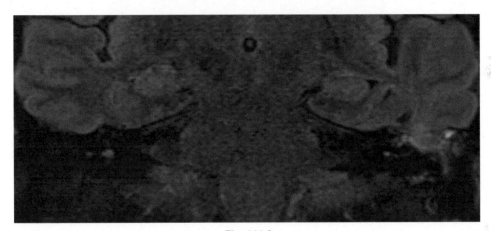

Fig. 111.3

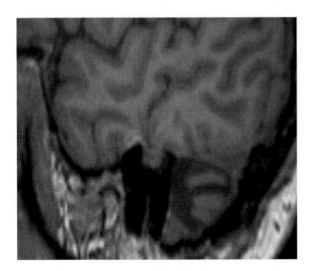

Fig. 111.4

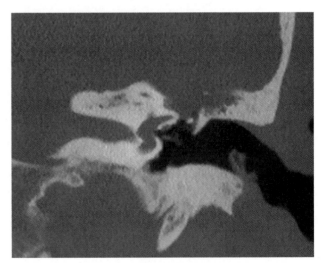

Fig. 111.5

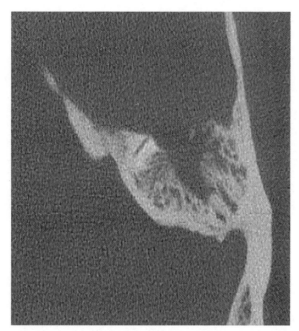

Fig. 111.6

Case 112

History: This is a 60-year-old male with metastatic grade 2 neuroendocrine tumor of the colon with right facial droop and numbness that started 6 days ago, which is now improving.

1. What is the most likely diagnosis?
   A. Metastases
   B. Perineural tumor spread
   C. Bell's palsy
   D. Tolosa–Hunt syndrome
2. What portions of the facial nerve normally enhance?
   A. Anterior genu
   B. Cisternal segment
   C. Meatal/canalicular segment
   D. Extracranial segment, beyond the stylomastoid foramen
3. What structure separates the internal auditory canal into superior and inferior portions?
   A. Crista galli
   B. Crista terminalis
   C. Crista falciformis
   D. Crista ampullaris
4. What cranial nerve runs in the anteroinferior portion of the internal auditory canal?
   A. Facial nerve
   B. Cochlear nerve
   C. Superior vestibular nerve
   D. Inferior vestibular nerve

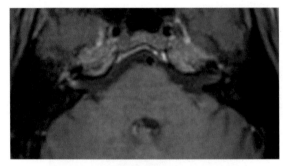

Fig. 112.1

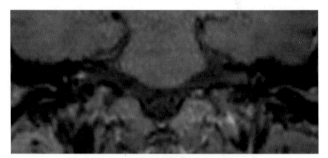

Fig. 112.2

Case 113

History: A 25-year-old right-handed female presents with localization-related epilepsy, functional MRI (f-MRI) for language lateralization.

1. f-MRI provides information about brain function by monitoring oxygen levels in the blood flow mostly dependent on which MRI parameter?
   A. T1
   B. T2
   C. T2*
   D. Mean transit time
2. Based on these task activation maps, what would you conclude?
   A. Study is inconclusive and hemispheric dominance cannot be assessed.
   B. Patient is left hemispheric dominant for language function.
   C. Patient is right hemispheric dominant for language function.
   D. Patient has codominance for language function.

3. Which of the following statement is correct regarding f-MRI and language localization?
   A. f-MRI is not yet good enough to replace intraoperative electrocortical stimulation but is useful for surgical mapping, thereby reducing the duration and extent of craniotomy.
   B. Validity of f-MRI in establishing hemispheric dominance has been proved in a large number of patients and studies, with a greater than 90% agreement between the invasive Wada test and f-MRI.
   C. Language f-MRI is currently being used as a substitute for the Wada test, since it is noninvasive and gives additional information on the spatial relationship between language areas and intracranial lesions.
   D. All of the above
4. Which anatomic region in the brain makes up the Broca's area?
   A. Supramarginal gyrus
   B. Angular gyrus
   C. Cingulate gyrus
   D. Pars opercularis coupled with pars triangularis

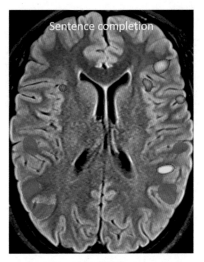

Fig. 113.1

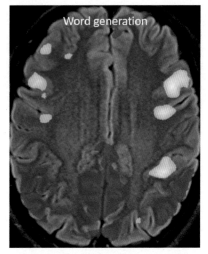

Fig. 113.2

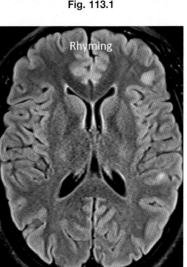

Fig. 113.3

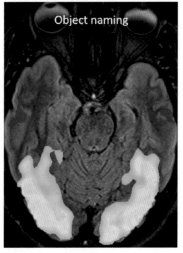

Fig. 113.4

Case 114

History: This 36-year-old female postpartum (vaginal delivery 7 days ago) presented with thunderclap headache.

1. What is the most common cause of acute subarachnoid hemorrhage?
   A. Pregnancy
   B. Recreational drug use
   C. Ruptured aneurysm
   D. Trauma
2. What is the diagnosis in this case?
   A. Posterior reversible encephalopathy syndrome (PRES)
   B. Primary angiitis of the CNS (PACNS)
   C. Reversible cerebral vasoconstriction syndrome (RCVS)
   D. Chronic lymphocytic inflammation with pontine perivascular enhancement responsive to steroids (CLIPPERS)
3. Which of the following is not associated with reversible cerebral vasoconstriction syndrome (RCVS)?
   A. Convexity subarachnoid hemorrhage
   B. Intraparenchymal hemorrhage
   C. Cerebral infarction
   D. Intracranial aneurysms
4. Which of the following entities can present with thunderclap headache?
   A. Aneurysmal subarachnoid hemorrhage
   B. Cerebral venous thrombosis
   C. Pituitary apoplexy
   D. Carotid or vertebral artery dissection
   E. Reversible cerebral vasoconstrictions syndrome
   F. Acute meningitis
   G. Acute hydrocephalus
   H. All of the above

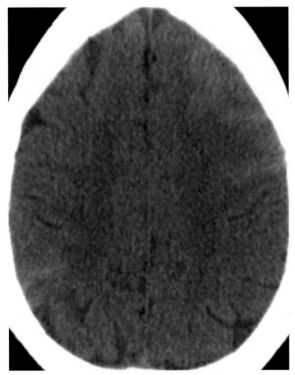

Fig. 114.1

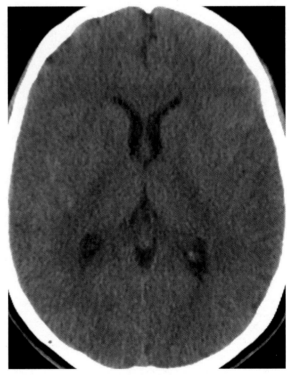

Fig. 114.2

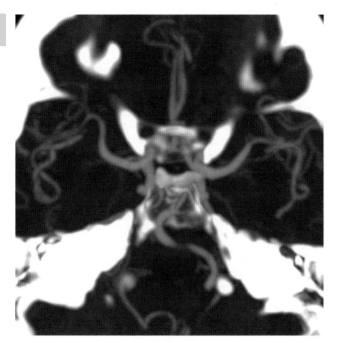

Fig. 114.3

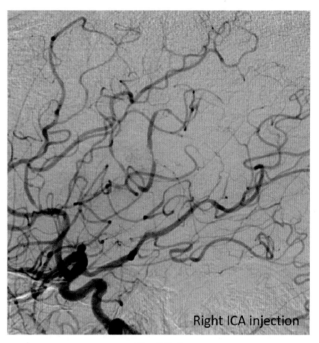

Right ICA injection

Fig. 114.4

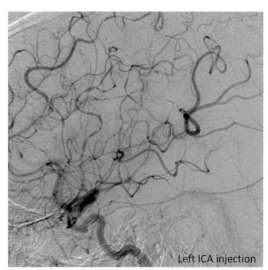

Left ICA injection

Fig. 114.5

Case 115

History: This is a 30-year-old female with seizures.

1. Which of the following tumors typically occur in the temporal lobes and present with seizures?
   A. Ganglioglioma
   B. Hemangioblastoma
   C. Glioblastoma
   D. Ependymoma

2. Which of the following is true regarding a ganglioglioma?
   A. Gangliogliomas are WHO grade 2 tumors most frequently found in the temporal lobe.
   B. Gangliogliomas can occasionally dedifferentiate into a GBM.
   C. Gangliogliomas present as a cystic mass with an enhancing mural nodule in ~95% of cases.
   D. Gangliogliomas do not have a BRAF V600E mutation.

3. Which of the following CNS tumors have BRAF V600E mutations?
   A. DNET
   B. Ganglioglioma
   C. Pleomorphic xanthoastrocytoma
   D. All of the above

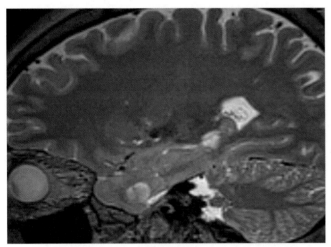

Fig. 115.1

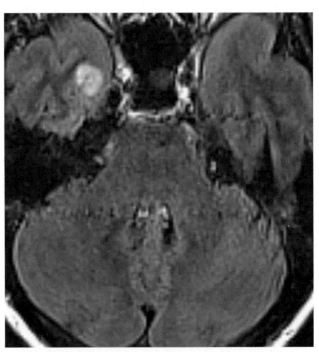

Fig. 115.2

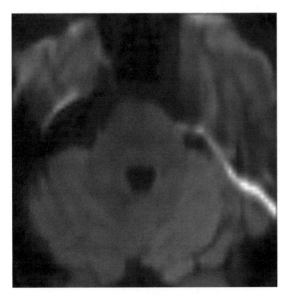

Fig. 115.3

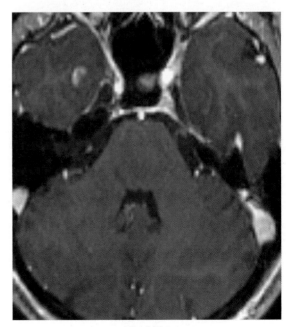

Fig. 115.4

Case 116

History: A 47-year-old male, a Tibetan immigrant working as a chef, presented with a ~4-week history of headaches, dizziness, and gait imbalance.

1. What is the most common fourth ventricular tumor in adults?
   A. Ependymoma
   B. Choroid plexus papilloma
   C. Pilocytic astrocytoma
   D. Hemangioblastoma
2. What is the most common location of choroid plexus papillomas in children?
   A. Fourth ventricle
   B. Lateral ventricle
   C. Third ventricle
   D. Spinal cord

3. Which of the following is the most common primary intra-axial infratentorial tumor in adults?
   A. Ependymoma
   B. Choroid plexus papilloma
   C. Pilocytic astrocytoma
   D. Hemangioblastoma
   E. Glioblastoma
4. What WHO grade are choroid plexus carcinomas?
   A. 1
   B. 2
   C. 3
   D. 4

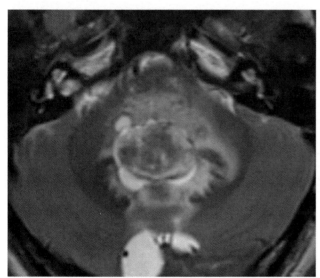

Fig. 116.1

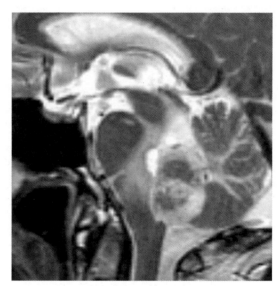

Fig. 116.2

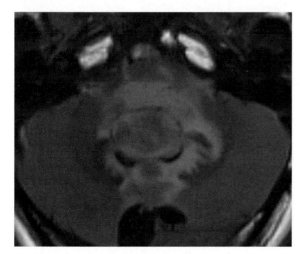

Fig. 116.3

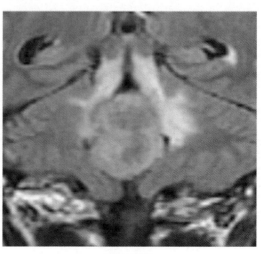

Fig. 116.4

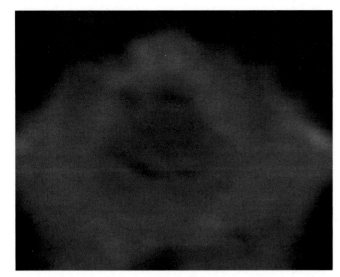

Fig. 116.5

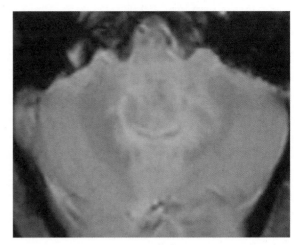

Fig. 116.6

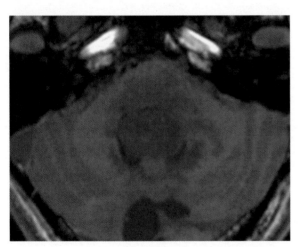

Fig. 116.7

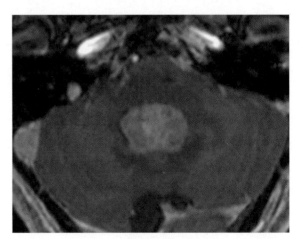

Fig. 116.8

Case 117

History: This 17-year-old girl presents with headaches and blurred vision.

1. What is the most likely diagnosis?
   A. Normal study
   B. Pineal cyst
   C. Aqueductal web
   D. Low-grade astrocytoma
2. The tectum, or roof, of the midbrain consists of what structures?
   A. Superior colliculus
   B. Inferior colliculus
   C. One superior and one inferior colliculus
   D. Paired superior and inferior collicli

3. Which of the following is correct regarding management of tectal gliomas?
   A. Surgical resection of these low-grade gliomas is often curative.
   B. Radiation therapy is the mainstay of treatment in preventing the growth of this lesion.
   C. Temozolamide chemotherapy usually has a good response.
   D. CSF diversion is often the only required intervention for long-term survival.
4. What congenital anomaly is usually associated with "beaking" of the tectum?
   A. Neurofibromatosis type-1 (NF1)
   B. Neurofibromatosis type-2 (NF2)
   C. Chiari I malformation
   D. Chiari II malformation

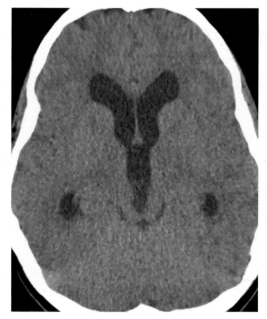

Fig. 117.1

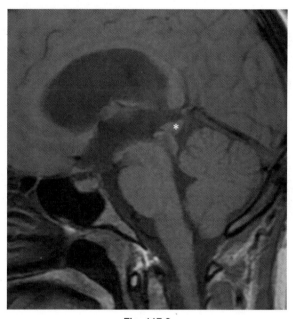

Fig. 117.2

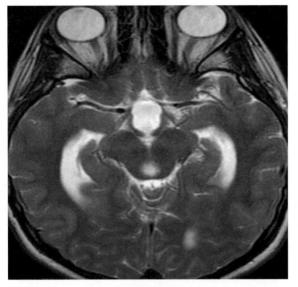

Fig. 117.3

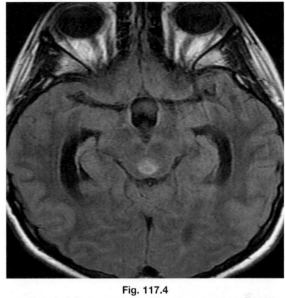

Fig. 117.4

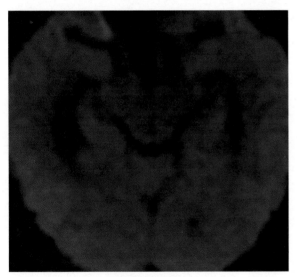

Fig. 117.5

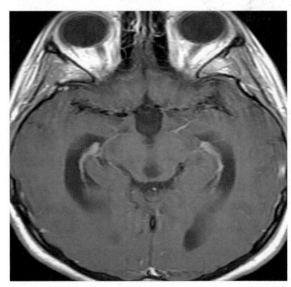

Fig. 117.6

Case 118

History: A 59-year-old male presents with a slowly enlarging lump over the right side of his skull at the site of remote surgery performed 29 years ago.

1. What is the most likely diagnosis?
   A. Calvarial hemangioma
   B. Adamantinoma
   C. Epidermoid cyst
   D. Langerhans cell histiocytosis
2. Which of the following is incorrect regarding intradiploic epidermoid cysts?
   A. Intradiploic epidermoids are more frequent than intradural epidermoid cysts.
   B. Restricted diffusion is characteristic of epidermoid cysts.
   C. Surgical resection is the standard treatment, but recurrence is not uncommon.
   D. Presence of contrast enhancement may indicate a giant cell reaction, coexistence of different histological types, and malignant transformation of the epidermoid cyst.
3. What are the proposed causes of epidermoid cysts of the skull?
   A. Congenital
   B. Acquired (posttraumatic)
   C. Postsurgical
   D. All of the above
4. Which is the most commonly involved bone in Langerhans cell histiocytosis in adults?
   A. Skull
   B. Vertebrae
   C. Long bones
   D. Mandible
   E. Ribs

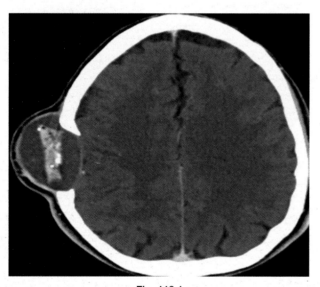

Fig. 118.1

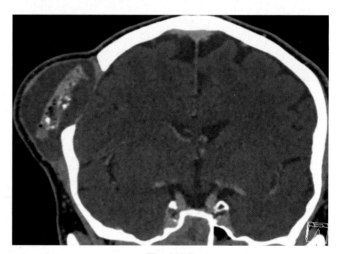

Fig. 118.2

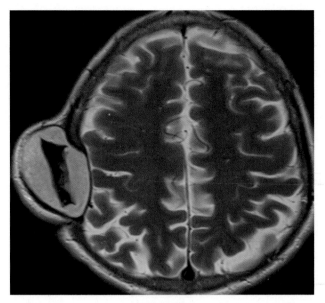

Fig. 118.3

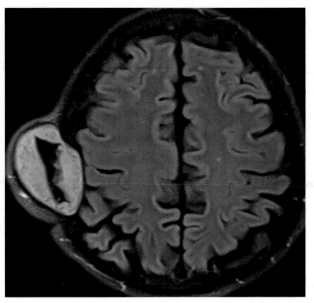

Fig. 118.4

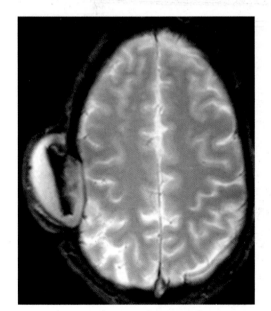

Fig. 118.5

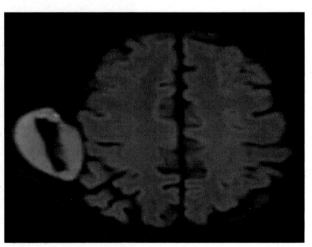

Fig. 118.6

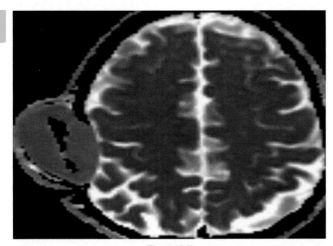

Fig. 118.7

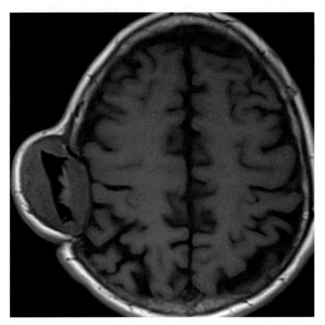

Fig. 118.8

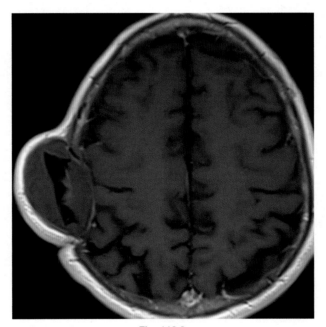

Fig. 118.9

Case 119

History: This 55-year-old man presents with new-onset left amaurosis fugax.

1. Which vessel is selected in Figure 119.5?
   A. Right common carotid artery
   B. Right vertebral artery
   C. Brachiocephalic artery
   D. Left common carotid artery
2. What is the pertinent finding on the brachiocephalic injection?
   A. Right vertebral artery occlusion
   B. Retrograde flow down the left vertebral artery
   C. Retrograde flow down the right vertebral artery
   D. Left vertebral artery occlusion
3. What is the name of this phenomenon, and is it more frequently found on the left or the right?
   A. Carotid stenosis and more frequently seen on the right
   B. Subclavian steal and more frequently seen on the left
   C. Takayasu's arteritis and more frequently seen on the right
   D. Preductal aortic coarctation
4. To confirm the diagnosis of "subclavian steal" on a two-dimensional time-of-flight MR angiography, what is the best place to position the stationary saturation pulse?
   A. Superior saturation pulse
   B. Inferior saturation pulse
   C. No saturation pulse
   D. Both B and C

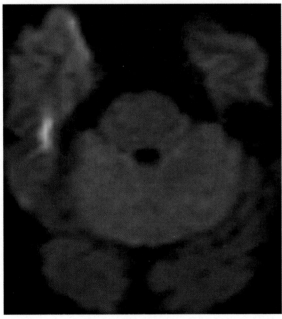

Fig. 119.1

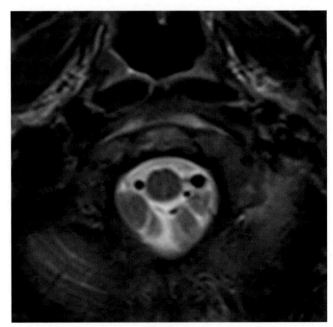

Fig. 119.2

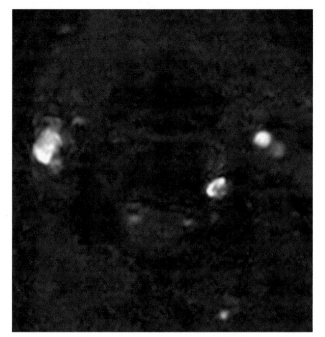

Fig. 119.3

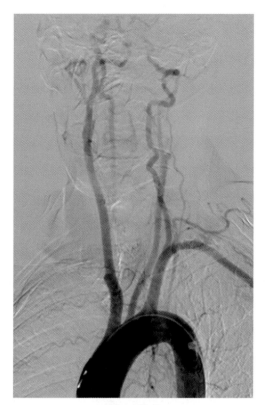

Fig. 119.4

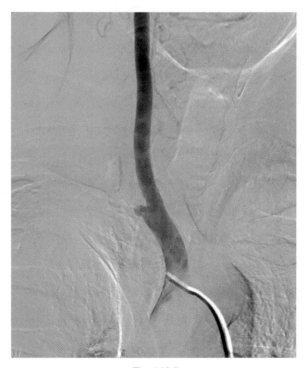

Fig. 119.5

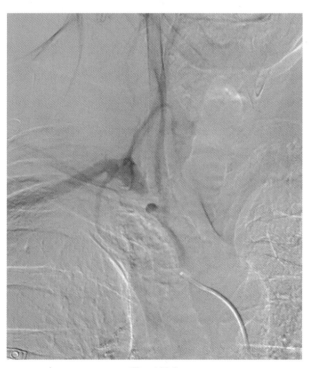

Fig. 119.6

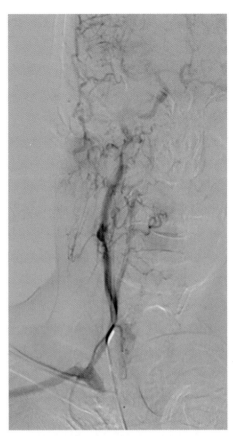

Fig. 119.7

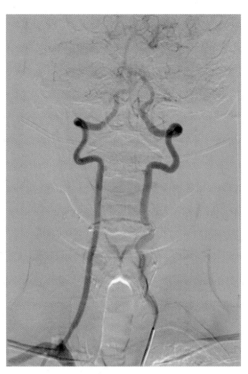

Fig. 119.8

Case 120

History: A 54-year-old male presents with progressive ambulatory dysfunction (cane → walker → wheelchair), worsening sensory loss, and bladder and bowel dysfunction. Also, intermittent weakness of the bilateral arms, two episodes of black spots in his left eye, and six episodes of gagging/choking on food.

1. Corpus callosum is the largest white matter tract in the brain with a rich vascular supply. Which of the following constitute the main sources of arterial supply to the corpus callosum?
   A. Pericallosal artery
   B. Anterior communicating artery, via the subcallosal artery or median callosal artery
   C. Posterior pericallosal artery
   D. All of the above
2. What is the most likely diagnosis based on these imaging findings?
   A. Multiple sclerosis
   B. CNS vasculitis
   C. Intravascular lymphoma
   D. Reversible cerebral vasoconstriction syndrome

3. Which of the following statements is incorrect regarding primary angiitis of the CNS (PACNS)?
   A. Imaging findings for PACNS are variable and nonspecific, with ischemic infarctions the most common finding.
   B. DSA remains the gold standard and demonstrates multifocal segmental narrowing of small and medium sized blood vessels.
   C. Intracranial vessel-wall MR imaging is an adjunct to conventional angiography and demonstrates concentric wall thickening and enhancement in patients with PACNS.
   D. MRI is almost 100% specific for PACNS, and a normal MRI essentially excludes this diagnosis.
4. What rare intracranial neoplasm may mimic CNS vasculitis?
   A. Intravascular lymphoma
   B. Masson's tumor
   C. Angiosarcoma
   D. Diffuse leptomeningeal glioneuronal tumor

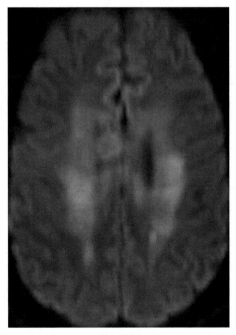

Fig. 120.1

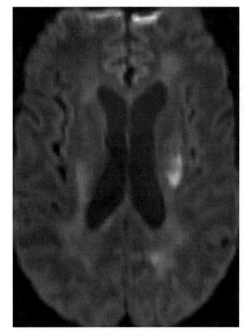

Fig. 120.2

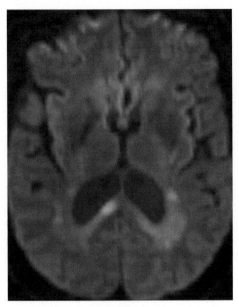

Fig. 120.3

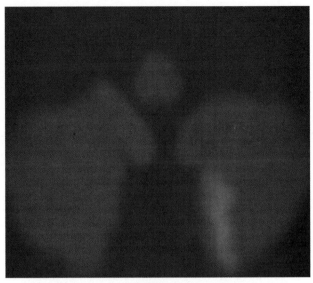

Fig. 120.4

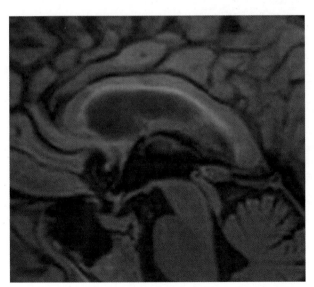

Fig. 120.5

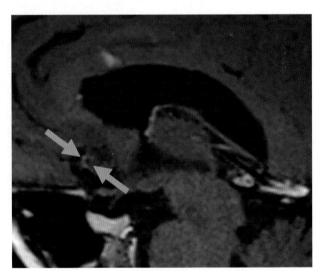

Fig. 120.6

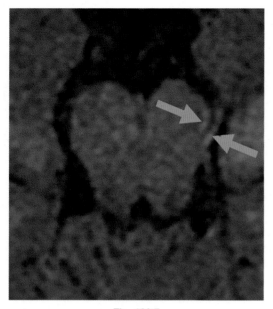

Fig. 120.7

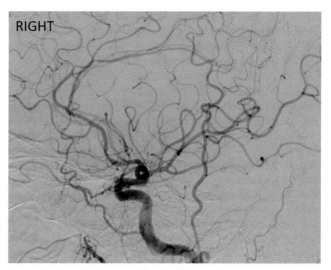

Fig. 120.8

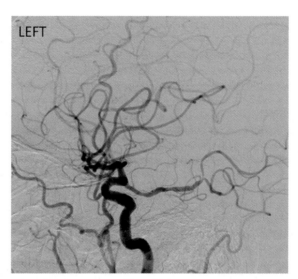

Fig. 120.9

Case 121

History: This is a 61-year-old male with a history of ESRD, stroke, and HTN was found obtunded following dialysis.

1. What does the asterisk (*) represent in Figure 121.3?
   A. Air
   B. Fat
   C. CSF
   D. Pus
2. What is the diagnosis?
   A. Abscesses
   B. Cerebral fat embolism
   C. Prominent perivascular spaces
   D. Cerebral air embolism

3. What is the preferred treatment for established neurological damage due to cerebral air embolism?
   A. Observation
   B. Trendelenburg position to induce air bubbles to leave the cerebral veins and return to the central circulation
   C. Hyperbaric oxygenation therapy
   D. Corticosteroids

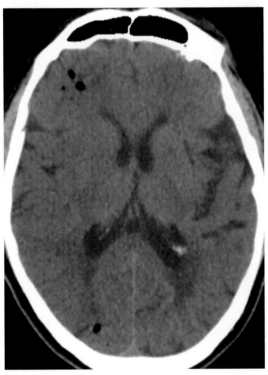

Fig. 121.1

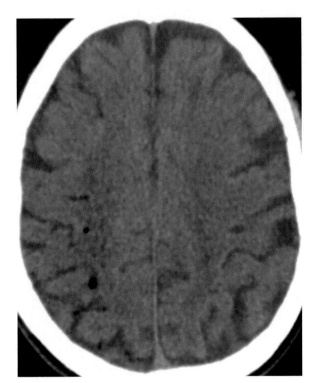

Fig. 121.2

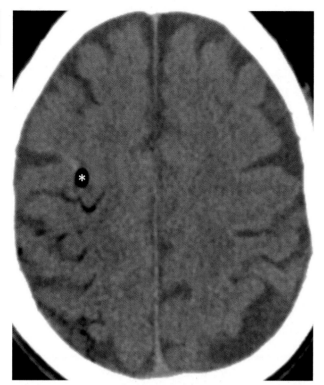

Fig. 121.3

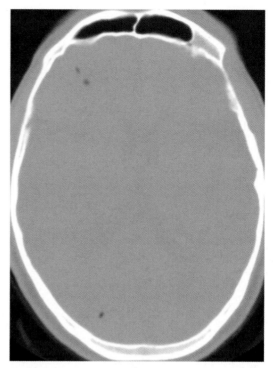

Fig. 121.4

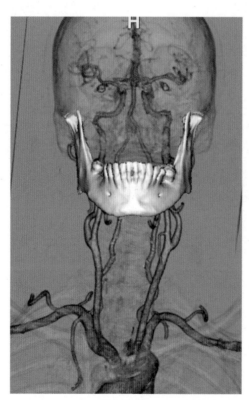

Fig. 121.5

Case 122

History: A 72-year-old woman presents with a history of hypertension and hyperlipidemia, prior repair of left middle cerebral artery aneurysm (2001), and recent right carotid endarterectomy presents with 2 weeks of altered mental status.

1. What is the most likely diagnosis?
   A. Sinonasal undifferentiated carcinoma
   B. Glioblastoma
   C. Nasal glioma
   D. Atypical meningioma
   E. Sinonasal mucosal melanoma
2. What is the most common histology of maxillary sinus malignancies?
   A. Sinonasal undifferentiated carcinoma
   B. Squamous cell carcinoma
   C. Adenocarcinoma
   D. Teratocarcinoma

3. What is the risk of malignant transformation of an inverted papilloma into squamous cell carcinoma?
   A. 5% to 10%
   B. 25% to 35%
   C. 50% to 60%
   D. 75% to 100%
4. Which of the following is true regarding a nasal glioma?
   A. Extranasal gliomas present as a firm, red to bluish skin-covered mass and typically exhibit pulsations or increase in size with the Valsalva maneuver.
   B. Nasal gliomas demonstrate rapid growth with high malignant potential.
   C. On imaging, these are isodense to the brain on CT, bright on T2, with a bifid crista galli and a prominent foramen cecum.
   D. Local recurrence is common despite aggressive surgical resection.

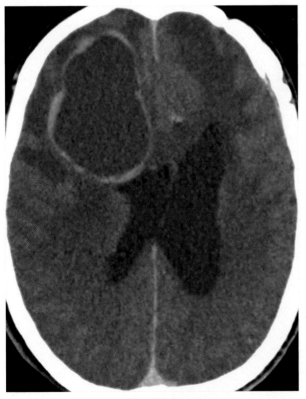

Fig. 122.1

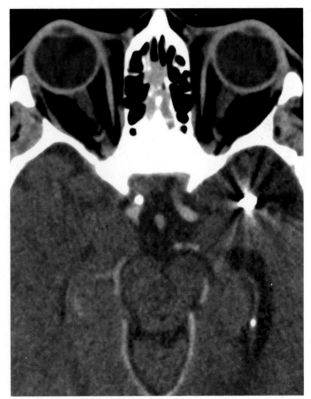

Fig. 122.2

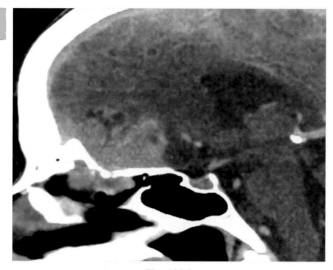

Fig. 122.3

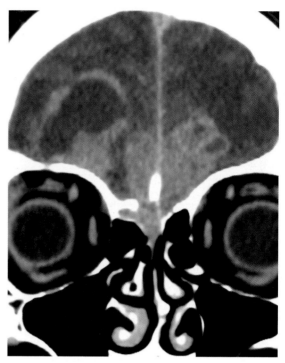

Fig. 122.4

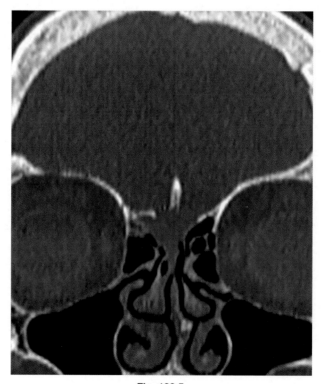

Fig. 122.5

Case 123

History: This 30-year-old male presents with hypogonadism.

1. What is the primary MR imaging finding?
   A. Normal study
   B. Hypophysitis
   C. Ectopic posterior pituitary gland
   D. Suprasellar Rathke's cleft cyst
2. What structure is not visualized?
   A. Anterior pituitary gland
   B. Optic chiasm
   C. Posterior pituitary gland
   D. Infundibulum

3. What is the most common clinical presentation in patients with ectopic posterior pituitary gland?
   A. Hypoglycemia
   B. Hyperglycemia
   C. Growth hormone deficiency
   D. Hyperprolactinemia
4. What is the cause of the focal hyperintense T1 signal frequently observed in the posterior aspect of the sella turcica?
   A. Calcification
   B. Flow artifact from adjacent arteries of the circle of Willis
   C. Magnetic susceptibility effect from the adjacent sphenoid sinus
   D. Storage of vasopressin

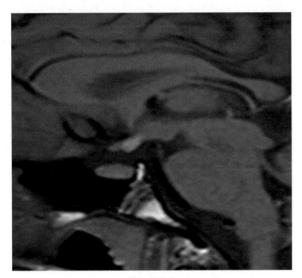

Fig. 123.1

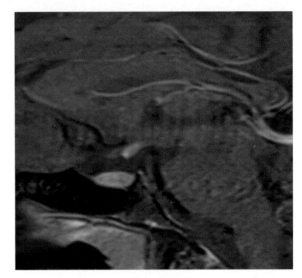

Fig. 123.2

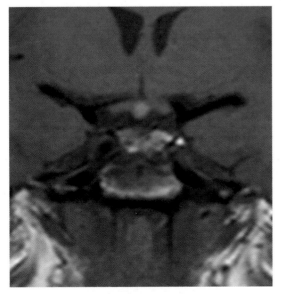

Fig. 123.3

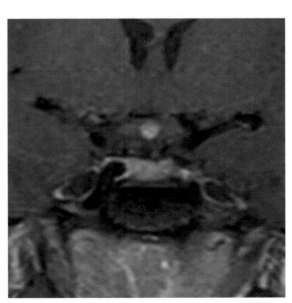

Fig. 123.4

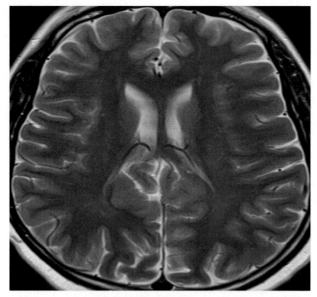

Fig. 123.5

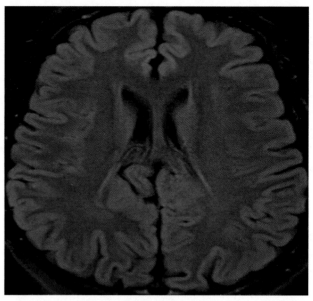

Fig. 123.6

Case 124

History: A 60-year-old male with right temporal lobe glioblastoma (IDH wild-type, MGMT unmethylated) underwent complete resection and finished standard of care chemoradiation therapy. Sequential follow-up scans demonstrated increasing heterogeneous enhancement in the resection bed.

1. What is the most likely diagnosis for this new enhancing lesion in this patient?
   A. Perioperative ischemia
   B. Radiation necrosis
   C. Pseudoresponse
   D. True tumor progression
2. When is the best time to image a patient after the initial resection of a brain tumor to assess for the extent of resection?
   A. Within 2 days
   B. Within 7 days
   C. Within 1 month
   D. Within 2 months

3. What is the current standard of care treatment options for a patient with newly diagnosed glioblastoma?
   A. Bevacizumab alone
   B. Bevacizumab plus temozolomide
   C. Temozolomide plus TTFields
   D. Immunotherapy
4. Which of the following is correct regarding IDH wild-type glioblastomas?
   A. IDH wild-type GBM patients carry a worse prognosis than IDH-1 mutant GBM patients.
   B. IDH wild-type GBM patients carry a better prognosis than IDH-1 mutant GBM patients.
   C. IDH mutation has no effect on prognosis in GBM patients.
   D. IDH mutation cannot be predicted on imaging.

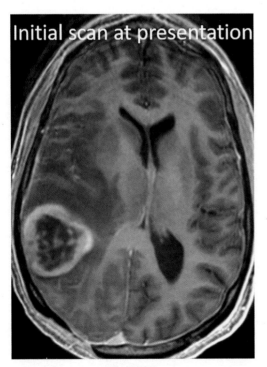

Fig. 124.1

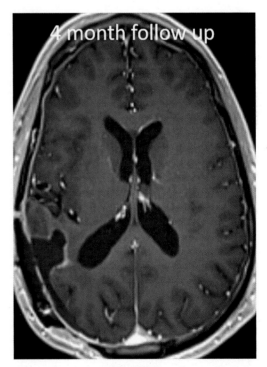

Fig. 124.2

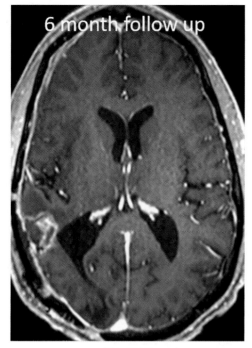

Fig. 124.3

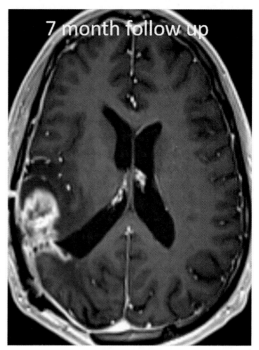

Fig. 124.4

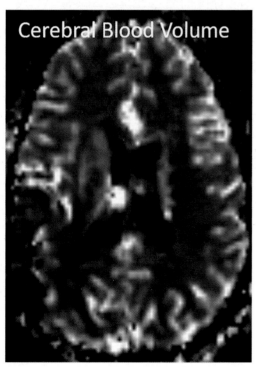

Fig. 124.5

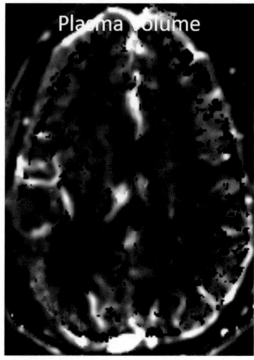

Fig. 124.6

Case 125

History: This 21-year-old male with bipolar disorder presents with 1 month of progressive numbness and tingling starting in his right hand, then his right foot, followed by right-hand weakness, difficulty walking, and a right facial droop.

1. What is the most likely diagnosis?
   A. Pilocytic astrocytoma
   B. Medulloblastoma
   C. Diffuse midline glioma, H3 K27M–mutant
   D. Glioblastoma
2. What part of the brainstem is most commonly affected by this entity?
   A. Pons
   B. Medulla
   C. Midbrain
   D. Cervico-medullary junction

3. Besides the pons, diffuse midline glioma H3 K27M–mutant can be found in which of the following locations?
   A. Thalamus
   B. Brainstem
   C. Medulla
   D. Spinal cord
   E. Cerebellum
   F. All of the above
4. Which of the following is correct regarding diffuse midline gliomas H3 K27M–mutant?
   A. They are usually WHO grade 1 tumors
   B. Most commonly located in the spinal cord
   C. These tumors generally have a poor prognosis
   D. Leptomeningeal spread is not a reported feature for these tumors

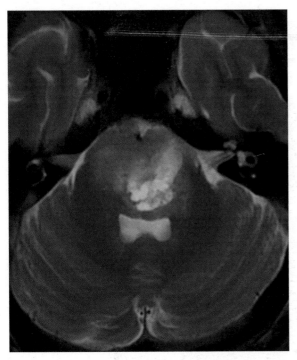

Fig. 125.1

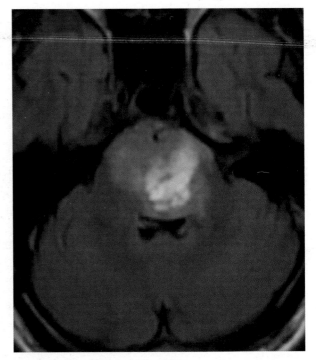

Fig. 125.2

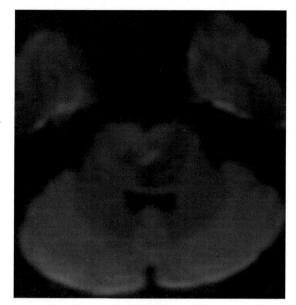

Fig. 125.3

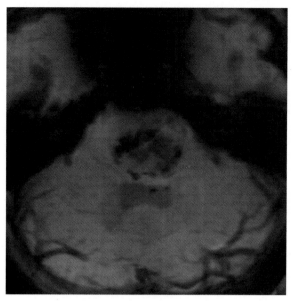

Fig. 125.4

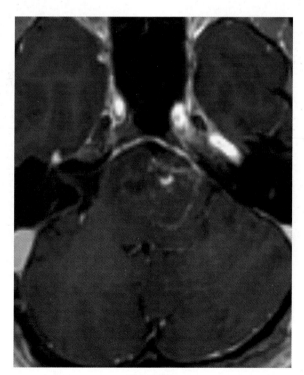

Fig. 125.5

Case 126

History: A 40-year-old man with a history of left temporal grade 2 astrocytoma (A, B) status-post complete resection (C, D). One year follow-up MRI demonstrates new peripherally enhancing lesions adjacent to the surgical cavity (E, F). Proton therapy had initially been planned, but the patient never received radiation therapy.

1. What is the most likely diagnosis?
   A. Radiation necrosis
   B. Transformation to glioblastoma
   C. Subacute infarction
   D. Textiloma
2. What may these foreign body reactions be mistaken for on CT or MR imaging?
   A. Recurrent tumor
   B. Radiation necrosis
   C. Abscess
   D. Hematoma
   E. All of the above

3. What is the typical imaging appearance of a gelatin–thrombin matrix (Floseal) on immediate postoperative imaging?
   A. Pseudoair appearance on CT
   B. Speckled hypointensity on T2
   C. Blooming susceptibility on GRE
   D. All of the above

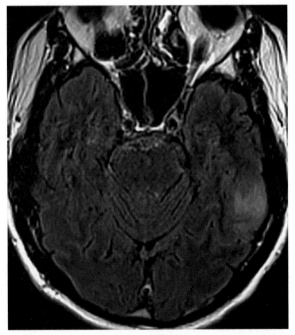

Fig. 126.1

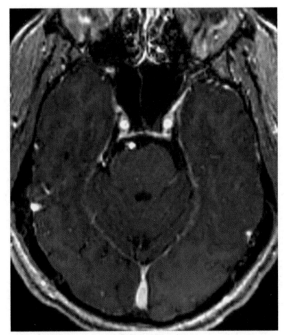

Fig. 126.2

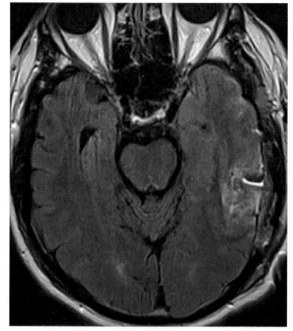

Fig. 126.3

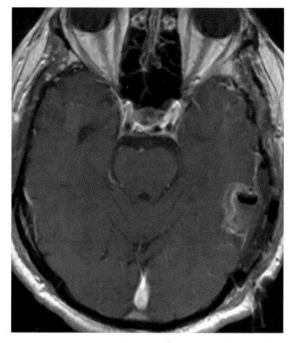

Fig. 126.4

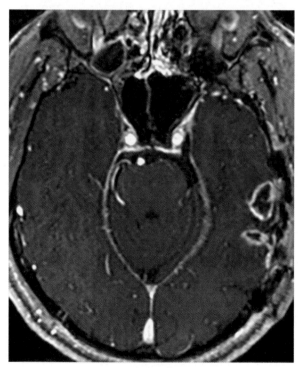

Fig. 126.5

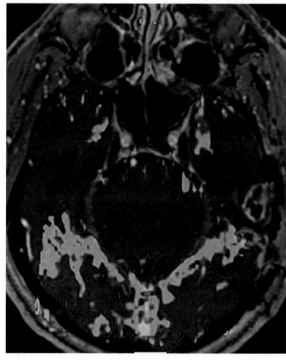

Fig. 126.6

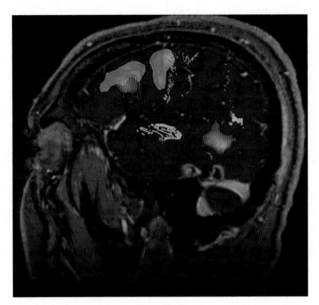

Fig. 126.7

Case 127

History: A 59-year-old woman presents with a history of seizures.

1. What is the anatomic location of this lesion?
   A. Masa intermedia
   B. Tuber cinereum
   C. Posterior pituitary
   D. Optic chiasm
2. What is the typical clinical presentation of this lesion?
   A. Asymptomatic
   B. Hyperprolactinemia
   C. Bitemporal hemianopia
   D. Gelastic seizures

3. Which of the following is incorrect regarding the typical imaging appearance of this entity?
   A. The lesion is usually isointense on T1 to the adjacent cerebral cortex.
   B. Contrast enhancement is not present.
   C. The lesion is always isointense on T2 to the adjacent cerebral cortex.
   D. Occasionally, calcifications may be seen on CT.
4. Which of the following can be considered in the differential diagnosis of this entity?
   A. Craniopharyngioma
   B. Pituitary macroadenoma
   C. Germ cell tumor
   D. All of the above

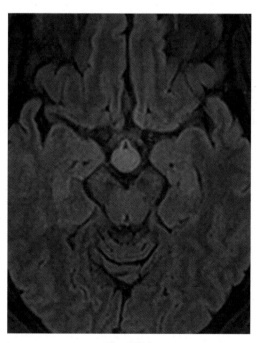

Fig. 127.1

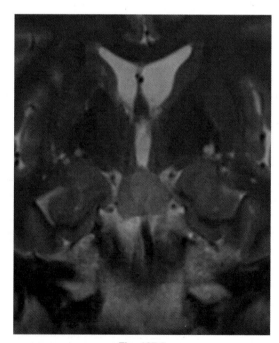

Fig. 127.2

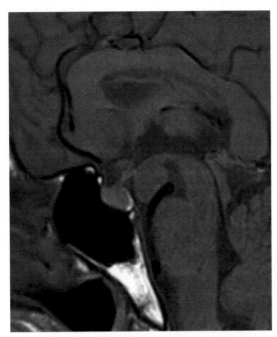

Fig. 127.3

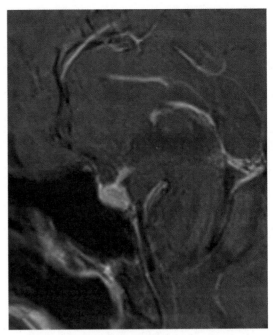

Fig. 127.4

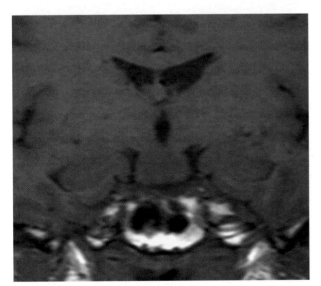

Fig. 127.5

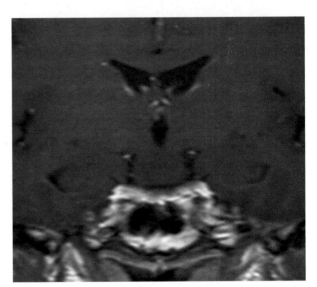

Fig. 127.6

Case 128

History: Withheld.

1. What is the most likely clinical presentation of this patient?
   A. 3rd nerve palsy
   B. 6th nerve palsy
   C. 7th nerve palsy
   D. 12th nerve palsy
2. Chordomas are most frequently found in what location?
   A. Clivus
   B. Cervical spine
   C. Thoracic spine
   D. Sacrum
3. Which imaging feature is most helpful in distinguishing skull base chordomas from chondrosarcomas?
   A. Contrast enhancement
   B. T2 hyperintensity
   C. Osseous destruction
   D. Midline location
4. Besides chordoma which other histologically benign tumor may have distant metastases?
   A. Schwannoma
   B. Pituitary adenoma
   C. Giant cell tumor
   D. Ecchordosis physaliphora

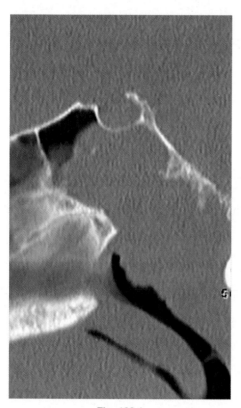

Fig. 128.1

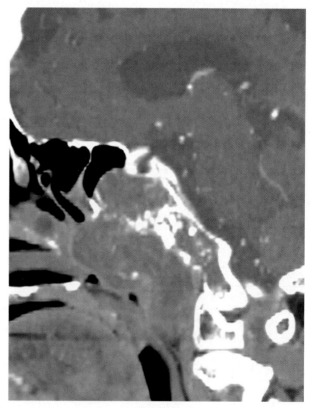

Fig. 128.2

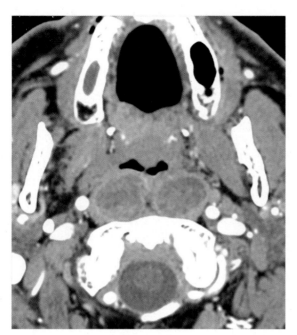

Fig. 128.3

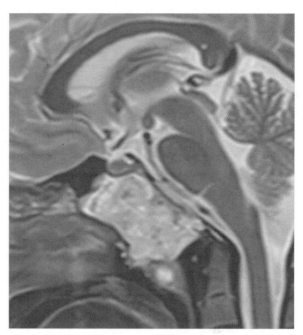

Fig. 128.4

Case 129

History: This is a 90-year-old male with a remote history of recurrent laryngeal tumor status-post partial laryngectomy and radiation therapy. Right neck dissection for a new right neck mass, and biopsy of the left posterior ear show squamous cell carcinoma. The patient now presents with right facial weakness and pain shooting down the neck and across the shoulder blades.

1. What is the diagnosis in this case?
   A. Radiation neuritis
   B. Salivary gland carcinoma
   C. Perineural tumor spread
   D. Neurosarcoidosis
2. Which of the following statements is incorrect regarding perineural tumor spread?
   A. Best appreciated on a noncontrast CT
   B. Imaging is necessary in many cases as clinical findings may be silent.
   C. Increasing in prevalence
   D. Contrast-enhanced MRI is the modailty of choice to evaluate perineural tumor spread.
3. What primary salivary tumor is notorious for its propensity for perineural spread?
   A. Pleomorphic adenoma
   B. Adenoid cystic carcinoma
   C. Mucoepidermoid carcinoma
   D. Warthins tumor
4. What branch of cranial nerve V3 (trigeminal nerve) transmits tumor to Meckel's cave through the foramen ovale?
   A. Auriculotemporal nerve
   B. Maxillary nerve
   C. Lacrimal nerve
   D. Zygomatic nerve

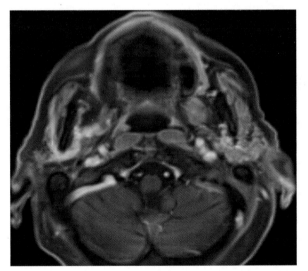

Fig. 129.1

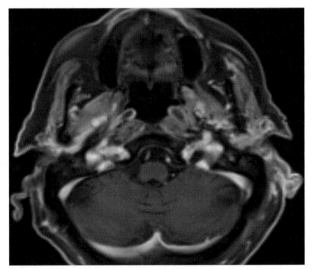

Fig. 129.2

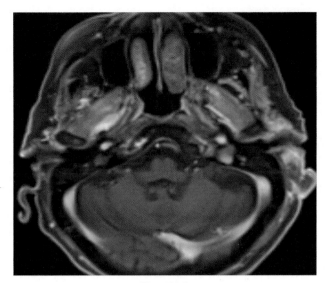

Fig. 129.3

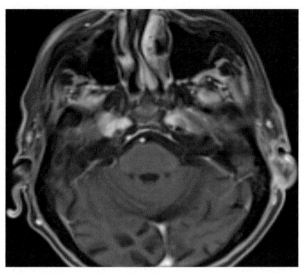

Fig. 129.4

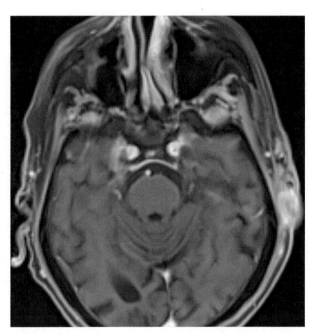

Fig. 129.5

Case 130

History: A 65-year-old right-handed African American female presents to the office bed bound from a skilled nursing facility with a several-year history of problems with her speech, coordination, and walking. She has a 55-year-old brother with a similar disorder, and her father also had a similar disorder and died at age 75. The patient denies any autonomic dysfunction.

1. What is the most common clinical presentation of patients with degenerative processes of the cerebellum?
   A. Urinary incontinence
   B. Ataxia
   C. Cognitive impairment
   D. Visual hallucinations
2. Which of the following is incorrect regarding multiple system atrophy cerebellar type (MSA-C)?
   A. MSA-C is also known as olivopontocerebellar degeneration and is one of the clinical manifestations of multiple systemic atrophy (MSA).
   B. There is a predominance of parkinsonian signs and symptoms.
   C. Cruciform T2 hyperintensity in the pons, "hot cross bun sign," is classically seen in patients with MSA-C.
   D. It is also a recognized cause of T2 hyperintensities in the middle cerebellar peduncles (middle cerebellar peduncle sign).

3. What are the common causes of acquired cerebellar degeneration?
   A. Alcohol
   B. Anticonvulsant drugs
   C. Paraneoplastic syndromes
   D. All of the above
4. Regarding Friedreich ataxia, what is the inheritance pattern and what chromosome is implicated?
   A. Autosomal recessive and chromosome 9
   B. Autosomal recessive and chromosome 16
   C. Autosomal recessive and chromosome 22
   D. X-linked and chromosome 9

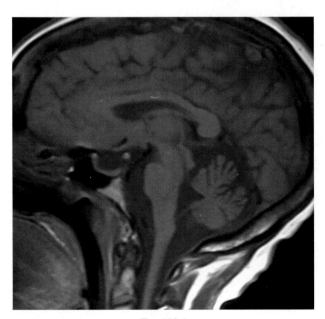

Fig. 130.1

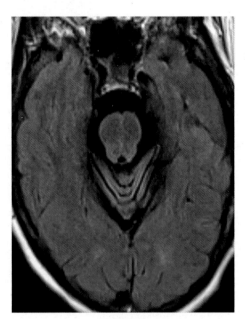

Fig. 130.2

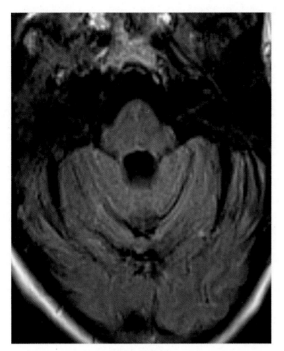

Fig. 130.3

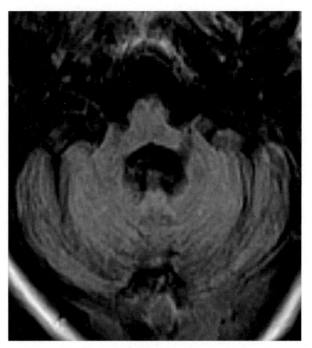

Fig. 130.4

Case 131

History: A 55-year-old male with a several year history of involuntary arm and face movements, clumsiness, and gradually progressive difficulty with speech and cognitive decline. The patient's mother died when she was 42 years old.

1. What is the most likely diagnosis?
   A. Wilson's disease
   B. Huntington's disease
   C. Hyperglycemia
   D. Hepatic encephalopathy
2. Which of the following deep gray nuclei are commonly involved in patients with Huntington's disease?
   A. Caudate nucleus and thalamus
   B. Globus pallidus and putamen
   C. Caudate nucleus and globus pallidus
   D. Caudate nucleus and putamen
3. Neurodegeneration with brain iron accumulation (NBIA), previously known as Hallervorden-Spatz, is an autosomal recessive disorder that results in the accumulation of iron products in which deep gray matter structures?
   A. Caudate nucleus and thalamus
   B. Globus pallidus and putamen
   C. Caudate nucleus and globus pallidus
   D. Globus pallidus and substantia nigra
4. In Wilson's disease (hepatolenticular degeneration), abnormal copper deposition is caused by a deficiency of what serum transport protein?
   A. Ceruloplasmin
   B. Ferritin
   C. Thyroglobulin
   D. Plasma retinol-binding protein

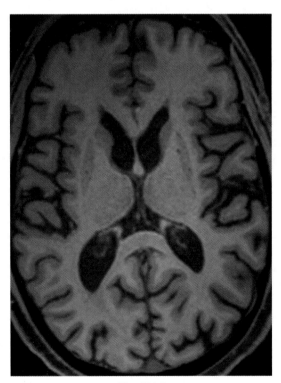

Fig. 131.1

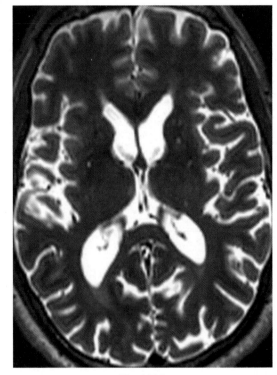

Fig. 131.2

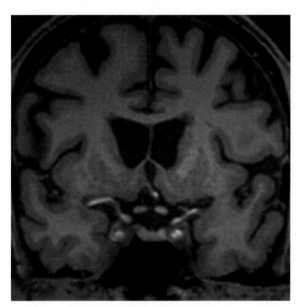

Fig. 131.3

Case 132

History: This 52-year-old man presents with a history of multiple sclerosis (baseline MRI, Figures 132.1-132.3) currently on immunomodulation therapy with Tysabri. Five-month follow-up MRI (Figures 132.4-132.7) shows a new large lesion.

1. What is the most likely diagnosis given elevated relative cerebral blood volume (rCBV) on perfusion imaging (Figure 132.7) in this patient?
   A. Tumefactive demyelinating lesion (TDL)
   B. Lymphoma
   C. High-grade glioma
   D. Progressive multifocal leukoencephalopathy (PML)
2. Which of the following is incorrect regarding a tumefactive demyelinating lesion (TDL)?
   A. Open or incomplete ring enhancement is a characteristic feature of TDL.
   B. Prominent surrounding vasogenic edema and mass effect are almost always present.
   C. On MR spectroscopy, elevation of choline and lactate is commonly seen.
   D. On MR perfusion, rCBV within a TDL is usually significantly less than in high-grade gliomas.

3. Progressive multifocal leukoencephalopathy (PML) is a dreaded complication particularly in patients treated with natalizumab (Tysabri) with positive JC virus serology. It is increasingly being recognized in which of these other conditions?
   A. HIV/AIDS
   B. Leukemia
   C. Post bone marrow or solid organ transplantation
   D. SLE
   E. All of the above

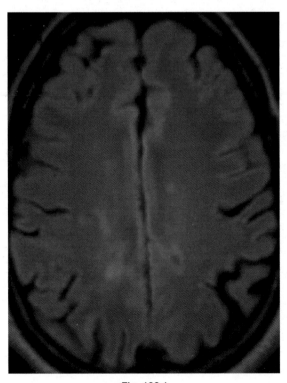

Fig. 132.1

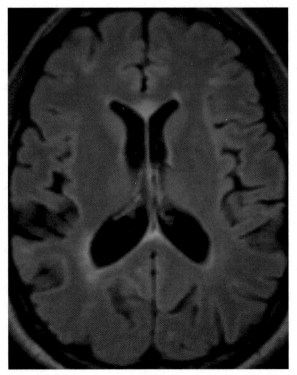

Fig. 132.2

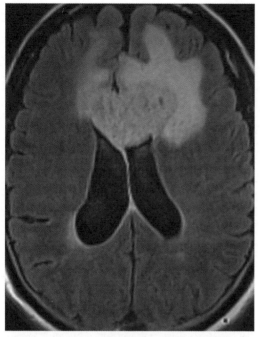

Fig. 132.3

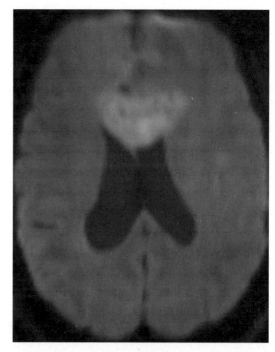

Fig. 132.4

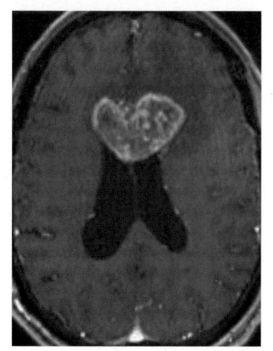

Fig. 132.5

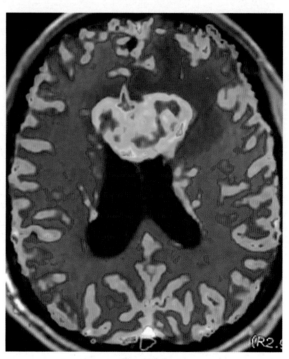

Fig. 132.6

Case 133

History: A 31-year-old male presents with a history of seizures and slowly progressive cognitive difficulties since childhood, and physical exam with upper motor neuron signs and pseudobulbar affect.

1. What is the most likely diagnosis in this case?
   A. Posterior reversible encephalopathy syndrome (PRES)
   B. Seizure-related changes
   C. Progressive multifocal leukoencephalopathy (PML)
   D. Adrenoleukodystrophy (ALD)
2. What do the areas of enhancement represent in this case?
   A. Active demyelination
   B. Gliosis
   C. Evolving subacute ischemia
   D. Seizure-related changes
3. How is adrenoleukodystrophy genetically transmitted?
   A. Autosomal dominant
   B. Autosomal recessive
   C. X-linked
   D. Complex inheritance pattern
4. Which leukodystrophy results from a deficiency in the enzyme *N*-acetylaspartoacylase?
   A. X-linked adrenoleukodystrophy
   B. Metachromatic leukodystrophy (MLD)
   C. Alexander disease
   D. Canavan disease

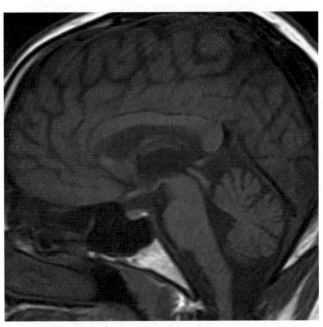

Fig. 133.1

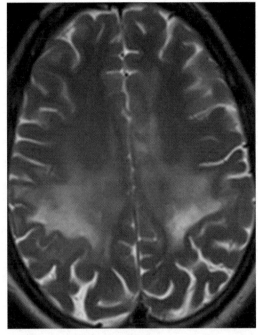

Fig. 133.2

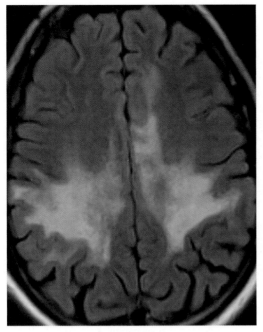

Fig. 133.3

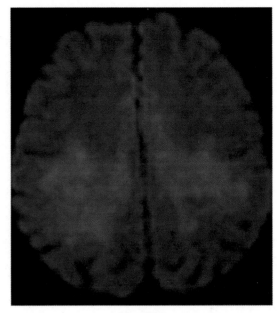

Fig. 133.4

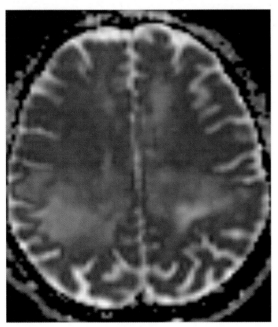

Fig. 133.5

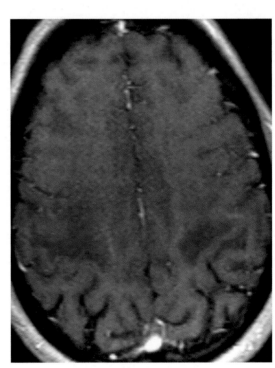

Fig. 133.6

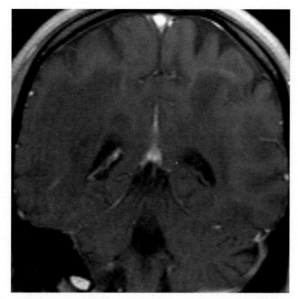

Fig. 133.7

Case 134

History: A 51-year-old patient with progressive memory loss, confusion, and left facial droop, recently diagnosed with HIV.

1. These imaging findings are most consistent with which of the following?
   A. Normal study
   B. Meningitis and ventriculitis
   C. Toxoplasmosis
   D. Lymphoma
2. What is the most common underlying condition responsible for ventriculitis?
   A. Trauma
   B. Brain abscess
   C. Iatrogenic
   D. Meningitis

3. Which of the following is incorrect regarding cytomegalovirus (CMV) meningitis and ventriculitis in a patient with HIV?
   A. Ventriculitis in the setting of profound immunosuppression is highly suggestive of CMV infection.
   B. It can affect the entire neuraxis.
   C. On imaging, it typically presents with mass effect and hydrocephalus.
   D. CMV infection can also present with meningoencephalitis with nonspecific increased foci of T2/FLAIR signal in the white matter.
4. What imaging findings are typical of CNS involvement in patients infected with cytomegalovirus (CMV) in utero?
   A. Bilateral ventricular subependymal calcifications
   B. Atrophy
   C. Migrational anomalies (pachygyria or polymicrogyria)
   D. All of the above

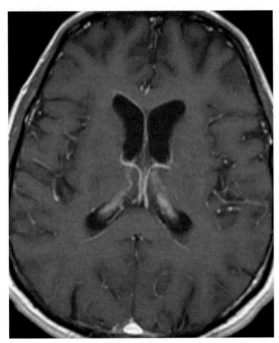

Fig. 134.1

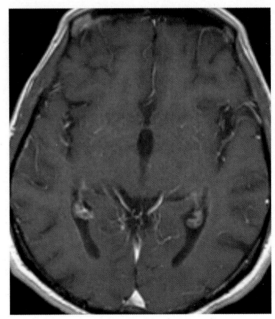

Fig. 134.2

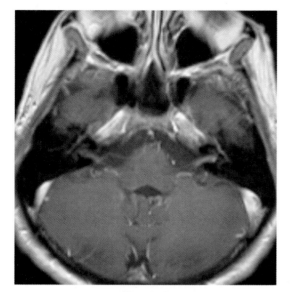

Fig. 134.3

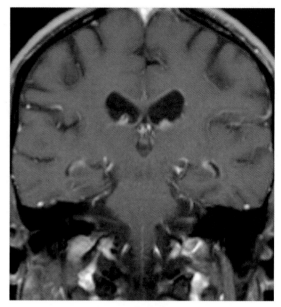

Fig. 134.4

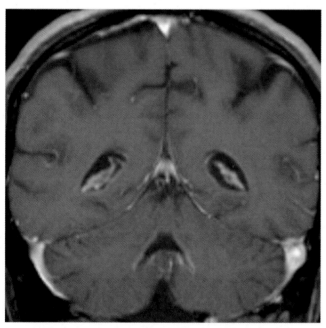

Fig. 134.5

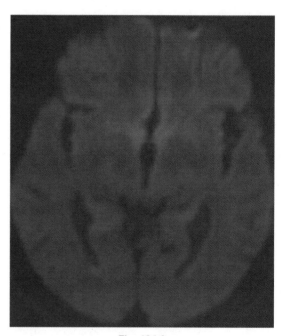

Fig. 134.6

Case 135

History: A 31-year-old male presents with headaches, blurry vision, dizziness, and tingling on the left side of his body.

1. What is the most likely diagnosis?
   A. Central neurocytoma
   B. Choroid plexus papilloma
   C. Cavernoma
   D. Meningioma
2. On conventional imaging and microscopic examination of pathology, central neurocytomas are frequently indistinguishable from what primary glial neoplasm?
   A. Oligodendroglioma
   B. Choroid plexus papilloma
   C. Meningioma
   D. Glioblastoma

3. What are the most common locations for choroid plexus papillomas in children and adults?
   A. In children, the atria of the lateral ventricles. In adults, the fourth ventricle.
   B. In children, the fourth ventricle. In adults, the atria of the lateral ventricles.
   C. In children, the third ventricle. In adults, the third ventricle as well.
   D. In children, the third ventricle. In adults, the fourth ventricle.
4. What is the most common site for intraventricular meningiomas?
   A. Atria of the lateral ventricles
   B. Fourth ventricle
   C. Third ventricle
   D. Septum pellucidum

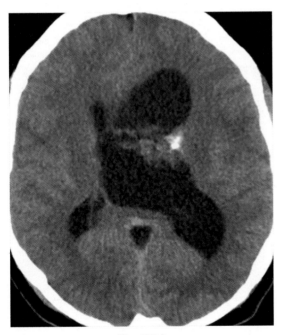

Fig. 135.1

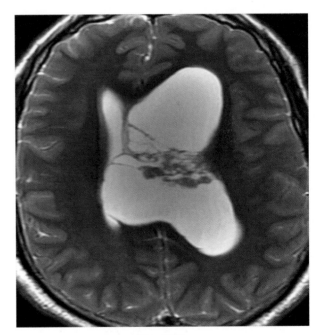

Fig. 135.2

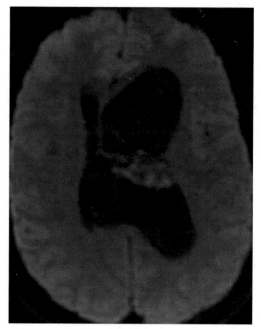

Fig. 135.3

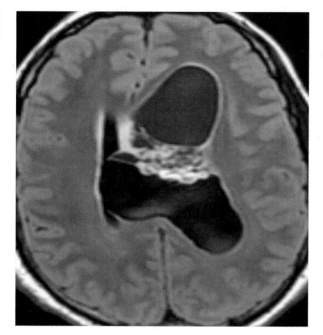

Fig. 134.4

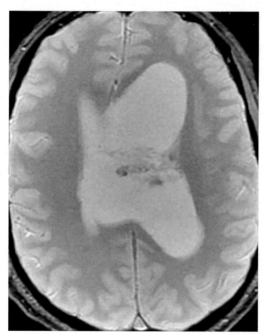

Fig. 134.5

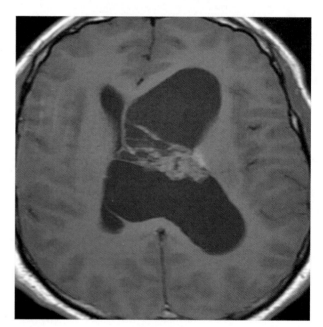

Fig. 134.6

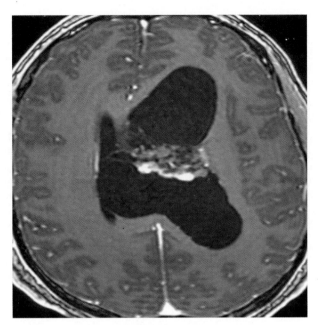

Fig. 134.7

Case 136

History: This 58-year-old female presents with severe COVID-19 infection, prolonged ICU stay and altered mental status.

1. What is the most likely diagnosis?
   A. Acute infarction of the corpus callosum
   B. Hypoxic-ischemic encephalopathy
   C. Marchiafava-Bignami disease (MBD)
   D. Acute disseminated encephalomyelitis (ADEM)
   E. Cytokine storm-related corpus callosal injury
2. What is the most likely mechanism of this insult?
   A. SARS-CoV-2-induced direct neuronal injury
   B. Immune-mediated process with markedly increased levels of cytokines and extracellular glutamate leading to cytotoxic edema
   C. Acute hypoxic insult from severe respiratory distress
   D. Acute demyelination

3. Which of the following is incorrect regarding Marchiafava-Bignami disease?
   A. It is most commonly seen in chronic alcoholics.
   B. It is a form of acute demyelination typically involving the central fibers of corpus callosum.
   C. It presents with hemispheric disconnection syndrome.
   D. Treatment includes rapid administration of vitamin C.
4. Which of the following conditions can present as Cytotoxic Lesion of the Corpus Callosum (CLOCC)?
   A. Seizures
   B. Osmotic demyelination
   C. SARS-CoV-2
   D. Antiepileptics
   E. All of the above

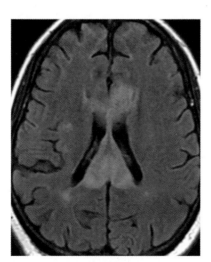

Fig. 136.1

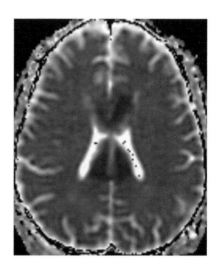

Fig. 136.2

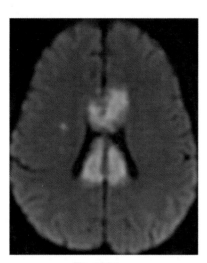

Fig. 136.3

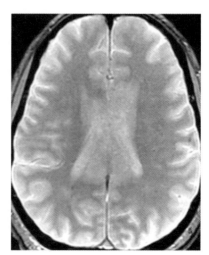

Fig. 136.4

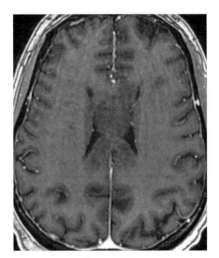

Fig. 136.5

Case 137

History: This is a 49-year-old with new proptosis.

1. Why is this the most likely diagnosis?
   A. Thyroid-associated orbitopathy
   B. Idiopathic orbital inflammation
   C. Orbital metastasis
   D. Infectious myositis
2. What is the classic presentation of idiopathic orbital inflammation (orbital pseudotumor)?
   A. Proptosis
   B. Pain
   C. Diplopia
   D. Chemosis

3. Which of the following primary tumors have a propensity to metastasize to the extraocular muscles?
   A. Neuroendocrine tumor (carcinoid)
   B. Breast cancer
   C. Lung cancer
   D. Melanoma
   E. All of the above
4. What characteristic imaging finding, when present, is highly suggestive of metastatic breast carcinoma to the orbit?
   A. Proptosis
   B. Enophthalmos
   C. Pain
   D. Diplopia

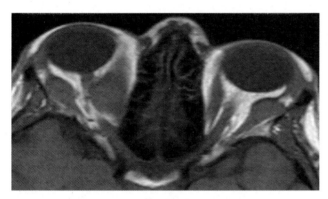

Fig. 137.1

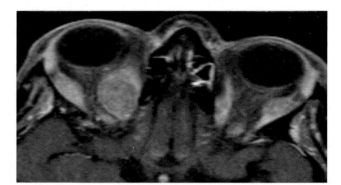

Fig. 137.2

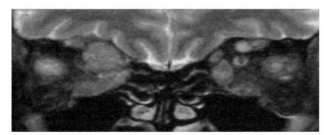

Fig. 137.3

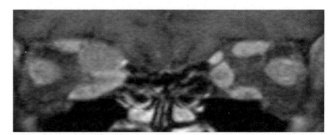

Fig. 137.4

Case 138

History: A 55-year-old male status-post liver transplant and aortic valve replacement with subacute change in mental status.

1. What is the most likely diagnosis?
   A. Embolic infarcts
   B. Mesial temporal sclerosis (MTS)
   C. Multiple sclerosis
   D. Human Herpesvirus-6 (HHV-6) Encephalitis
2. Which of the following differentiates HHV-6-associated encephalopathy from herpes simplex encephalitis (HSE)?
   A. In HHV-6 encephalopathy, there is usually exclusive involvement of the mesial temporal lobes.
   B. HHV-6 usually responds to acyclovir.
   C. Head CT is usually abnormal in the early stages of HHV-6 infection.
   D. DWI is usually negative in acute HHV-6 infection.

3. What group of patients are at an increased risk for HHV-6 infection?
   A. Hematopoietic cell transplant
   B. Solid organ transplantation
   C. High-dose chemotherapy
   D. All of the above
4. What is the arterial supply to the hippocampus?
   A. Posterior cerebral artery
   B. Anterior choroidal artery
   C. Both A and B
   D. Vertebral artery

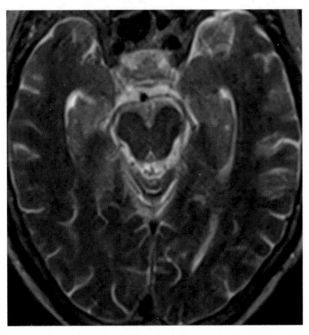

Fig. 138.1

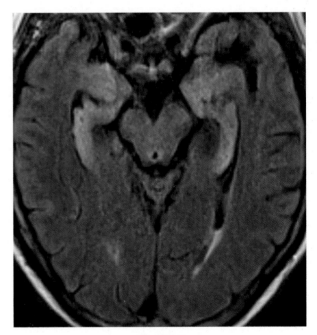

Fig. 138.2

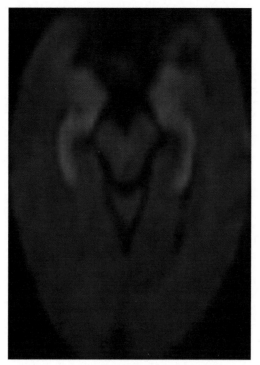

Fig. 138.3

Case 139

History: This 61-year-old female with unwitnessed mechanical fall down multiple steps while intoxicated, presents with worsening bilateral periorbital edema.

1. The * on Figure 139.5 represents what anatomic structure?
   A. Superior ophthalmic veins
   B. Facial veins
   C. Internal carotid arteries
   D. Vertebral arteries
2. What is the diagnosis in this case?
   A. Carotid-cavernous fistula
   B. Cavernous carotid aneurysm
   C. Cavernous sinus thrombosis
   D. Cavernous sinus meningioma
3. What is the most common type of carotid cavernous fistula according to Barrow classification?
   A. Type A
   B. Type B
   C. Type C
   D. Type D
4. Cavernous sinus schwannomas most commonly arise from which of the following cranial nerves?
   A. CN3
   B. CN4
   C. CN5
   D. CN6

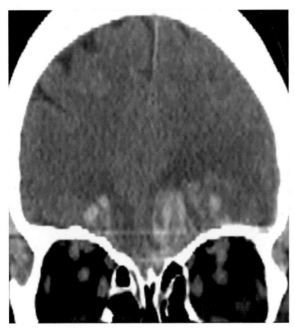

Fig. 139.1

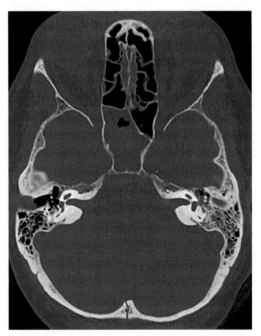

Fig. 139.2

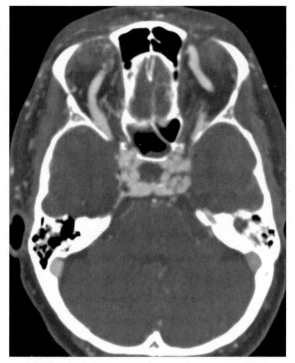

Fig. 139.3

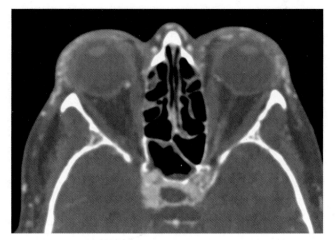

Fig. 139.4

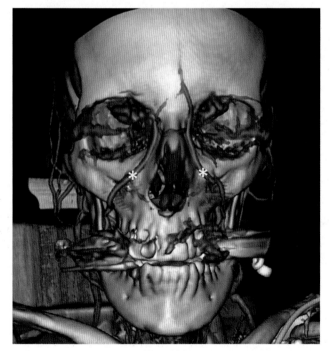

Fig. 139.5

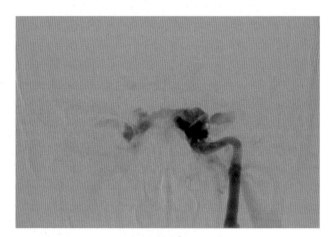

Fig. 139.6

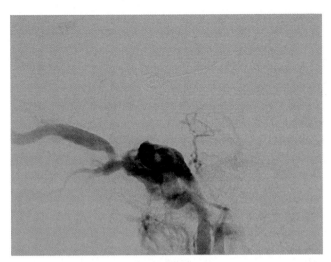

Fig. 139.7

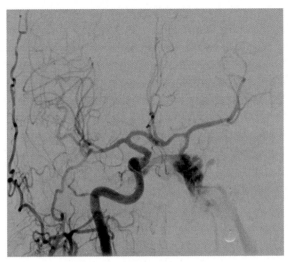

Fig. 139.8

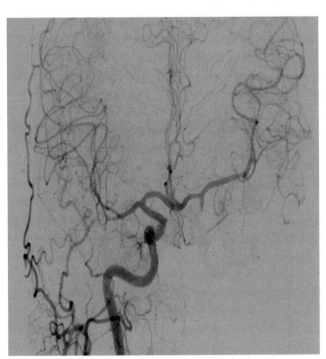

Fig. 139.9

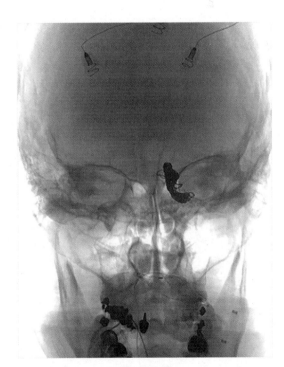

Fig. 139.10

Case 140

History: A 46-year-old male presents with slowly progressive personality changes.

1. What is the most likely diagnosis?
   A. Progressive multifocal leukoencephalopathy (PML)
   B. Subacute infarction
   C. Viral encephalitis
   D. Astrocytoma
2. According to the 5th Edition (2021) update to the WHO classification of CNS tumors, which of the following term(s) have been retired?
   A. Hemangiopericytoma
   B. Gliomatosis cerebri
   C. Primitive neuroectodermal tumor (PNET)
   D. All of the above

3. Gliomatosis cerebri was previously recognized as a distinct entity. Since 2016, it has been redefined as a pattern of tumor growth that can be displayed by any infiltrating glioma that involves at least_____cerebral lobes.
   A. One
   B. Two
   C. Three
   D. Four
4. According to the 5th Edition (2021) update to the WHO classification of CNS tumors, an IDH-wild-type astrocytoma with low-grade histologic features, presence of EGFR amplification, TERT promoter mutation and the combined gain of chromosome 7 and loss of chromosome 10 will be classified as:
   A. Astrocytoma, IDH-mutant, CNS WHO grade 3
   B. Astrocytoma, IDH-mutant, CNS WHO grade 2
   C. Astrocytoma, IDH-mutant, CNS WHO grade 4
   D. Glioblastoma, IDH-wild-type, CNS WHO grade 4

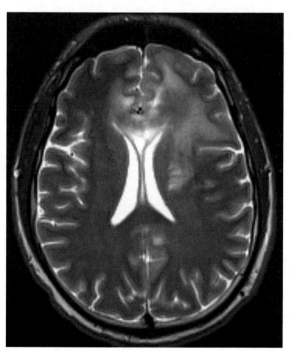

Fig. 140.1

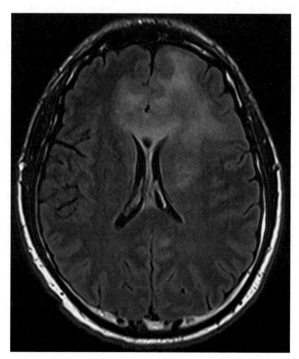

Fig. 140.2

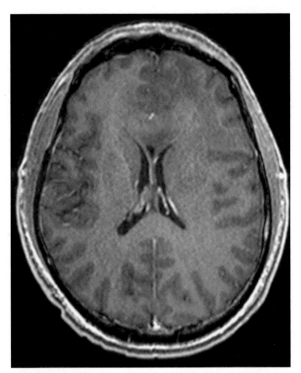

Fig. 140.3

Case 141

History: 33-year-old male transferred from China with left hemiplegia, multiple left-sided cranial nerve deficits, progressive gait ataxia, somnolence, and hydrocephalus.

1. Which of the following posterior fossa tumors commonly demonstrate low ADC values?
   A. Ependymoma
   B. Pilocytic astrocytoma
   C. Subependymoma
   D. Atypical teratoid/rhabdoid tumor (AT/RTs)
2. Primary AT/RTs can occur at which of the following sites within the CNS?
   A. Infratentorial and intra-axial
   B. Extra-axial situated at the cerebellopontine angle
   C. Both infra- and supratentorial
   D. All of the above

3. Which of the following genetic alterations is the hallmark of an AT/RT?
   A. SMARCB1
   B. NF1
   C. IDH1
   D. NF2

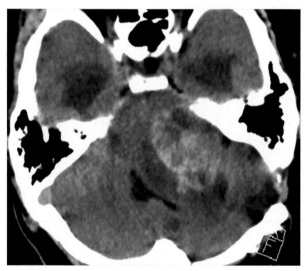

Fig. 141.1

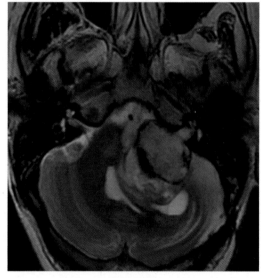

Fig. 141.2

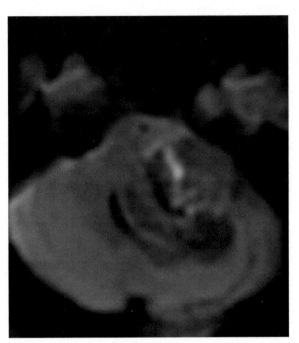

Fig. 141.3

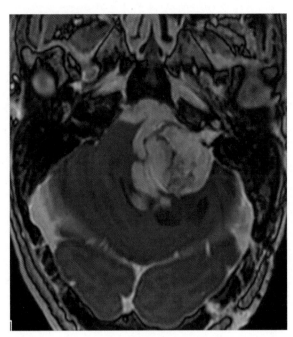

Fig. 141.4

Case 142

History: A 46-year-old male presents with progressive intermittent dysarthria, slurred speech, difficulty communicating in French, Hindi, and English. Family members are unable to understand him.

1. What is the most likely diagnosis?
   A. Normal MRI scan
   B. Huntington's disease
   C. Amyotrophic lateral sclerosis
   D. Alzheimer's disease
2. This specific diagnosis involves degeneration of what CNS structures?
   A. Caudate nucleus
   B. Hippocampus
   C. Corticospinal tracts
   D. Substantia nigra

3. In what part of the brainstem does the pyramidal decussation occur?
   A. Midbrain
   B. Pons
   C. Medulla
   D. Upper cervical spinal cord
4. What is the most common cause of death in these patients?
   A. Stroke
   B. Respiratory failure
   C. Road traffic accidents
   D. Drug overdose

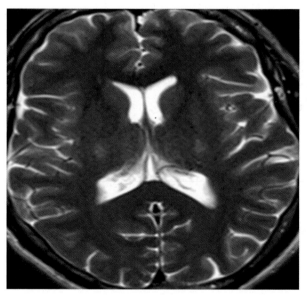

Fig. 142.1

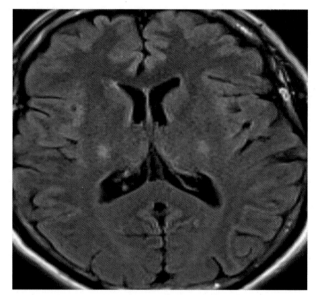

Fig. 142.2

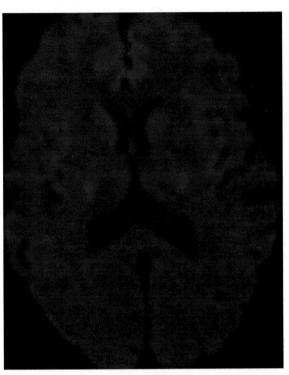

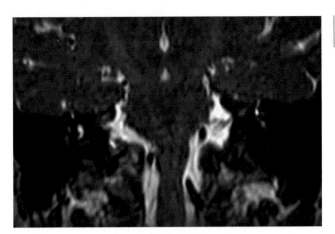

Fig. 142.4

Fig. 142.3

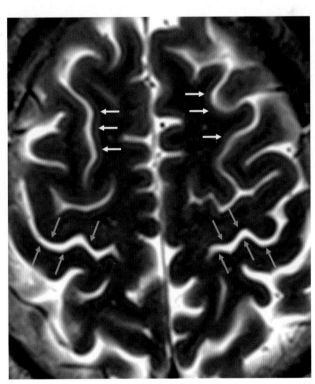

Fig. 142.5

Case 143

History: This 22-year-old woman with two episodes of transient left body numbness.

1. What is the most likely diagnosis?
   A. Dysembryoplastic neuroepithelial tumor (DNET)
   B. Dysplastic gangliocytoma
   C. Multinodular and vacuolating neuronal tumor (MVNT)
   D. Pleomorphic xanthoastrocytoma (PXA)
2. What is the most common location of a pleomorphic xanthoastrocytoma (PXA)?
   A. Temporal lobe
   B. Frontal lobe
   C. Parietal lobe
   D. Cerebellum
3. What is the most common clinical presentation of tumors located in the temporal lobe?
   A. Numbness
   B. Headache
   C. Hemiplegia
   D. Seizures
4. Which of the following is the most frequently found mutation in PXAs?
   A. EGFR amplification
   B. BRAF V600E
   C. p53 and p16
   D. Loss of heterozygosity of chromosome 10

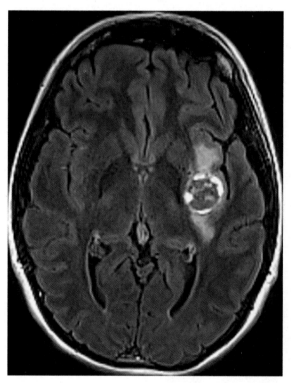

Fig. 143.1

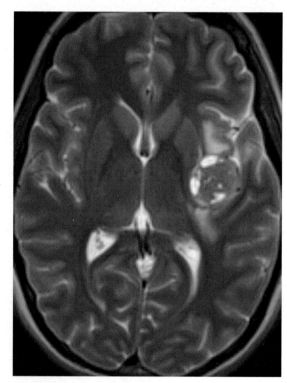

Fig. 143.2

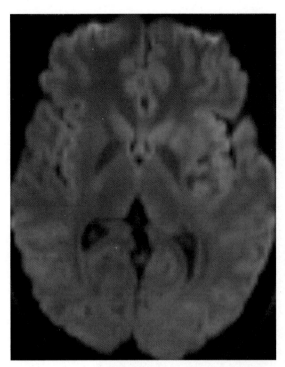

Fig. 143.3

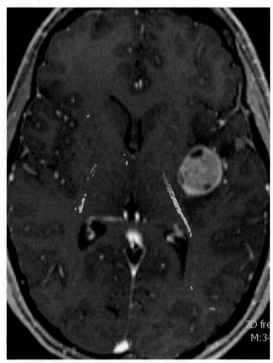

Fig. 143.4

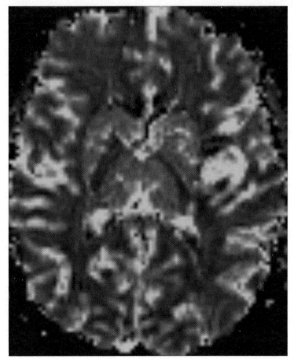

Fig. 143.5

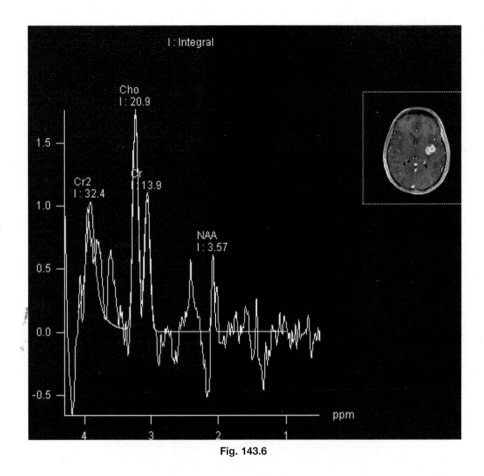

Fig. 143.6

Case 144

History: This 72-year-old female with a remote history of breast cancer (32 years ago) presents with progressive confusion, imbalance, and headaches.

1. Which of the following will not show blooming/susceptibility artifact on susceptibility-weighted imaging (SWI)?
   A. Melanin
   B. Air
   C. Metal
   D. Hemosiderin
2. What is the likely cause of the increased T1 signal in the subarachnoid spaces in Figures 144.1 and 144.3?
   A. Melanin
   B. Artifact
   C. Increased FiO_2
   D. Hemosiderin

3. Based on these images, what is the most likely diagnosis?
   A. Neurosarcoidosis
   B. Leptomeningeal melanomatosis
   C. Primary leptomeningeal lymphoma
   D. Superficial siderosis

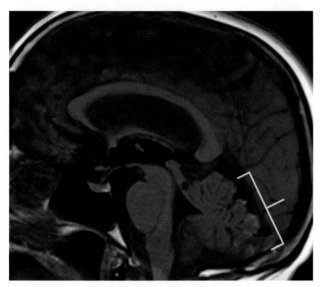

Fig. 144.1

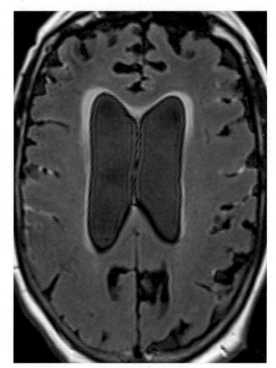

Fig. 144.2

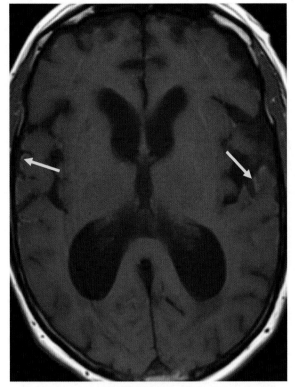

Fig. 144.3

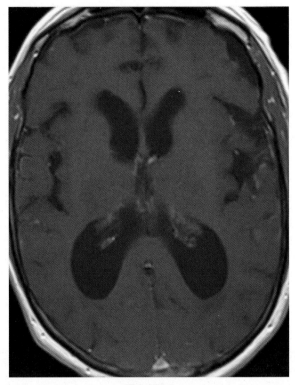

Fig. 144.4

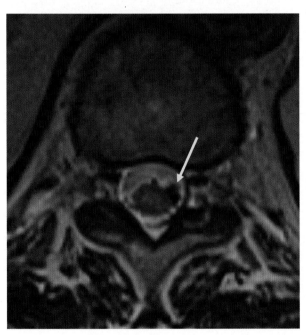

Fig. 144.5

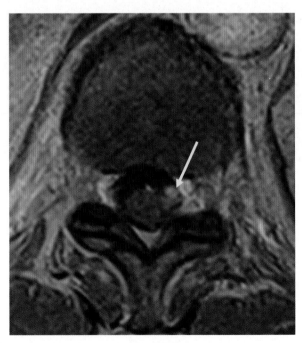

Fig. 144.6

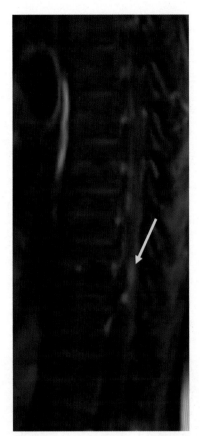

Fig. 144.7

Case 145

History: A 52-year-old man with no significant past medical history presents acutely with depressed mental status. The patient has recently been abusing cocaine and other illicit drugs.

1. What is the most likely cause of bithalamic signal abnormality?
   A. Venous congestion
   B. Arterial ischemia
   C. Osmotic demyelination
   D. Viral infection
2. What are the findings on the angiographic images, and what is the diagnosis?
   A. AV shunting in an infiltrating glioma
   B. Artery of Percheron infarction
   C. Tentorial dural AVF
   D. Tumor blush in a diffuse midline glioma
3. The artery of Davidoff-Schechter is a branch of?
   A. Internal carotid artery
   B. Posterior communicating artery
   C. P1 segment of the PCA
   D. A1 segment of ACA
4. Which of the following is not known to cause bithalamic lesions?
   A. Artery of Percheron infarction
   B. Tentorial dural AVF
   C. Cocaine abuse
   D. Wernicke's encephalopathy
   E. Deep cerebral vein thrombosis

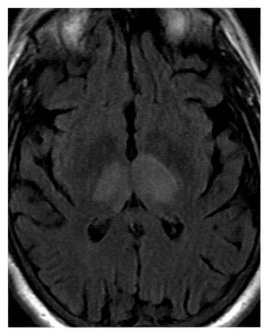

Fig. 145.1

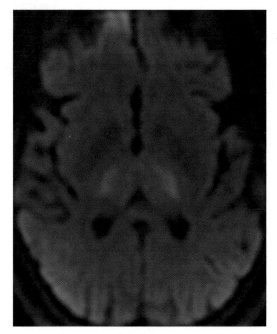

Fig. 145.2

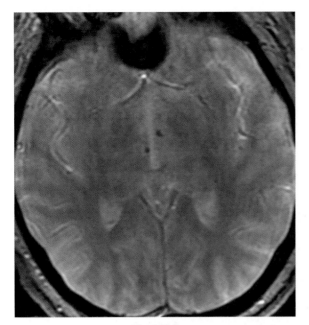

Fig. 145.3

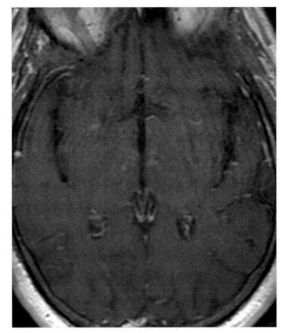

Fig. 145.4

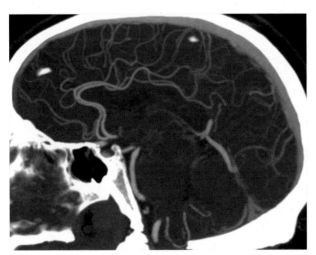

Fig. 145.5

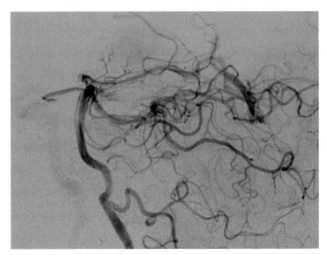

Fig. 145.6

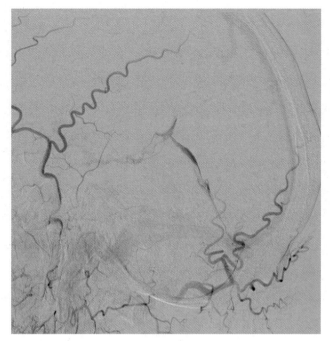

Fig. 145.7

Case 146

History: This 30-year-old male with Tetralogy of Fallot repair, presents with headache, nausea, vomiting, and a witnessed seizure.

1. What is the most likely cause of intracranial hemorrhage in this patient?
   A. Hypertensive hemorrhage with "spot sign" on CT angiography
   B. Arteriovenous malformation
   C. Mycotic aneurysm
   D. Hemorrhagic infarct
2. What is the most common location of intracranial mycotic aneurysms?
   A. Branch points of circle of Willis vessels
   B. Distal middle cerebral artery
   C. Cavernous internal carotid artery
   D. Posterior inferior cerebellar artery

3. What percentage of intracranial mycotic aneurysms are multiple?
   A. 50%
   B. 90%
   C. 5%
   D. 25%
4. Which of the following is incorrect regarding intracranial mycotic aneurysms?
   A. Right-sided infective endocarditis is the primary risk factor in over 75% of cases.
   B. Ruptured mycotic aneurysms present with subarachnoid or intraparenchymal hemorrhage.
   C. DSA remains the gold-standard imaging modality for the evaluation of intracranial mycotic aneurysms.
   D. Treatment usually involves a combination of antibiotics, surgical, and/or endovascular repair.
   E. Unruptured mycotic aneurysms have a mortality of up to 30%, while ruptured mycotic aneurysms have a mortality of up to 80%.

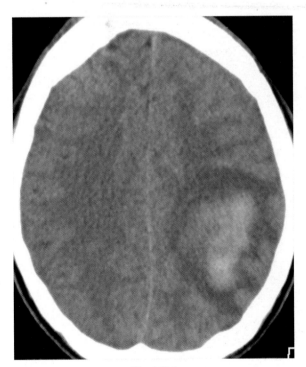

Fig. 146.1

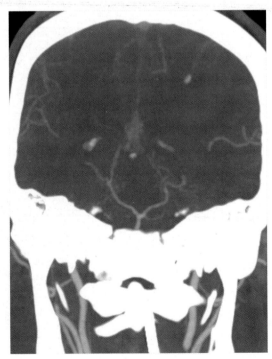

Fig. 146.2

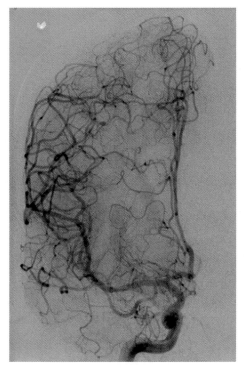

Fig. 146.3

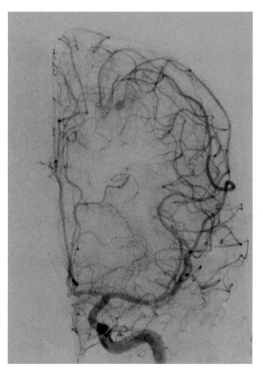

Fig. 146.4

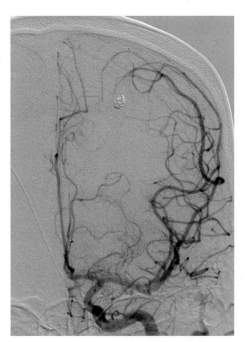

Fig. 146.5

Case 147

History: This 75-year-old male presents with a history of ocular myasthenia gravis and multiple prior primary cancers presents now with amnesia.

1. What is the most likely diagnosis?
   A. Seizure-related changes
   B. Autoimmune limbic encephalitis
   C. Rasmussen encephalitis
   D. Diffuse astrocytoma
2. What is the most common location of CNS involvement in autoimmune encephalitis?
   A. Frontal lobes
   B. Cerebellum
   C. Mesial temporal lobes and limbic systems
   D. Bilateral thalami

3. What malignancy is most commonly associated with autoimmune limbic encephalitis and which is the associated antibody?
   A. Mesothelioma, anti-VGKC antibody
   B. Small cell carcinoma of the lung, anti-Hu antibody
   C. Thymoma, anti-Ma
   D. Breast cancer, anti-Ri antibody
4. Autoimmune encephalitis is divided based on whether the antibodies are against intracellular antigens or cell surface antigens. As a rule, antibodies targeted against intracellular antigens are more frequently associated with which of the following?
   A. Memory impairment
   B. Psychiatric symptoms
   C. Underlying tumor
   D. Seizures

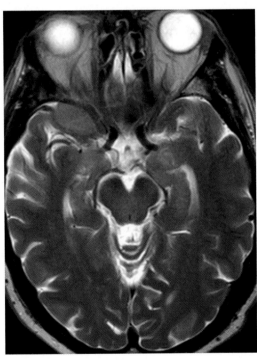

Fig. 147.1

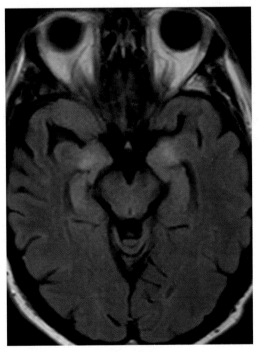

Fig. 147.2

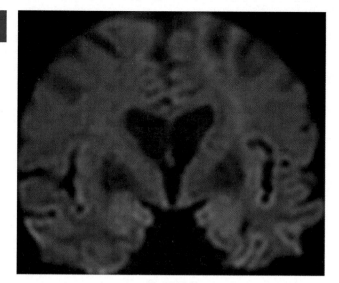

Fig. 147.3

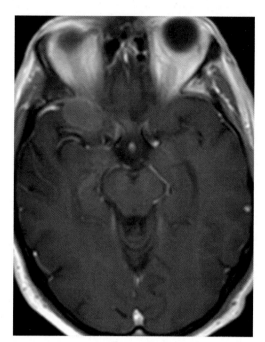

Fig. 147.4

Case 148

History: A 39-year-old with skin cancer on treatment, presents with headache and sensitivity to light.

1. What is the most likely etiology of these imaging findings?
   A. Pituitary metastasis
   B. Pituitary apoplexy
   C. Drug-induced hypothyroidism
   D. Drug-induced hypophysitis
2. Hypophysitis is a well-known adverse effect of which class of anticancer drugs?
   A. Immune checkpoint inhibitor immunotherapy
   B. Chimeric antigen receptor (CAR) T-cell immunotherapy
   C. Dendritic cell vaccine (DCVax) immunotherapy
   D. Anti-angiogenic therapy
3. What is the treatment of choice for immune checkpoint inhibitor–induced hypophysitis?
   A. Continuation of therapy as it is self-limiting and represents successful treatment
   B. Cessation of therapy
   C. Cessation of therapy with the addition of corticosteroids
   D. Cessation of therapy, addition of corticosteroids, and supplementation of deficient hormones
4. Which of the following is incorrect regarding immune checkpoint inhibitor–induced hypophysitis?
   A. Normal MRI essentially excludes the diagnosis
   B. No significant remodeling of the bony sella
   C. Often has a low signal on T2W images
   D. Often involves the pituitary infundibulum

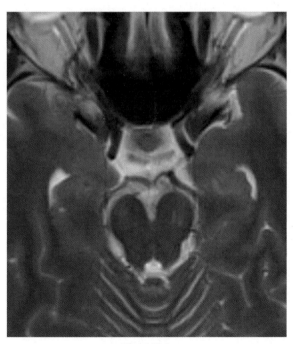
Fig. 148.1

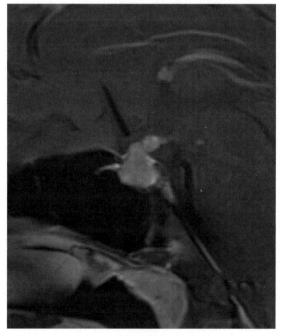
Fig. 148.2

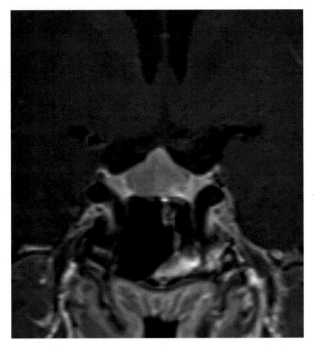

Fig. 148.3

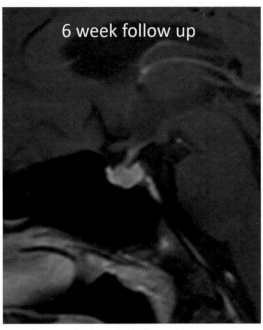

Fig. 148.4

Case 149

History: A 46-year-old woman with systemic lupus erythematosus, status post rectal biopsy, developed bilateral eye swelling, pain, and vision loss.

1. What is the most likely diagnosis?
   A. Bilateral orbital metastases
   B. Spontaneous subperiosteal hematomas
   C. Extramedullary hematopoiesis
   D. Bilateral encephaloceles
2. Spontaneous subperiosteal hematomas can be seen in which of the following circumstances?
   A. Bleeding disorders
   B. Acute sinusitis
   C. Severe vomiting
   D. Child birth
   E. Scuba diving
   F. All of the above

3. Which of the following is incorrect about spontaneous subperiosteal hematomas of the orbit, presenting with pain and vision loss, as in this case?
   A. The superior orbit is the most common location as the periosteal attachment in this location is relatively loose.
   B. Usually result of rupture of subperiosteal veins
   C. Well-defined biconvex high-attenuation masses on CT
   D. No specific treatment is necessary as they are known to resorb spontaneously

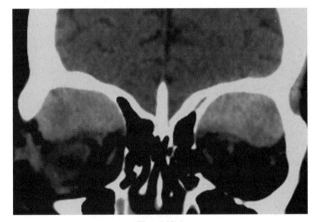

Fig. 149.1

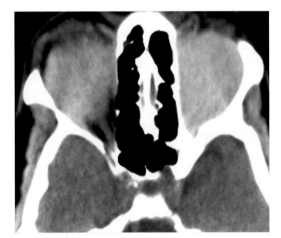

Fig. 149.2

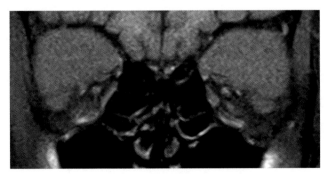

Fig. 149.3

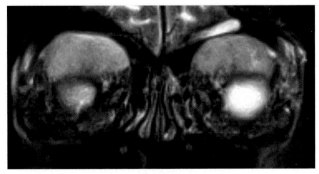

Fig. 149.4

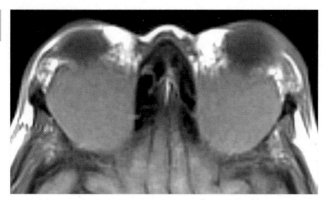

Fig. 149.5

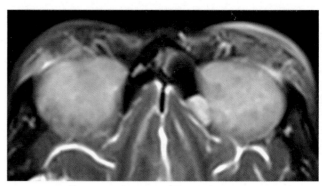

Fig. 149.6

Case 150

History: A 57-year-old patient presents with frequent falls and hydrocephalus.

1. What is the diagnosis?
   A. Joubert syndrome
   B. Dandy–Walker malformation
   C. Agenesis of corpus callosum
   D. Rhombencephalosynapsis
2. Which of the following abnormalities are associated with this condition?
   A. Fusion of cerebellar hemispheres
   B. Fusion of dentate nuclei
   C. Fusion of the superior cerebellar peduncles
   D. Fusion of inferior colliculi
   E. Hydrocephalus from aqueductal stenosis
   F. Agenesis of the posterior lobe of the pituitary
   G. All of the above

3. What other posterior fossa anomalies are associated with vermian dysgenesis or agenesis?
   A. Joubert syndrome
   B. Dandy–Walker malformation
   C. Chiari 2 malformation
   D. Both A and B
   E. Both A and C
   F. A, B, and C
4. Which of the following is incorrect regarding an absent septum pellucidum?
   A. Cavum septum pellucidum should always be visualized between 18 and 37 weeks of gestation.
   B. Isolated septal deficiency is rare but is considered a variant of normal.
   C. Absent septum pellucidum is commonly associated with a variety of conditions.
   D. Prenatal imaging can differentiate between isolated absent septum pellucidum and septo-optic dysplasia.

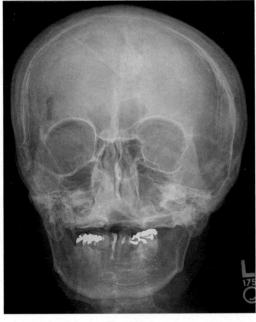

Fig. 150.1

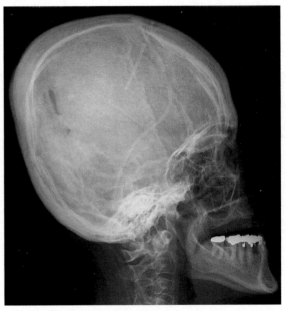

Fig. 150.2

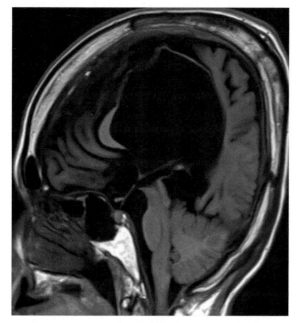

Fig. 150.3

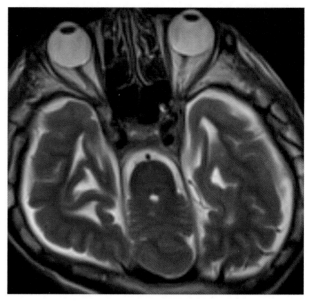

Fig. 150.4

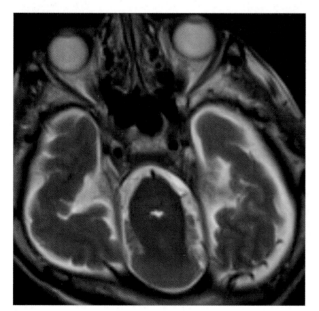

Fig. 150.5

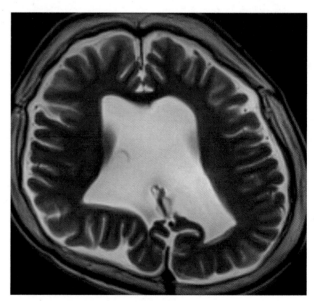

Fig. 150.6

Opening Round

CASE 1

Acute Left Anterior Cerebral Artery (ACA) Infarct

1. **D.** ACA supplies the medial part of the frontal and the parietal lobes, the anterior portion of the corpus callosum, basal ganglia, and internal capsule. ACA territory infarcts comprise ~2% of all ischemic strokes and typically present as dysarthria, aphasia, and contralateral motor weakness.
2. **A.** Recurrent artery of Heubner, also known as the medial striate artery, arises near the A1-ACOM-A2 junction of the ACA, from the proximal A2 in 90% of cases, and from the distal A1 in 10% of cases. It then curves back sharply on itself, parallel to the A1 and is at risk from ACOM aneurysm clipping.
3. **B.** The recurrent artery of Heubner supplies the head and anteromedial caudate nucleus as well as the anterior limb of the internal capsule. The olfactory bulb and tracts are supplied by the A2 segment of the ACA, while the posterior limb of the internal capsule is supplied by the anterior choroidal artery. The corpus callosum and medial cerebral surface are supplied by the pericallosal artery.
4. **A.** The medial lenticulostriate arteries arise from the A1 segment (the most proximal segment) of the ACA. The *lateral* lenticulostriate arteries branch instead from the M1 segment of the MCA.

Comment

This case shows the characteristic appearance of an acute left anterior cerebral artery territory infarct. On CT **(A)**, there is hypodensity in the medial left frontal lobe extending to the left parietal lobe, with corresponding T2 **(B)** and FLAIR **(C)** hyperintensity and restricted diffusion demonstrated on diffusion-weighted imaging **(D)** and apparent diffusion coefficient (ADC) **(E)** maps.

REFERENCES

Deguchi I, Dembo T, Fukuoka T, et al. Usefulness of MRA-DWI mismatch in neuroendovascular therapy for acute cerebral infarction. *Eur J Neurol*. 2012;19(1):114-120.
Kang SY, Kim JS. Anterior cerebral artery infarction: stroke mechanism and clinical-imaging study in 100 patients. *Neurology*. 2008;70(24):2386-2393.
Neuroradiology: THE REQUISITES. 4th ed. pp 31-32, 109-111.

CASE 2

Hemorrhagic Metastases—Renal Cell

1. **B.** Metastases are the most common posterior fossa tumor in adults. In a child, the most common posterior fossa tumor is a pilocytic astrocytoma, followed by medulloblastoma and ependymoma.
2. **A.** Acute hemorrhage, high cellularity, high protein concentration, and the presence of calcification are all hyperdense on CT and hypointense on T2W images. On the other hand, fat, edema, and extracellular methemoglobin are hyperintense on T2.
3. **D.** Hemorrhagic metastases classically originate from melanoma, renal cell carcinoma, choriocarcinoma, papillary thyroid carcinoma, lung carcinoma, breast carcinoma, and hepatocellular carcinoma. A useful mnemonic to remember is MR CT BB.
4. **D.** In adults, the most common "mass" lesion in the posterior fossa is a subacute stroke, whereas the most common neoplastic lesion in the posterior fossa is cerebellar metastasis (intra-axial) or vestibular schwannoma (extra-axial).

Comment

Metastatic disease is among the most common causes of intracranial masses in adults. Metastases are frequently multiple; however, in 30% to 50% of cases, they may occur as an isolated lesion on imaging. Enhanced MR imaging is clearly more sensitive than CT in detecting cerebral metastases. Metastases are typically circumscribed masses that demonstrate variable enhancement patterns (solid, peripheral, or heterogeneous). Metastases are often associated with a disproportionate amount of surrounding edema, manifested on T2-weighted (T2W) images as increased signal intensity in the adjacent white matter.

Metastases typically occur at the gray–white matter interface because tumor cells lodge in the small-caliber vessels in this location. Metastatic deposits may also involve the cortex. With cortical metastases in particular, edema may be absent or minimal such that metastatic lesions could be missed on T2W imaging. Therefore, it is essential to administer intravenous contrast to patients with suspected brain metastases. Studies examining the role of double- and triple-dose gadolinium have shown that although higher doses of contrast reveal more lesions than does a single dose, this often occurs in patients whose standard-dose study already shows more than one metastasis. Therefore, management in these patients is not affected, and multidose gadolinium is neither indicated nor recommended. In patients with no or a single metastasis on single-dose gadolinium, higher doses of contrast material yield additional metastases in fewer than 10% of cases.

Hypointensity (T2W shortening) may be seen with blood products, as a result of the paramagnetic effects of melanin, and when lesions have calcification, hypercellularity, or proteinaceous material. In the case shown here, the patient has hemorrhagic metastatic renal cell carcinoma, hypointense on T2 **(A)** and FLAIR **(B)** with surrounding vasogenic edema, isointense on T1W **(C)** and heterogenous post-contrast enhancement on **(D)**.

REFERENCES

Hill Jr KL, Lipson AC, Sheehan JM, et al. Brain magnetic resonance imaging changes after sorafenib and sunitinib chemotherapy in patients with advanced renal cell and breast carcinoma. *J Neurosurg*. 2009;111(3):497-503.
Shih RY, Smirniotopoulos JG. Posterior fossa tumors in adult patients. *Neuroimaging Clin N Am*. 2016;26(4):493-510. doi:10.1016/j.nic.2016.06.003.
Neuroradiology: THE REQUISITES. 4th ed. pp 72-74.

CASE 3

Penetrating Brain Injury—Bow and Arrow Injury

1. **B.** This was a case of a self-inflicted bow and arrow injury with intraparenchymal hemorrhage in the left frontal lobe, intraventricular extension, with a retained bow and arrow.
2. **D.** A self-inflicted injury, with likely entrance under the mandible (submental) and then through the anterior cranial fossa.
3. **C.** A noncontrast head CT is the most expedient way to assess a penetrating brain injury. It can rapidly determine whether a surgical emergency is present, such as an acute hemorrhage with mass effect necessitating acute surgical decompression. It also shows the location and the extent of retained foreign bodies.
4. **D.** Intracranial air or pneumocephalus refers to the presence of intracranial gas and is most commonly encountered following trauma or surgery.

Comment

Penetrating injuries cause lacerations of the brain and its coverings (dura), and these are associated with gunshot wounds, stab wounds (in this case, a self-inflicted bow and arrow injury), or displaced bone fragments. With penetrating wounds, there is a risk of injury to critical structures that are in the trajectory of the penetrating object. Brain injury may result in functional and cognitive losses, depending on the region of the brain injured. Injury to the intracranial arteries may result in dissection, occlusion, hemorrhage, or pseudoaneurysm formation. Pseudoaneurysms must always be considered because they have a very high incidence of delayed hemorrhage. Computed tomography is the most efficient and effective way to assess a penetrating brain injury rapidly. It can determine whether a surgical emergency is present, such as an acute hemorrhage with mass effect necessitating acute surgical decompression. It also shows the location and the extent of retained foreign bodies.

Computed tomography also identifies intracranial air that is due to communication with the extracranial compartment (open fracture) or may indicate an associated fracture through an adjacent paranasal sinus or the temporal bone. Trapped intracranial air may result in tension pneumocephalus "Mount Fuji sign" related to a one-way ball valve mechanism that causes gradual expansion of the intracranial air and mass effect on the adjacent brain. Mount Fuji sign refers to the presence of subdural pneumocephalus causing compression and separation of the frontal lobes with widening of the interhemispheric space giving the silhouette-like appearance of Mount Fuji. It suggests that the pressure of the gas is greater than that of the surface tension of cerebrospinal fluid between the frontal lobes and often warrants immediate surgery to prevent permanent neurological damage.

REFERENCES

Bodanapally UK, Shanmuganathan K, Boscak AR, et al. Vascular complications of penetrating brain injury: comparison of helical CT angiography and conventional angiography. *J Neurosurg*. 2014;121(5):1275-1283.

Kriet JD, Stanley Jr RB, Grady MS. Self-inflicted submental and transoral gunshot wounds that produce nonfatal brain injuries: management and prognosis. *J Neurosurg*. 2005;102(6):1029-1032. doi:10.3171/jns.2005.102.6.1029.

Neuroradiology: THE REQUISITES. 4th ed. pp 159.

CASE 4

Acute Epidural Hematoma and Associated Linear Fracture of the Frontal Bone

1. **D.** The CT swirl sign is recognized as an area of low attenuation within an extra-axial hyperattenuating collection. The swirl sign is an ominous sign in patients with epidural hematoma and represents unclotted fresh blood which is of lower attenuation than clotted blood which is of higher attenuation. It represents acute extravasation of blood into the hematoma and results from leakage of serum from the epidural clot or active bleeding. This may also be seen in coagulopathic patients or in patients receiving anticoagulation therapy.
2. **B.** Typically, epidural hematomas are seen in younger patients who have sustained trauma and are usually associated with a skull fracture.
3. **A.** Epidural hematoma is a collection of blood between the periosteum of the inner calvarium and the dura mater. Subdural hematoma is a collection of blood between the duramater and the arachnoid mater.
4. **A.** The most common source of hemorrhage is an injury to the middle meningeal artery.

Comment

There are two anatomic types of extra-axial collections or hematomas, namely, subdural and epidural. On CT imaging, acute epidural hematomas (EDHs) are hyperdense extra-axial collections that can usually be distinguished from acute subdural hematomas (SDHs) based on their shape and location relative to the calvarial sutures. EDHs are usually confined by the cranial sutures because the dura is adherent to the periosteum of the inner calvarium. This results in the biconvex or lenticular shape of these collections, which occur between the dura and the periosteum. In comparison, SDH cross-sutures boundaries occur deep to the duramater, occupying the space between the dura and the pia arachnoid along the surface of the brain. As a result, subdural collections or hematomas tend to be crescentic in shape, similar to a sliver of the moon.

In the vast majority of cases (75%–80%), EDHs are secondary to a direct laceration of the meningeal arteries, most commonly the middle meningeal artery by an overlying skull fracture. In a small percentage of cases (<20%), EDHs occur due to tearing of meningeal arteries in the absence of a fracture. This is most commonly seen in children and may be related to transient depression of the incompletely ossified soft calvarium, resulting in laceration of a meningeal artery. Most arterial EDHs occur in the temporal region, although they may be seen in the frontal or temporoparietal regions.

EDHs due to venous rather than arterial injury are much less common. Venous epidural hematomas are usually due to tearing of a dural venous sinus related to an underlying calvarial fracture. They are most common in the posterior fossa as a result of injury to the transverse or sigmoid sinuses and are most frequently seen in the pediatric population. Unlike arterial EDH, venous epidural hematomas may extend across the tentorium cerebelli and involve both the supratentorial and infratentorial compartments. These may also occur in a paramedian location over the cerebral convexities or in the middle cranial fossa as the result of a tear in the superior sagittal or sphenoparietal sinus, respectively.

Acute EDH isolated to the anterior aspect of the middle cranial fossa constitutes a unique subgroup of traumatic EDHs with a benign natural history. It is postulated that they arise from venous bleeding due to disruption of the sphenoparietal sinus and no active intervention is necessary. A follow-up single CT scan at 24 to 36 hours after injury is recommended to document stability, and patients with good neurologic condition can then be discharged.

Other traumatic sequelae that may occasionally be seen in the setting of epidural hematomas include pseudoaneurysms of the meningeal artery (most commonly, the middle meningeal artery) and arteriovenous fistulas if a fracture lacerates both the middle meningeal artery and vein, resulting in their communication.

REFERENCES

Nakahara K, Shimizu S, Utsuki S, et al. Linear fractures occult on skull radiographs: a pitfall at radiological screening for mild head injury. *J Trauma*. 2011;70(1):180-182.

Talbott JF, Gean A, Yuh EL, Stiver SI. Calvarial fracture patterns on CT imaging predict risk of a delayed epidural hematoma following decompressive craniectomy for traumatic brain injury. *AJNR Am J Neuroradiol*. 2014;35(10):1930-1935.

Neuroradiology: THE REQUISITES. 4th ed. pp 153-154.

CASE 5

Acute Hydrocephalus Secondary to Carcinomatous Meningitis

1. **A.** The primary imaging finding is dilatation of the lateral and third ventricles with enlargement of the temporal horns which is considered the best indicator for hydrocephalus. Note that the temporal horns have the greatest capacitance of the ventricular system, and enlargement is the earliest sign of hydrocephalus.
2. **C.** Presence of transependymal edema, or periventricular seepage may be seen as areas of high T2 signal on MRI or low density on CT around the ventricles.
3. **C.** It is a type of interstitial edema seen in acute obstructive hydrocephalus. It is thought to reflect some combination of CSF trapped within the periventricular white matter, not able to flow into the high-pressure ventricles, as well as some degree of outward, transependymal flow from the high-pressure ventricles into the brain parenchyma, as CSF secretion continues.
4. **B.** The primary treatment of obstructive hydrocephalus is a ventricular shunt or by endoscopic third ventriculostomy (ETV), a procedure that creates a fenestration of the third ventricular floor. Note that it is critical to report the location of the basilar artery in relation to the floor of the third ventricle to prevent accidental trauma to the basilar artery.

Comment

Obstructive Hydrocephalus

Obstructive hydrocephalus can be categorized as communicating or noncommunicating. Noncommunicating hydrocephalus is usually related to the obstruction of CSF flow at some level within the ventricular system and is commonly related to neoplasms; however, infection, hemorrhage, cysts, or congenital lesions (synechiae, webs, arachnoid cysts) may be responsible. Communicating hydrocephalus typically results from obstruction of the arachnoid villi, foramen magnum, or tentorial incisura. Common causes of communicating hydrocephalus include inflammation of the meninges, or meningitis (as in this case, the patient has bacterial meningitis); ventriculitis; subarachnoid hemorrhage; and carcinomatous meningitis. Obstruction of the arachnoid villi in these situations is usually related to high protein concentrations, hemorrhage, or hypercellularity of the CSF. In bacterial meningitis, purulent exudate in the subarachnoid spaces over the cerebral convexities and in the basilar cisterns, where CSF flow is more sluggish, results in impairment of CSF absorption by the arachnoid villi.

Imaging

On imaging, dilation of the temporal horns is the earliest sign of hydrocephalus. Elevation and thinning of the corpus callosum, best appreciated on sagittal MR imaging, is present in more than 75% of cases of hydrocephalus. Acute hydrocephalus may manifest with hypodensity around the ventricles on CT scans or hyperintensity on MR T2W images in the periventricular white

matter due to transependymal flow of CSF. Compensated longstanding hydrocephalus usually does not present with this finding. Treatment of noncommunicating and communicating hydrocephalus is different. Noncommunicating hydrocephalus often requires surgery (e.g., resection of a neoplasm), whereas communicating hydrocephalus is usually treated with shunting.

REFERENCES

Rekate HL, Blitz AM. Hydrocephalus in children. *Handb Clin Neurol*. 2016;136:1261-1273.

Singh P, Paliwal VK, Neyaz Z, et al. Clinical and magnetic resonance imaging characteristics of tubercular ventriculitis: an under-recognized complication of tubercular meningitis. *J Neurol Sci*. 2014;342 (1-2):137-140.

Yuan W, McKinstry RC, Shimony JS, et al. Diffusion tensor imaging properties and neurobehavioral outcomes in children with hydrocephalus. *AJNR Am J Neuroradiol*. 2013;34(2):439-445.

Neuroradiology: THE REQUISITES. 4th ed. pp 230-238.

CASE 6

Pineal Cyst

1. **B.** The imaging findings are most consistent with a pineal cyst which are common, usually asymptomatic, and incidentally detected.
2. **D.** The vast majority of pineal cysts are small (<10 mm) and are asymptomatic. Larger cysts can present with a mass effect over the tectum leading to compression of the superior colliculi and Parinaud syndrome. These can also compress the cerebral aqueduct and result in obstructive hydrocephalus. Rarely, hemorrhage into a pineal cyst can cause rapid expansion, the so-called "pineal apoplexy."
3. **A.** Parinaud syndrome is characterized by a classic triad of upward gaze palsy, pupillary light-near dissociation (pupils respond to near stimuli, but not to light), and convergence-retraction nystagmus. These symptoms localize pathology to the tectal plate, most frequently due to a posterior commissure or pineal region mass (more commonly solid tumors rather than pineal cysts). Argyll Robertson pupil presents with bilateral miotic and irregular pupils, which constrict briskly with accommodation but do not react to bright light, is a highly specific sign of late neurosyphilis; however, it can also occur in diabetic neuropathy, multiple sclerosis, alcoholic midbrain degeneration, and stroke. Wernicke-Korsakoff syndrome presents with ophthalmoplegia, horizontal nystagmus, and ataxia. Horner's syndrome presents with ptosis, miosis, and anhidrosis.
4. **C.** Pineal gland lies below the fornix, velum interpositum, and internal cerebral veins, and masses in any of these structures will displace the pineal gland downward. Masses in the tectal plate or midbrain will displace the pineal gland superiorly.

Comment

The pineal gland develops during the second month of gestation as a diverticulum in the diencephalic roof of the third ventricle. Pineal cysts are common incidental findings on MR imaging of the head obtained for unrelated indications, and are seen in 1% to 4% of patients. In autopsy series, cystic lesions of the pineal gland have been found in 20% to 40% of specimens. Masses of the pineal gland may cause mass effect on the tectum and the aqueduct, resulting in paralysis of upward gaze (Parinaud's syndrome) and hydrocephalus or headache, respectively. However, even large pineal cysts are rarely symptomatic. Pineal cysts are variable in size, and 50% of cysts identified on MR imaging are larger than 1 cm. Studies have shown that, overall, the majority of cysts do not change in size; however, small changes in size (increases and decreases) have been noted. Enlargement of these cysts may be due to increased cyst fluid or intracystic hemorrhage. Rare cases of pineal apoplexy have been reported in which there may be sudden death as a result of intracystic hemorrhage and acute hydrocephalus.

Pineal cysts are less common in young children and are usually seen in middle-aged adults, suggesting that these cysts may develop in late childhood or adolescence and later involute. Pineal cysts are homogeneous on MR imaging. They are typically well demarcated and are round or oval, and they have a thin or imperceptible wall. On FLAIR imaging (as in this case), the cyst contents are frequently hyperintense relative to cerebrospinal fluid. Nodular enhancement of the wall should not be present with cysts. Asymptomatic, larger cysts may cause tectal deformity.

REFERENCES

Fang AS, Meyers SP. Magnetic resonance imaging of pineal region tumours. *Insights Imaging*. 2013;4(3):369-382.
Pu Y, Mahankali S, Hou J, et al. High prevalence of pineal cysts in healthy adults demonstrated by high-resolution, noncontrast brain MR imaging. *AJNR Am J Neuroradiol*. 2007;28(9):1706-1709.
Neuroradiology: THE REQUISITES. 4th ed. pp 80.

CASE 7

Hemorrhagic Contusions—Closed Head Injury

1. **D.** There are multiple regions of intraparenchymal high density consistent with hemorrhage, and associated surrounding edema. The pattern of intracranial hemorrhage is consistent with multiple contusions in the setting of closed head injury.
2. **D.** Cerebral hemorrhagic contusions are common in the setting of significant head injury and have a predilection for certain locations such as frontal lobes adjacent to the floor of the anterior cranial fossa, temporal poles, and portions of the brain located at the site of impact (coup injury) and on the opposite side (contrecoup injury).
3. **B.** Hemorrhage in the deep gray nuclei (basal ganglia and thalami) is common in the setting of hypertension; also see Case 10. All other locations are common in closed head injury.

Comment

Hemorrhagic contusions (brain bruising) are among the most common traumatic brain injuries. Contusions represent petechial hemorrhages in the cortex that may extend into the adjacent white matter and are frequently associated with adjacent subarachnoid hemorrhage. They tend to occur along the superficial surfaces of the brain and are the result of acceleration (boxing) and deceleration forces (motor vehicle accident with head impact, such as against the steering wheel or side window or where the head strikes the ground) that cause the brain to rub along surfaces where there are prominent osseous ridges or dural reflections. The anterior and inferior portions of the temporal and frontal lobes, the posterolateral temporal lobes, and the occipital poles are typically contused in acceleration–deceleration injuries, as in this case. The surfaces of these portions of the brain rub against the floor and anterior walls of the anterior and middle cranial fossae, sphenoid wings, temporal bones, and petrous ridges. Hemorrhagic contusions may also occur in the setting of penetrating trauma (gun and knife club-type injuries, depressed skull fractures, or iatrogenic causes). Contusions may also occur along the convexities of the cerebral hemispheres adjacent to the midline as a result of the brain rubbing against the rigid falx or the surface of the inner table of the calvaria.

Imaging findings will depend on when the patient is imaged relative to the time of injury. In the acute setting, hemorrhages are hyperdense and are frequently associated with surrounding hypodensity that represents edema. Hemorrhagic contusions can become more apparent on follow-up imaging (blossoming). Acute hemorrhagic contusions are hypointense on T2W, FLAIR, and gradient echo MR imaging, with surrounding high signal intensity due to edema. Long-term follow-up shows resolution of the hemorrhage, encephalomalacia in the area of the traumatized brain, and hemosiderin staining in the contusion bed.

REFERENCES

Anderst JD, Carpenter SL, Abshire TC, et al. Evaluation for bleeding disorders in suspected child abuse. *Pediatrics*. 2013;131(4):1314-1322.
Hayashida Y, Kakeda S, Hiai Y, et al. Diagnosis of intracranial hemorrhagic lesions: comparison between 3D-SWAN (3D T2*-weighted imaging with multi-echo acquisition) and 2D-T2*-weighted imaging. *Acta Radiol*. 2014;55(2):201-207.
Juratli TA, Zang B, Litz RJ, et al. Early hemorrhagic progression of traumatic brain contusions: frequency, correlation with coagulation disorders, and patient outcome: a prospective study. *J Neurotrauma*. 2014;31(17):1521-1527.
Neuroradiology: THE REQUISITES. 4th ed. pp 159.

CASE 8

Cerebral Embolic Infarcts—Arterial

1. **B.** Multiple small foci of reduced diffusion scattered throughout the brain parenchyma within all major vascular territories, including the brainstem (not shown) and cerebellar hemispheres in keeping with a shower of emboli from a central source. Given the known aortic dissection, this was considered the most likely source.
2. **E.** Cardioembolic stroke is a potentially devastating condition and accounts for 15%–20% of all ischemic strokes. High-risk cardioembolic origins carry a relatively high risk for an initial stroke and for recurrent stroke. The findings that indicate a high risk for a cardioembolic stroke include left atrial thrombus with atrial fibrillation, left ventricular thrombus with acute myocardial infarction, dilated cardiomyopathy, myxoma, and prosthetic valve vegetation. Specifically, 6% of all patients with Type A aortic dissection presented with stroke at hospital admission.
3. **A.** ADC pseudonormalization is encountered in the subacute stage of ischemic stroke and represents an apparent return to normal healthy brain values on ADC maps. It does not, however, represent the true resolution of ischemic damage and is seen typically around 1 week following ischemic stroke and is thought to be due to a combination of cell wall breakdown and an increase in extracellular edema resulting in facilitated diffusion with increased ADC values.
4. **E.** All of these represent hypercoagulable conditions and can present with ischemic stroke. Screening for prothrombotic conditions is recommended in several current guidelines and is often part of the diagnostic workup for people experiencing ischemic stroke.

Comment

Approximately 80% of strokes are ischemic. They can develop in major blood vessels, which are referred to as "large vessel infarcts," or in small blood vessels, perforating arteries deep in the brain, which are referred to as "lacunar infarcts." Types of ischemic stroke include embolic infarct, thrombotic infarct, and lacunar infarct. Infarcts of undetermined etiology may account for as many as 30% of cases of stroke.

Cardiac embolism, in which a blood clot forms in the heart and travels to a vessel supplying the brain, accounts for about 20% to 30% of ischemic strokes. Recurrent strokes are most common in patients with a cardioembolic source, and these strokes have the highest 1-month mortality rate. Thrombotic infarcts account for 10% to 15% of strokes and occur when a blood clot forms in an artery that supplies the brain, causing tissue death. These usually occur as a result of plaque buildup from atherosclerosis and develop over time. Lacunar infarctions account for 20% of strokes, and usually occur as a result of small arterial blockage, most often caused by high blood pressure. Lacunar infarcts have a predilection for the basal ganglia, internal capsule, thalamus, pons, and corona radiata. This type of stroke has the best prognosis.

Prothrombotic disorders can induce venous, arterial, or microvascular thrombosis. Factor V Leiden mutation is one of the most common prothrombotic disorders that causes ischemic infarction in young adults. Oral contraceptive use has been seen in association with ischemic stroke in 19% of young female patients. This risk is potentiated by smoking.

REFERENCES

Bossone E, Corteville DC, Harris KM, et al. Stroke and outcomes in patients with acute type A aortic dissection. *Circulation*. 2013;128(11 suppl 1):S175-S179.

Cho AH, Kwon SU, Kim JS, Kang DW. Evaluation of early dynamic changes of intracranial arterial occlusion is useful for stroke etiology diagnosis. *J Neurol Sci*. 2012;312(1-2):127-130.

Neuroradiology: THE REQUISITES. 4th ed. pp 88-90.

CASE 9

Vestibular Schwannomas of the Internal Auditory Canal

1. **B.** Bilateral vestibular schwannomas are rare and strongly associated with neurofibromatosis type 2 (NF2).
2. **C.** Vestibular schwannomas are benign tumors (WHO grade 1) that arise from the intracanalicular segment of the vestibular portion of the vestibulocochlear nerve (CN VIII).
3. **A.** Crista falciformis is a horizontal ridge that divides the lateral portion of the internal acoustic canal (IAC) into superior and inferior portions. The facial nerve (CN VII) and superior vestibular nerve run in the superior portion of the IAC with the facial nerve anterior to the superior vestibular nerve and are separated from it in the lateral portion by Bill's bar.

Comment

Intracranial schwannomas most commonly arise from the vestibulocochlear nerve (CN VIII) and represent ~80% of cerebellopontine angle (CPA) masses. In over 90% of cases, these tumors arise from the inferior division of the vestibular nerve, with less than 5% of cases arising from the cochlear component of the CN VIII. The vestibular branches run in the superior and inferior portions of the posterior IAC, whereas the cochlear division runs in the anteroinferior portion of the IAC. When masses involve the IAC or the CPA, the role of the radiologist is usually in distinguishing a schwannoma from a meningioma as it affects management. Imaging findings favoring a schwannoma are masses that involve both the CPA and IAC, associated flaring or widening of the porus acusticus (the opening of the IAC/trumpeted IAM sign); a small "CSF cap" typically remains, separating intracanalicular tumor from the cochlea; however, growth laterally through the cochlea may occasionally occur as is seen on the right side in this case.

Meningiomas infrequently (5%) extend into the IAC, and when they do, the IAC is not expanded and may have an associated dural tail (although not diagnostic of a meningioma) and are usually centered superior or inferior and anterior or posterior to the porus acusticus. In this case, the patient had NF2 with bilateral vestibular schwannomas. Left vestibular schwannoma causes a mass effect on the left pons and brachium pontis. Right fundal schwannoma demonstrates an intracochlear component. On MR imaging, schwannomas have variable signal intensity, depending on their cellularity, water content, and the presence of necrosis or cystic degeneration. Small lesions (<2 cm) are typically isointense to white matter, and enhancement is often homogeneous, as on the right side in this case. Lesions larger than 2 cm frequently undergo necrosis or cystic degeneration, resulting in heterogeneous enhancement, as is seen on the left side.

Note that an important pitfall in diagnosing intracanalicular vestibular schwannoma is the vestibular ganglion, also known as "Scarpa's ganglion," which is a focal enlargement of the vestibular nerve within the IAC. These are occasionally demonstrated on high-resolution T2W sequences and can mimic small schwannomas. Most of the vestibular ganglia present as tiny nodules (<3 mm) along the vestibular nerve with a fusiform shape along the axis of the nerve, compared to schwannoma that is more spherical.

REFERENCES

Borden JA, Tsai JS, Mahajan A. Effect of subpixel magnetic resonance imaging shifts on radiosurgical dosimetry for vestibular schwannoma. *J Neurosurg*. 2002;97(5):445-449.

Kocaoglu M, Bulakbasi N, Ucoz T, et al. Comparison of contrast-enhanced T1-weighted and 3D constructive interference in steady state images for predicting outcome after hearing-preservation surgery for vestibular schwannoma. *Neuroradiology*. 2003;45(7):476-481.

Wu YW, Karandikar A, Goh JP, Tan TY. Imaging features differentiating vestibular ganglion from intracanalicular schwannoma on single-sequence non-contrast magnetic resonance imaging study. *Ann Acad Med Singap*. 2020;49(2):65-71.

Yong RL, Westerberg BD, Dong C, Akagami R. Length of tumor-cochlear nerve contact and hearing outcome after surgery for vestibular schwannoma. *J Neurosurg*. 2008;108(1):105-110.

Neuroradiology: THE REQUISITES. 4th ed. pp 45.

CASE 10

Acute Hypertensive Thalamic Hemorrhage

1. **A.** Hypertension is the most common cause of nontraumatic intracerebral hemorrhage, commonly seen (in order of frequency) in the basal ganglia (putamen), thalami, pons, and cerebellum.
2. **D.** The properties of a hematoma that have been shown to be effective for predicting patient prognosis include the location, size, and associated IVH and hydrocephalus.
3. **B.** Blooming artifact is a susceptibility artifact encountered in the presence of paramagnetic substances that affect the local magnetic milieux. MRI sequences that maximize blooming artifacts are susceptibility-weighted imaging (SWI) and Gradient-Recalled Echo (GRE). Low B-value diffusion-weighted imaging may also be useful in the absence of a dedicated SWI or GRE sequence (poor man's GRE sequence).
4. **B.** Duret hemorrhages are small hemorrhages in the brainstem of patients who are rapidly developing brain herniation. The classical appearance of a Duret hemorrhage is a single small, round hemorrhage located in the midline of the medulla or pons that can also be multiple or extend into the cerebellar peduncles.

Comment

This case shows a typical acute left thalamic hypertensive hemorrhage with intraventricular extension. The hematoma is mildly hyperintense to the brain on T1W imaging and hypointense on T2W imaging. Also noted are extensive sequelae of chronic small vessel ischemic disease in the periventricular white matter and in the deep gray nuclei. In adults, the most common cause of intracerebral hemorrhage is hypertension, which accounts for approximately 80% of nontraumatic hemorrhages. Hemorrhages related to high blood pressure have a predilection to involve the deep gray matter (basal ganglia and thalamus) and brainstem, which are supplied by perforating vessels arising from the cerebral and basilar arteries. Rupture of microaneurysms (Charcot-Bouchard) arising from the deep perforating vessels may be the basis of hypertensive hemorrhages in a subset of patients. Rupture into the ventricular system, as in this case, may be present in up to one-half of these patients and is associated with a poorer prognosis.

The MR imaging evaluation of intracerebral hemorrhage is complex, and the imaging appearance is related to a multitude of factors. In hyperacute hemorrhage (within the first 6 hours), hemorrhage is hypointense on T1W imaging and hyperintense on T2W imaging due to oxyhemoglobin in intact red blood cells. In the acute setting (hours to a few days), hemorrhage may be isointense to hypointense on T1W and is markedly hypointense on T2W images because of increasing deoxyhemoglobin. In the early subacute phase (2 days to 1 week), hemorrhage is hyperintense on T1W imaging and hypointense on T2W imaging as a result of high protein concentrations and intracellular methemoglobin. In the late subacute phase (1 week to months), hemorrhage is hyperintense on both T1W and T2W imaging. Finally, in the chronic setting (months to years), hemorrhage is hypointense due to susceptibility effects of hemosiderin and ferritin.

REFERENCES

Boulouis G, Dumas A, Betensky RA, et al. Anatomic pattern of intracerebral hemorrhage expansion: relation to CT angiography spot sign and hematoma center. *Stroke.* 2014;45(4):1154-1156.
Dylewski D, Demchuk AM, Morgenstern LB. Utility of magnetic resonance imaging in acute intracerebral hemorrhage. *J Neuroimaging.* 2000;10(2):78-83.
Neuroradiology: THE REQUISITES. 4th ed. pp 132.

CASE 11

Arachnoid Cyst

1. **B.** Large well-circumscribed cysts, with an imperceptible wall, displacing adjacent structures, and following the CSF pattern, hypodense on CT (A), and hyperintense on T2 (C), with FLAIR suppression (D), and adjacent osseous remodeling on CT bone windows (B), findings most consistent with an arachnoid cyst
2. **C.** A near-CSF intensity mass with high signal on DWI is the characteristic of an epidermoid cyst.
3. **A.** Arachnoid cysts are most frequently (50%–60%) located in the middle cranial fossa followed by the retrocerebellar location which accounts for 30%–40% of all arachnoid cysts.

Comment

Most intracranial arachnoid cysts are congenital and are derived from the meninx primitiva, which envelops the developing CNS. As CSF fills the subarachnoid spaces, the meninx is resorbed. At the same time, a cleft may develop between layers of the arachnoid membrane and may behave as a one-way ball-valve mechanism. There is preferential flow of CSF into this cleft, resulting in the formation of a cyst. Less commonly, arachnoid cysts may be acquired as a result of adhesions in the subarachnoid space related to a previous inflammatory process or hemorrhage.

The most common location for an arachnoid cyst is the middle cranial fossa. Other common locations include the retrocerebellar location, cerebral convexities, basal cisterns, suprasellar, cistern, and cerebellopontine angle (as in this case). On CT and MR imaging, arachnoid cysts usually follow the density or intensity of CSF, respectively. When large, cysts may cause smooth remodeling of the adjacent osseous structures, as is seen along the posterior central skull base in this case. There may also be hypogenesis of the underlying brain parenchyma (most commonly described in the temporal lobe with middle cranial fossa cysts). Calcification and hemorrhage are unusual, and enhancement should not be present.

The major differential consideration is an epidermoid cyst. On unenhanced T1W images, an internal matrix, although subtle, is typically evident in epidermoid cysts. On FLAIR images, arachnoid cysts follow the signal intensity characteristics of CSF, whereas epidermoid cysts tend to be hyperintense relative to CSF. In addition, on diffusion-weighted images, arachnoid cysts are hypointense (similar to the CSF), resulting from an increased apparent diffusion constant, whereas epidermoid cysts demonstrate decreased diffusion with low apparent diffusion coefficient (ADC) values.

REFERENCES

Li Y, Chen X, Xu B. The efficacy of neuroendoscopic treatment for middle cranial fossa arachnoid cysts assessed by MRI 3D segmentation and modeling. *Childs Nerv Syst.* 2014;30(6):1037-1044.
Yikilmaz A, Durak AC, Mavili E, et al. The role of diffusion-weighted magnetic resonance imaging in intracranial cystic lesions. *Neuroradiol J.* 2009;21(6):781-790.
Yildiz H, Erdogan C, Yalcin R, et al. Evaluation of communication between intracranial arachnoid cysts and cisterns with phase-contrast cine MR imaging. *AJNR Am J Neuroradiol.* 2005;26(1):145-151.
Neuroradiology: THE REQUISITES. 4th ed. pp 55, 280-289.

CASE 12

Subdural Empyema—Complicated by Cerebritis

1. **C.** Crescentic hyperintense subdural collection (A), with marked meningeal enhancement (B) and restricted diffusion (C&D) suggestive of a subdural empyema.
2. **C.** Reduced diffusion in an empyema differentiates it from sterile subdural effusions.
3. **A.** Sinusitis is the primary cause of subdural empyema in 50% to 80% of patients, and otitis media is the primary cause in 10% to 20%.
4. **C.** Subdural empyema is a medical and neurosurgical emergency with mortality approaching 10%. Successful treatment is centered on prompt diagnosis, followed by surgical evacuation and administration of appropriate antibiotics.

Comment

Interruption of the arachnoid meningeal barrier by infection leads to the formation of subdural empyemas. Mechanisms by which subdural empyemas may develop include rupture of a distended arachnoid villus into the subdural compartment, thrombophlebitis of a bridging cortical vein, hematogenous spread, and direct spread of an extracranial infection such as otomastoiditis, sinusitis, and frontal osteomyelitis, as in this case. These serious infections may also occur as a complication after craniotomy or in patients with meningitis. Epidural abscesses are most frequently caused by direct extension of infection from the paranasal sinuses or mastoid air cells. Of the conditions affecting the paranasal sinuses, frontal sinusitis is probably the most common cause of intracranial epidural abscesses and subdural empyemas.

On imaging, these lesions share the common appearance of other extracerebral collections. Epidural abscesses (such as hematomas) are contained by the cranial sutures and may cross the midline. In contrast, subdural hematomas do not spread across the midline because they are confined by the falx, allowing differentiation from epidural collections. On MR imaging, these extracerebral infections are usually hypointense to isointense on T1W imaging (depending on the protein concentration and the cellular content) and hyperintense relative to the brain on FLAIR and T2W imaging. Empyemas are typically hyperintense on diffusion-weighted imaging (DWI) and have low apparent diffusion coefficients (ADCs), as seen in this case, whereas sterile subdural effusions are hypointense on DWI. There is usually a prominent enhancement of a thickened dura or a dural membrane. Epidural and subdural empyemas may be complicated by cerebritis and intraparenchymal abscess formation. In addition, dural venous or cortical vein thrombosis with venous infarction may occur. In the presence of suspected epidural abscess or subdural empyema, the radiologist (and the clinician!) should search for a site of origin of the infection, as well as its contiguous spread into the intracranial compartment.

REFERENCES

Mohan S, Jain KK, Arabi M, Shah GV. Imaging of meningitis and ventriculitis. *Neuroimaging Clin N Am.* 2012;22(4):557-583.
Wong AM, Zimmerman RA, Simon EM, et al. Diffusion-weighted MR imaging of subdural empyemas in children. *AJNR Am J Neuroradiol.* 2004;25(6):1016-1021.
Neuroradiology: THE REQUISITES. 4th ed. pp 175-177.

CASE 13

Ocular Trauma—A: Ectopia Lentis (Lens Dislocation) and B: Globe Rupture

1. **C.** Ectopia lentis (traumatic lens subluxation or dislocation). Notice a right periorbital hematoma and a small amount of retrobulbar hemorrhage.
2. **B.** Trauma is the most common cause of lens subluxation or dislocation. The most common atraumatic etiologies are Marfan syndrome and homocystinuria.
3. **A.** Disrupted right globe with the presence of intraocular gas in keeping with globe rupture.

Comment

On CT imaging, lens dislocation (Case A) may be differentiated from other intraocular foreign bodies by identifying that the intraocular density has the configuration of a lens and, importantly, observing that the lens in that eye is not located in its normal position. Lens dislocation may be confirmed on physical examination. CT is the imaging modality of choice in the initial assessment of patients with orbital trauma due to its availability as well as the ease and rapidity with which the examination can be performed. In addition, CT readily establishes the presence of orbital foreign bodies, delineates orbital fractures, and assesses for retrobulbar complications of trauma.

Subluxation or dislocation of the lens may be unrelated to trauma. It may be spontaneous or related to infection. There are also hereditary disorders that affect the connective (mesodermal) tissues that may be associated with lens dislocation, such as Marfan syndrome, Ehlers–Danlos syndrome, and homocystinuria. In Marfan syndrome, lens subluxation or dislocation is superior and at the periphery of the globe (and usually bilateral), whereas in homocystinuria, subluxations are inferior ("down and out").

Globe rupture indicates that the integrity of the outer membranes of the eye is disrupted. Globe rupture may occur when a blunt object impacts the orbit, causing anterior–posterior compression of the globe and raising intraocular pressure such that the sclera tears. Ruptures from blunt trauma usually occur at the sites where the sclera is thinnest, at the insertions of the extraocular muscles, at the limbus, and around the optic nerve. Sharp objects or those traveling at high velocity may perforate the globe directly. Globe rupture represents an ophthalmologic emergency and requires surgical intervention. Damage to the posterior segment of the eye is associated with a very high frequency of permanent visual loss. Early recognition and ophthalmologic intervention are critical to maximizing functional outcomes. On CT imaging, the presence of vitreous hemorrhage suggests an associated globe rupture. An enlarged anterior chamber and retraction of the lens are indicative of rupture of the posterior sclera. Other findings of globe rupture are collapsed misshapen globe ("flat tyre" or "mushroom" appearance).

REFERENCES

Betts AM, O'Brien WT, Davies BW, Youssef OH. A systematic approach to CT evaluation of orbital trauma. *Emerg Radiol.* 2014;21(5):511-531.
Kubal WS. Imaging of orbital trauma. *Radiographics.* 2008;28(6):1729-1739.
Neuroradiology: THE REQUISITES. 4th ed. pp 316-324.

CASE 14

Persistent Trigeminal Artery

1. **D.** Persistent trigeminal artery (PTA) arises from the proximal cavernous ICA and is the most common persistent carotid-vertebrobasilar anastomosis.
2. **D.** An easy mnemonic to remember the persistent carotid and vertebrobasilar communications is "*HOT Pepper.*" H: hypoglossal artery, O: otic artery, T: trigeminal artery, P: proatlantal intersegmental artery.
3. **A.** PTA is associated with intracranial aneurysms and vascular malformations.
4. **A.** PTA is usually unilateral and is seen in 0.1%–0.6% of cerebral angiograms.

Comment

Persistent carotid-vertebrobasilar anastomoses are variant anatomical communications between the anterior and posterior circulations due to abnormal embryological development of the vertebrobasilar system. They are named, with the exception of the proatlantal artery, using the cranial nerves with which they run: trigeminal, otic, and hypoglossal arteries. PTA is the most common embryonic carotid–vertebrobasilar anastomosis to persist into adulthood, reported in as many as 0.1% to 0.6% of cerebral arteriograms. PTA may be associated with hypoplasia or absence of the ipsilateral posterior communicating artery, or with hypoplasia of both posterior communicating arteries. In addition, the proximal basilar artery and the distal vertebral arteries are often hypoplastic.

PTA usually arises from the precavernous internal carotid artery and is of two types: Saltzman type I: PTA supplies the distal vertebrobasilar arteries. The posterior communicating artery is absent, and the caudal basilar artery is absent or hypoplastic with hypoplastic distal vertebral arteries.

Saltzman type II: PTA supplies the superior cerebellar arteries with the posterior cerebral arteries supplied by the posterior communicating artery.

In some cases, trigeminal arteries may course through the sella turcica before joining the basilar artery (knowledge of this variant is critical in patients before transsphenoidal surgery). PTAs are associated with a variety of intracranial vascular abnormalities, including aneurysms and arteriovenous malformations, as well as a spectrum of clinical syndromes, such as tic douloureux (cranial nerve V), other cranial neuropathies, and vertebrobasilar insufficiency. Accurate identification and an understanding of this anatomic variation are important because interventional neuroradiologic and neurosurgical procedures (often performed to treat an associated vascular abnormality) may need to be modified appropriately.

REFERENCES

Bai M, Guo Q, Li S. Persistent trigeminal artery/persistent trigeminal artery variant and coexisting variants of the head and neck vessels diagnosed during 3 T MRA. *Clin Radiol.* 2013;68(11):578-585.
Meckel S, Spittau B, McAuliffe W. The persistent trigeminal artery: development, imaging anatomy, variants and associated vascular pathologies. *Neuroradiology.* 2013;55(1):5-16.
Neuroradiology: THE REQUISITES. 4th ed. pp 29-30.

CASE 15

Cavum Septum Pellucidum and Cavum Vergae

1. **D.** A common anatomical variant with fluid-filled space between the leaflets of the septum pellucidum extending posteriorly accompanies a cavum vergae and is referred to as cavum septum pellucidum et vergae.
2. **B.** Anomalies of the corpus callosum and septum pellucidum are both disorders of prosencephalic midline development.
3. **B.** The roof of the third ventricle has five layers: the body of the fornix, the superior layer of the tela choroidea, the vascular layer, the inferior layer of the tela choroidea, and the choroid plexus of the third ventricle. The bilaminar tela choroidea stretches beneath the body of the fornix, is closed anteriorly at the foramen of Monro, and contains the vascular layer of the third ventricle roof. The vascular layer is synonymous with the velum interpositum and contains the internal cerebral veins and the medial posterior choroidal arteries, bathed in cerebrospinal fluid (CSF). When the posterior aspect of the vascular layer is open, it communicates with the quadrigeminal cistern and is known as the cavum velum interpositum.
4. **D.** Approximately 75 mL is distributed around the spinal cord, 25 mL is in the ventricular system, and 50 mL is in the subarachnoid spaces around the brain.

Comment

The cavum septum pellucidum (CSP) is a CSF space between the leaflets of the septum pellucidum. CSP is bordered superiorly by the corpus callosum and posteriorly by the body of the fornix. The cavum extending posterior to the columns of the fornix and the foramen of Monro is called the cavum vergae (CV). Historically, CSP has also been called the *fifth ventricle*, and CV the *sixth ventricle*, which is inaccurate as these have no direct communication with the ventricular system.

During embryologic development, these spaces obliterate posteroanteriorly, CV followed by CSP; hence, a CSP almost always accompanies a CV and is referred to as "cavum septum pellucidum et vergae," and it represents a normal anatomic variant, as seen in this case. On antenatal ultrasound, the CSP is present in essentially all normal fetuses between 18 and 37 weeks gestation. During the latter half of gestation, the CSP decreases in size. At birth, approximately 50% to 80% of term infants have a small residual CSP that continues to decrease in size with age.

Autopsy studies have also shown significant variability (range, 3%–30%). They are usually asymptomatic. Cysts may arise in this location and exert mass effect. In addition, enlargement of the CSP, with intermittent obstruction of the foramen of Monro, resulting in hydrocephalus, has rarely been reported. Cysts may be treated with surgical resection, shunting, or fenestration.

The velum interpositum is a potential space just above and anterior to the pineal gland that can become enlarged to form a cavum velum interpositum.

REFERENCES

Glastonbury CM, Osborn AG, Salzman KL. Masses and malformations of the third ventricle: normal anatomic relationships and differential diagnoses. *Radiographics.* 2011;31(7):1889-1905.
Saba L, Anzidei M, Raz E, et al. MR and CT of brain's cava. *J Neuroimaging.* 2013;23(3):326-335.
White SF, Brislin S, Sinclair S, et al. The relationship between large cavum septum pellucidim and antisocial behavior, callous-unemotional traits and psychopathy in adolescents. *J Child Psychol Psychiatry.* 2013;54(5):575-581.
Neuroradiology: THE REQUISITES. 4th ed. pp 162-164, 265-266.

CASE 16

Cerebral Arteriovenous Malformation

1. **C.** Right occipital arterial venous malformation with nidus measuring 2 × 1.5 cm.
2. **B.** Parieto-occipital branches of the right posterior and middle cerebral arteries.
3. **A.** Only superficial venous drainage into cortical veins including the right vein of Trolard, right superior sagittal and right transverse sinuses, confirmed by conventional angiography.
4. **D.** Lack of angiographic visualization of a surgically proven arteriovenous malformation (AVM) may be due to a very small AVM, thrombosis of the AVM, or mass effect related to an associated parenchymal hemorrhage that compresses the AVM and prevents its filling.

Comment

An AVM is a vascular nidus made up of a core of entangled vessels fed by one or more enlarged feeding arteries. Blood is shunted from the nidus to enlarged draining vein(s), which terminate in the deep or superficial venous system. This case shows a right occipital lobe AVM. Time-of-flight MR angiography shows that the right posterior cerebral artery is enlarged because it supplies feeding arteries to the small AVM.

Spetzler and Martin proposed a grading scheme for AVMs that accurately predicts the outcome after surgical resection; however, its application to radiosurgery is limited because it does not accurately reflect lesion volume and location. AVMs are graded on a scale of I to VI, determined by the size (<3 cm, 3–6 cm, >6 cm), pattern of drainage (superficial or deep), and involvement of the cortex (noneloquent or eloquent). Grade I lesions are small and superficial and do not involve the eloquent cortex. On the opposite end of the spectrum, Grade VI lesions are usually inoperable.

On unenhanced CT scans, the vascular nidus of an AVM and the enlarged draining veins are usually isodense or hyperdense to gray matter as a result of pooling of blood. Calcification may be present. AVMs enhance and have characteristic serpentine flow voids on MR imaging related to fast flow in dilated arteries, and arterialized flow in dilated draining veins. The estimated annual hemorrhage rate of cerebral AVMs is 2% to 4%. The mean interval between hemorrhagic events is approximately 7 to 8 years.

In lesions associated with an acute parenchymal hemorrhage, phase-contrast magnetic MR angiography best demonstrates the AVM (it subtracts out the signal intensity of the blood products in the hematoma, in contrast to time-of-flight MR angiography). Cerebral angiography shows enlarged feeding arteries, the vascular nidus, and early draining veins. In cases of very small AVMs, early venous filling should be sought on careful evaluation of the angiographic images.

Gliosis in the affected brain may result in focal neurologic symptoms or seizures from "steal" phenomenon, in which there is parasitization of the blood supply from the normal brain preferentially to the AVM.

REFERENCES

O'Connor TE, Friedman WA. Magnetic resonance imaging assessment of cerebral arteriovenous malformation obliteration after stereotactic radiosurgery. *Neurosurgery.* 2013;73(5):761-766.
Raoult H, Bannier E, Robert B, et al. Time-resolved spin-labeled MR angiography for the depiction of cerebral arteriovenous malformations: a comparison of techniques. *Radiology.* 2014;271(2):524-533.
Neuroradiology: THE REQUISITES. 4th ed. pp 146-148.

CASE 17

Pyogenic Brain Abscess

1. **C.** Peripherally enhancing lesions with central restricted diffusion should be considered abscesses until proven otherwise.
2. **A.** Necrotic adenocarcinoma can mimic cerebral abscesses.
3. **A.** Intracavitary projections are a distinguishing feature of fungal abscesses. These arise from the wall of the abscess, which are usually iso-hypointense on T2-weighted images and do not enhance.
4. **A.** The most common locations for pyogenic brain abscesses are frontal and parietal lobes at gray–white matter junction in the distribution of the anterior or middle cerebral arteries.

Comment

The development of a pyogenic brain abscess may be divided into four stages: early cerebritis (1–3 days), late cerebritis (4–9 days), early capsule formation (10–13 days), and late capsule formation (14 days and after). In the mature abscess, there is a collagen capsule that is slightly thinner on the ventricular side than on the cortical margin (this may be related to differences in perfusion). The presence of a dimple or small evagination pointing toward the ventricular margin from a ring-enhancing lesion should raise suspicion for an abscess. This is also important because intraventricular rupture and ependymitis may occur and are associated with a very poor prognosis. In the presence of a mature abscess, there is relatively little surrounding cerebritis and edema compared with the early stages of abscess formation. A circumferential rim that is isointense to slightly hyperintense to white matter on unenhanced T1-weighted (T1W) images and hypointense on T2-weighted (T2W) images may be present around a brain abscess. This appearance may be related to the presence of collagen, free radicals within macrophages, or small areas of hemorrhage. Diffusion-weighted imaging may be very helpful because the high signal intensity of the pus-filled necrotic center may show restricted diffusion (low apparent diffusion coefficient, usually less than 40%), differentiating an abscess from a necrotic neoplasm, as in this case. The "dual-rim sign" is seen in approximately 75% of brain abscesses and is helpful in distinguishing an abscess from a glioblastoma. It consists of two concentric rims surrounding the abscess cavity, the outer one of which is hypointense, and

the inner one relatively more hyperintense on both susceptibility-weighted imaging (SWI) and T2WI.

The management of a brain abscess is surgical drainage and antibiotic therapy. Cerebritis and early abscesses may be managed with antibiotics and should be followed closely both with MR imaging and clinically for signs of improvement or deterioration. Successful management monitored with serial MR imaging examinations will show a decrease in the surrounding edema, mass effect, and associated enhancement. It is important to remember that radiologic findings lag behind clinical improvement, and enhancement may persist for months. Resolution of an abscess may result in an area of gliosis with small calcifications.

REFERENCES

Hsu SH, Chou MC, Ko CW, et al. Proton MR spectroscopy in patients with pyogenic brain abscess: MR spectroscopic imaging verses single-voxel spectroscopy. *Eur J Radiol.* 2013;82(8):1299-1307.
Luthra G, Parihar A, Nath K, et al. Comparative evaluation of fungal, tubercular, and pyogenic brain abscesses with conventional and diffusion MR imaging and proton MR spectroscopy. *AJNR Am J Neuroradiol.* 2007;28(7):1332-1338.
Reiche W, Schuchardt V, Hagen T, et al. Differential diagnosis of intracranial ring enhancing cystic mass lesions – role of diffusion-weighted imaging (DWI) and diffusion-tensor imaging (DTI). *Clin Neurol Neurosurg.* 2010;112(3):218-225.
Neuroradiology: THE REQUISITES. 4th ed. pp 179-182.

CASE 18

Acute Left Middle Cerebral Artery Infarction

1. **B.** The middle cerebral artery (MCA) territory is the most commonly affected vascular territory in cerebral infarctions, due to the large size of the territory and the direct inflow from the internal carotid artery into the MCA.
2. **E.** All of these are signs of early ischemia on a noncontrast head CT.
3. **D.** The law of cerebral dominance states that in the vast majority of right-handed individuals (note that more than 90% of people are right-handed), the left hemisphere controls language-related functions. In left-handed individuals, only about 75% have language functions predominantly controlled by the left hemisphere. The remainder of left-handed individuals have language functions controlled by the right hemisphere. A right hemispheric MCA territory infarct would typically present with left-sided hemiplegia, left hemisensory loss, hemianopia, and hemineglect. Since the vast majority of individuals are left hemispheric dominant, language function is located in the left hemisphere and should, therefore, be spared.
4. **D.** The mTICI grading is used to predict prognosis after mechanical thrombectomy procedures. Grade 0 represents no perfusion; Grade 1, minimal perfusion; Grade 2, partial perfusion, and Grade 3 represents complete perfusion.

Comment

An unenhanced head CT scan is the first imaging study for the emergent evaluation of acute ischemic stroke as it is readily available, rapidly performed, and sensitive in identifying acute intracranial hemorrhage. Some of the early signs of acute ischemia in the MCA distribution are as follows: (1) **dense MCA sign**, which represents thromboembolic occlusion of the artery, (2) subtle blurring and hypoattenuation with poor delineation of gray–white matter, (3) **lentiform nucleus sign**, which causes obscuration of the basal ganglia due to cytotoxic edema in proximal M1 occlusion involving the lenticulostriate arteries, (4) **insular ribbon sign**, loss of normal gray–white differentiation in the insular cortex, and

(5) **MCA dot sign**, which represents thromboembolism within a segmental branch of the MCA within the Sylvian fissure, generally the M2 segment. Note that all of these signs were present in this case, A–D (stroke window) from extensive internal carotid artery (ICA) dissection extending from proximal left ICA to the terminus with left MCA occlusion (E). Emergent mechanical thrombectomy with placement of overlapping stents from proximal cervical ICA to petrous segment with mechanical thrombectomy of left MCA was performed with TICI 3 reperfusion (F).

CT angiography may identify intracranial vascular occlusion and guide therapy. CT perfusion has emerged as a critical tool in selecting patients for reperfusion therapy, by allowing the detection of ischemic core (dead tissue that will never recover regardless of reperfusion), matched defects in cerebral blood volume (CBV) and mean transit time (MTT) as well as ischemic penumbra (potentially salvageable tissue), with prolonged MTT but preserved CBV.

Multiple practice changing randomized clinical trials showed improved clinical outcomes in patients with acute ischemic stroke due to Large vessel occlusion (LVO) undergoing thrombectomy compared to conservative treatment alone. As a result, mechanical thrombectomy has now become the standard of care in patients with intracranial LVO and a large ischemic penumbra.

Contraindications to mechanical thrombectomy include the presence of intracranial hemorrhage on initial noncontrast CT and a large infarct core with no significant penumbra.

MRI with diffusion imaging is more sensitive than CT in detecting acute infarcts which demonstrate increased DWI signal and reduced apparent diffusion coefficient (ADC) values within minutes after an acute arterial occlusion.

REFERENCES

Albers GW, Marks MP, Kemp S, et al. Thrombectomy for stroke at 6 to 16 hours with selection by perfusion imaging. *N Engl J Med.* 2018; 378(8):708-718. doi:10.1056/NEJMoa1713973.

Goyal M, Menon BK, van Zwam WH, et al. Endovascular thrombectomy after large-vessel ischaemic stroke: a meta-analysis of individual patient data from five randomised trials. *Lancet.* 2016;387(10029):1723-1731. doi:10.1016/S0140-6736(16)00163-X.

Riedel CH, Jensen U, Rohr A, et al. Assessment of thrombus in acute middle cerebral artery occlusion using thin-slice nonenhanced computed tomography reconstructions. *Stroke.* 2010;41(8):1659-1664.

Neuroradiology: THE REQUISITES. 4th ed. pp 32-33, 102-110, 114.

CASE 19

Multiple Sclerosis

1. **C.** Balo's concentric sclerosis is a rare demyelinating disorder, considered a subtype of multiple sclerosis (MS) characterized on MR imaging and pathologically as lesions with a laminated appearance that reflect alternating regions of demyelinated and myelinated tissue. Concentric or laminated contrast enhancement is noted around the lesion with a core that is more similar to CSF in signal with a characteristic "onion bulb" appearance.

2. **D.** Dissemination in space assesses the presence of lesions in the following four regions: periventricular, cortical or juxtacortical, infratentorial, and spinal cord. Lesions in the optic nerve cannot be used in fulfilling the 2017 revised McDonald criteria. Note that subcortical lesions are also not counted.

3. **B.** Approximately 8% to 12%. In patients presenting with myelopathy and an MR imaging study that reveals a cord lesion, MS should be considered. Evaluation should include complete spinal cord and brain MR imaging.

4. **D.** Anti-MOG-associated encephalomyelitis represents a distinct group of inflammatory demyelinating disorders characterized by the presence of IgG antibodies to myelin oligodendrocyte glycoprotein (MOG) with overlapping features with acute disseminated encephalomyelitis (ADEM), neuromyelitis optica spectrum disorder (NMOSD), and MS. There are no specific clinical or imaging features with no single set of accepted diagnostic criteria at this time.

Comment

This case shows numerous white matter lesions with a periventricular predominance. Lesions are also noted at the callososeptal interface (D) as well in the subcortical white matter (A). The largest lesion in the right frontal white matter has a demarcated central region that follows the signal characteristics of CSF on all pulse sequences, with a peripheral rim, or "halo," that has restricted diffusion (B) and enhancement (C) consistent with active demyelination.

Most acquired diseases involving the white matter have similar MR imaging findings. Patient age, history, and physical examination are of paramount importance in limiting the differential diagnosis, which may include vasculopathies (small vessel ischemic disease, vasculitis, hypertension, migraines), demyelinating disease, and inflammatory processes (sarcoid).

MS is a chronic inflammatory disease characterized by relapsing or progressive demyelinating plaques in the brain and spinal cord. MS affects the oligodendrocytes. In the acute stage, plaques have an inflammatory reaction with edema, cellular infiltration, and a spectrum of demyelination. Plaques tend to be perivenular in distribution. Chronic lesions show astrocytic hypoplasia, resolution of cellular infiltration, and loss of myelin. The diagnosis of MS was established by the McDonald criteria revised in 2017. On T1W images, plaques may be isointense to hypointense to the brain. Hypointense lesions are chronic and most likely are associated with gliosis and significant myelin loss. FLAIR imaging is particularly helpful in identifying lesions in the periventricular white matter or along CSF interfaces because suppression of water results in increased lesion conspicuity. Lesions at the callososeptal interface are highly suggestive of MS, as seen in this case. Contrast administration allows separation of lesions with an abnormal blood–brain barrier (enhancing lesions) from those with an intact blood–brain barrier (nonenhancing lesions). A lesion that has restricted diffusion also indicates active demyelination. MR imaging is also more sensitive than clinical examination in detecting active disease in clinically silent areas of the brain.

REFERENCES

Cappellani R, Bergsland N, Kennedy C, et al. Subcortical deep gray matter pathology in patients with multiple sclerosis is associated with white matter lesion burden and atrophy but not with cortical atrophy: a diffusion tensor MRI study. *AJNR Am J Neuroradiol.* 2014;35(5):912-919.

Crombe A, Saranathan M, Ruet A, et al. MS lesions are better detected with 3D T1 gradient-echo than with 2D T1 spin-echo gadolinium-enhanced imaging at 3T. *AJNR Am J Neuroradiol.* 2015;36(3):501-507.

Hodel J, Outteryck O, Ryo E, et al. Accuracy of postcontrast 3D turbo spin-echo MR sequence for the detection of enhanced inflammatory lesions in patients with multiple sclerosis. *Am J Neuroradiol.* 2014;35(3):519-523.

Thompson AJ, Banwell BL, Barkhof F, et al. Diagnosis of multiple sclerosis: 2017 revisions of the McDonald criteria. *Lancet Neurol.* 2018; 17(2):162-173. doi:10.1016/S1474-4422(17)30470-2.

Neuroradiology: THE REQUISITES. 4th ed. pp 206-216.

CASE 20

Atypical Meningioma

1. **B.** Meningioma. These are the most common radiation-induced CNS neoplasms (70%), followed by gliomas (20%) and sarcomas (10%).

2. **A.** The alanine peak at 1.48 ppm helps in distinguishing meningiomas from mimics.
3. **D.** The dural tail sign is not pathognomonic of meningiomas and can be seen in many other conditions.
4. **B.** Arterial narrowing is typically seen in meningiomas that encase arteries. It is a useful sign in suprasellar or parasellar tumors in distinguishing it from a pituitary macroadenoma that does not narrow vessels.

Comment

Meningiomas are the most common intracranial, extra-axial neoplasm, with a variety of histologic subtypes. Large meningiomas occurring over the cerebral convexities may be treated with embolization when necessary, followed by surgery without neurologic deficits; in contrast, meningiomas as small as 1 cm involving the cavernous sinus may be very symptomatic and present a more challenging treatment dilemma. Meningiomas occur most commonly in middle-aged women; however, they are also found frequently in men. Most meningiomas are sporadic, isolated lesions. Multiple meningiomas may be familial or may be seen in patients with a history of radiation therapy to the brain (as seen in this case), neurofibromatosis type 2, and basal cell nevus (Gorlin–Goltz) syndrome.

On unenhanced CT, more than 50% of meningiomas are hyperdense. Approximately 20% to 25% are associated with calcification or a reaction in the adjacent bone (hyperostosis is more common than osteolysis). On MR imaging, meningiomas are often isointense to gray matter on T1W and T2W sequences; however, they may be hyperintense on T2W imaging. Meningiomas typically have avid, homogeneous enhancement. The most important clue to making the diagnosis of a meningioma is establishing that the mass is extra-axial. One finding consistent with an extra-axial location is the presence of a pseudocapsule, which may represent CSF, dura, or vessels along the pia-arachnoid. Although the presence of an enhancing dural tail is highly suggestive of meningioma, this is a nonspecific finding and may be seen in other disease processes. On imaging, it is not possible to confidently distinguish benign (WHO Grade 1) from atypical (WHO Grade 2), as in this case, and anaplastic (WHO Grade 3) meningiomas.

REFERENCES

Chen TY, Lai PH, Ho JT, et al. Magnetic resonance imaging and diffusion-weighted images of cystic meningioma: correlating with histipathy. *Clin Imaging.* 2004;28(1):10-19.
Sanai N, Sughrue ME, Shangari G, et al. Risk profile associated with convexity meningioma resection in the mode neurosurgical era. *J Neurosurg.* 2010;112(5):913-919.
Neuroradiology: THE REQUISITES. 4th ed. pp 370.

CASE 21

Acute Actively Bleeding Subdural Hematoma—Subfalcine Herniation and Acute Anterior Cerebral Artery (ACA) Infarction

1. **D.** There is a large, actively bleeding left convexity subdural hematoma with a mass effect including left-to-right subfalcine herniation, hydrocephalus, and acute left ACA infarction.
2. **B.** The swirl sign refers to the noncontrast CT appearance of acute extravasation of blood into a hematoma. It represents unclotted fresh blood that is of lower attenuation than the clotted surrounding blood.
3. **C.** Subfalcine herniation, also known as midline shift, is herniation of the cingulate gyrus beneath the anterior free edge of the falx and is the most common cerebral herniation

pattern. It can cause hydrocephalus due to obstruction of the foramen of Monro and ACA territory infarct due to compression of ACA branches, specifically the pericallosal artery.
4. **A.** Approximately 85% of SDHs are unilateral in adults and commonly seen along frontoparietal convexities and in the middle cranial fossa. On the other hand, 75%–85% of SDHs are bilateral in infants. Note: isolated interhemispheric/para-falcine SDHs are seen more commonly in children and are common in cases of nonaccidental trauma.

Comment

Acute subdural hematomas in young patients are usually the result of closed head injury (e.g., motor vehicle accident), as in this case. This case shows a large left convexity, acute, actively bleeding subdural hematoma with left-to-right subfalcine herniation complicated by an acute left anterior cerebral artery infarct due to compression of this vessel and hydrocephalus. The heterogeneous "swirling" appearance within the subdural hematoma is due to active bleeding in this case, but such an appearance can also be related to leakage of serum from the clot in coagulopathic patients or patients receiving anticoagulation therapy. Also, note the small amount of subarachnoid blood.

Subdural hematomas are typically caused by tearing of the bridging veins that cross the subdural compartment, extending from the pia to the venous sinuses. Tearing of these veins is due to motion of the brain relative to the fixed dural sinuses. Most subdural hematomas are located along the supratentorial convexities; however, they may also occur in the posterior fossa and along the tentorium cerebelli.

The imaging features of subdural hematomas on CT scans depend on their age. Acute (hours to days old) hematomas are typically hyperdense "crescentic" extracerebral collections. Subacute (days to weeks old) hematomas tend to be isodense to gray matter; therefore, it is easy to miss them on a quick glance at a CT scan. To avoid missing this finding, compare the size of the sulci over the left and right cerebral convexities. The absence of sulci or asymmetric sulci should raise suspicion. Always check that the sulci extend to the inner table of the calvarium, and evaluate the gray–white matter interface for inward buckling. Chronic (weeks to months old) hematomas are usually hypodense. Fluid levels within these hematomas may be caused by interval bleeding. Calcification along the dural membrane may also occur.

REFERENCES

Besenski N. Traumatic injuries: imaging of head injuries. *Eur Radiol.* 2002;12(6):1237-1252.
Dalfino JC, Boulos AS. Visualization of an actively bleeding cortical vessel into the subdural space by CT angiography. *Clin Neurol Neurosurg.* 2010;112(8):737-739.
Neuroradiology: THE REQUISITES. 4th ed. pp 154-157.

CASE 22

Acute Subarachnoid Hemorrhage—Rupture of an Anterior Communicating Artery Aneurysm

1. **D.** Acute subarachnoid hemorrhage from ruptured anterior communicating artery aneurysm.
2. **D.** The most common clinical presentation of an acute subarachnoid hemorrhage from aneurysmal rupture is "the worst headache of my life," and "thunderclap headache."
3. **D.** All of the previous statements are correct. Approximately 70% of patients with vasospasm experienced improvement in their symptoms after initiation of "Triple-H therapy"

(hypertension, hemodilution, and hypervolemia). Calcium-channel antagonists and other investigational agents have also been used with variable benefits and outcomes.

4. **D.** Oculomotor nerve palsies result in pupillary dilation, ptosis, and diplopia, suggesting compression of CN III, because the parasympathetic pupillary fibers are located peripherally and are more likely affected by external compression from posterior communicating artery aneurysm with or without SAH. Note: ischemic involvement of CNIII will usually be pupil sparing!

Comment

Saccular (berry) aneurysms represent focal vascular dilations most commonly found at branching points of parent vessels. Approximately 90% are seen in the anterior circulation, and the most frequent sites for ruptured aneurysms include, in descending order of frequency, the anterior communicating artery complex (30%–40%), the origin of the posterior communicating artery, the middle cerebral artery, and the vertebrobasilar circulation. Multiple aneurysms may be present in up to 15% to 20% of cases. Although most aneurysms are sporadic in nature, there is an increased incidence in certain conditions, such as connective tissue disorders or collagen vascular disease (fibromuscular dysplasia, moyamoya disease, Ehlers–Danlos syndrome, and polycystic kidney disease).

The most common clinical presentation of acute subarachnoid hemorrhage is "the worst headache of life." Acute high-density subarachnoid blood is present on CT in 90% to 95% of cases in the first 24 hours. The sensitivity of CT in detecting acute subarachnoid hemorrhage decreases with time. Detection drops to 80% within 3 days, and to only 30% by 2 weeks. If CT is negative and acute subarachnoid hemorrhage is suspected, a lumbar puncture is performed. Evaluation of a patient with suspected acute subarachnoid hemorrhage should always begin with an unenhanced CT head study.

Patterns of intracranial hemorrhage seen with rupture of anterior communicating artery aneurysms include bilaterally symmetric subarachnoid hemorrhage, hemorrhage within the interhemispheric fissure, frontal lobe hematoma, or septal or intraventricular hemorrhage. This case shows acute subarachnoid hemorrhage, most notably in the interhemispheric fissure, right olfactory sulcus, extending into Sylvian cisterns, a pattern consistent with rupture of an anterior communicating artery aneurysm. There is intraventricular blood and early hydrocephalus. The CT angiography axial maximum intensity projection images show a 7.5 × 6 mm anterior–inferior pointing ruptured anterior communicating artery aneurysm with right dominant A1 and hypoplastic left A1 segment.

REFERENCES

Inoue T, Takada S, Shimizu H, et al. Signal changes on T2*-weighted magnetic resonance imaging from the acute to chronic phases in patients with subarachnoid hemorrhage. *Cerebrovasc Dis*. 2013;36(5-6):421-429.

Wani AA, Phadke R, Behari S, et al. Role of diffusion-weighted MRG in predicting outcome in subarachnoid hemorrhage due to anterior communicating artery aneurysms. *Turk Neurosurg*. 2008;18(1):10-16.

Neuroradiology: THE REQUISITES. 4th ed. pp 138-141.

CASE 23

Glioblastoma of the Corpus Callosum—"Butterfly Glioma"

1. **D.** Glioblastoma (GBM). It is the most common primary malignant brain tumor in adults.

2. **D.** Neoplasms (glioblastoma multiforme, lymphoma, and much less commonly, metastatic disease), demyelinating disease, and traumatic shear injury.

3. **C.** Standard of care treatment includes maximal safe surgical resection, followed by radiation therapy plus concomitant and maintenance temozolomide (TMZ). The addition of bevacizumab to standard treatment with TMZ revealed no improvement in overall survival (OS). Tumor-treating fields (TTFields) plus TMZ represent a major advance for the treatment of GBM, with recent clinical trials demonstrating improvement in OS as well as progression-free survival (PFS) with no deleterious effects on the quality of life (QOL), and is considered a standard for patients with newly diagnosed GBM with no contraindications.

4. **A.** GBMs are formally subdivided by the presence or absence of mutation in the isocitrate dehydrogenase (IDH) gene.

Comment

This case demonstrates findings characteristic of a butterfly glioma. There is a complex heterogeneous mass with an expansion of the genu of the corpus callosum with extension in bilateral frontal lobes (A and B). Enhanced images better reveal the marked internal areas of necrosis (C). There is a significant elevation in relative cerebral blood volume (D) as well as plasma volume (E) with elevated choline to creatine and choline to NAA ratios on MR spectroscopy (F).

It may occasionally be difficult to distinguish such gliomas from metastases on imaging. Assessment of peritumoral regions can be extremely helpful in distinguishing infiltrative gliomas from metastases. When separate lesions are identified, it is important to evaluate the presence of continuity between the separate lesions on the basis of abnormal T2W signal intensity. However, the connection may not be apparent on imaging and may be seen only on pathologic evaluation. Of the infiltrative astrocytic tumors, GBM is most commonly associated with subependymal and ependymal spread.

Glioblastoma (GBM) is the most common primary malignant brain tumor in adults. In newly diagnosed GBM, methylation of the O6-methylguanine-DNA methyltransferase (MGMT) promoter has been shown to predict the response to temozolomide. Tumor-treating fields (TTFields) plus TMZ represent a major advance for the treatment of GBM, with recent clinical trials demonstrating improvement in overall survival (OS) as well as progression-free survival (PFS) with no deleterious effects on the quality of life (QOL). GBM is a disease with an extremely poor prognosis and hence treatment paradigms go beyond improving survival to preserve and improve the quality of life of these patients.

REFERENCES

Gonçalves FG, Chawla S, Mohan S. Emerging MRI techniques to redefine treatment response in patients with glioblastoma. *J Magn Reson Imaging*. 2020;52(4):978-997.

Stupp R, Taillibert S, Kanner A, et al. Effect of tumor-treating fields plus maintenance temozolomide vs maintenance temozolomide alone on survival in patients with glioblastoma: a randomized clinical trial [published correction appears in *JAMA*. 2018;319(17):1824]. *JAMA*. 2017;318(23):2306-2316. doi:10.1001/jama.2017.18718.

Neuroradiology: THE REQUISITES. 4th ed. pp 59-62.

CASE 24

Abusive Head Trauma — Child Abuse

1. **B.** Abusive Head Trauma (AHT). Note the diffuse loss of gray–white differentiation, cerebral swelling (A, B), bilateral retinal and vitreous hemorrhages (C), as well as hemorrhage extending in the upper cervical spinal canal (D).

2. **B.** Subdural hemorrhages of different ages. These findings are highly suspicious of Abusive Head Trauma.
3. **B.** Whenever a skeletal survey is to be performed in infants (under the age of 1 year), it should always include a CT head, regardless of associated neurological findings. Skull X-rays are performed in children over the age of 1 who have a skeletal survey. When MRI imaging is performed, initial imaging should always be performed with an MRI brain and spine. This is also required when the neurological exam is abnormal, or there is an abnormality on the head CT.
4. **I.** All of these can cause retinal hemorrhages in an infant. However, note that retinal hemorrhages in infancy are believed to be an important sign of nonaccidental injury (may occur in up to 89% of infants). They may result from direct head trauma or the acceleration and deceleration forces generated by the shaking of the head. Terson syndrome refers to vitreous/retinal hemorrhage usually associated with intracranial subarachnoid hemorrhage.

Comment

The presence of skull fractures or intracranial hemorrhage, particularly in children younger than the age of 2 years, in the absence of known trauma to explain such injuries, should raise the suspicion of Abusive Head Trauma (AHT; child abuse). Nearly 700,000 children are abused in the United States each year, and closed head injury is among the leading causes of morbidity and death in these children. Approximately 10% of neurologic developmental delays can be attributed to AHT. Brain injury may be the result of direct trauma, aggressive shaking, strangulation, or suffocation. There is often little or no evidence of external trauma.

The following are the two major categories of AHT: (1) shaking mechanisms, where repetitive acceleration–deceleration forces generally result in subdural hematomas, retinal hemorrhages, and global parenchymal damage (as seen in these two cases); and (2) direct-impact trauma, which results in skull fractures and coup/contrecoup parenchymal injuries. Noncontrast head CT followed by MRI is widely considered to be the first step in evaluating suspected AHT, noting that serial imaging may be necessary in some cases.

In addition to brain imaging, increasing emphasis has been placed on imaging of the orbits and cervical spine. The most common type of intracranial hemorrhage in the setting of child abuse is a subdural hematoma (Case 2), although subarachnoid hemorrhage, epidural hematoma, intraventricular hemorrhage, hemorrhagic cortical contusion, diffuse axonal injury, and cytotoxic edema are all manifestations of AHT.

Bilateral retinal hemorrhages are highly suggestive of child abuse (shaken baby syndrome), as seen in Case 1. In the absence of significant head trauma, the presence of skull fractures (especially bilateral, depressed, or occipital fractures), which are found in as many as 45% of AHT cases, should raise suspicion for child abuse. Because it is not fully developed, the infant skull is extremely pliable and relatively resistant to fracture. In the worst case, diffuse cerebral edema resulting in mass effect and herniation may occur. Cerebral infarction may occur as a result of strangulation or anoxic-hypoxic injury, and vascular compromise may be caused by intracranial mass effect. Infarctions in multiple vascular territories should be viewed with suspicion.

The radiologist plays an important role in identifying AHT. The clinical presentation can be nonspecific and thus investigations always warrant a thorough, multidisciplinary approach including skeletal surveys and ophthalmologic exams. Neuroimaging is vital in the evaluation of suspected cases, potentially offering insight into the mechanisms of injury and long-term prognosis. More recently, other advanced MRI techniques, such as DWI, DTI, SWI, and MRS, have been used to predict long-term outcomes and identification of those at high risk, offering opportunities for earlier intervention.

REFERENCES

Aaen GS, Holshouser BA, Sheridan C, et al. Magnetic resonance spectroscopy predicts outcomes for children with nonaccidental trauma. *Pediatrics.* 2010;125(2):295-303.

Colbert CA, Holshouser BA, Aaen GS, et al. Value of cerebral microhemorrhages detected with susceptibility-weighted MR imaging for prediction of long-term outcome in children with nonaccidental trauma. *Radiology.* 2010;256(3):898-905.

Neuroradiology: THE REQUISITES. 4th ed. pp 165-166, 169-170.

CASE 25

Developmental Venous Anomaly

1. **D.** Developmental venous anomaly in the right frontal lobe.
2. **A.** A mixed vascular malformation is a common congenital cerebral vascular malformation, composed of a developmental venous anomaly and a cavernous malformation.
3. **D.** DVA thrombosis may lead to venous ischemic infarction, parenchymal hemorrhage, venous congestive edema, or subarachnoid hemorrhage.
4. **C.** Sturge–Weber syndrome. This represents a more extensive venous malformation that results from failure of development of the normal venous system, often covering a large portion of a cerebral hemisphere. Large cerebral malformations may also be seen in Klippel-Trénaunay–Weber syndrome.

Comment

Developmental venous anomalies (DVAs), previously referred to as venous angiomas, are the most common cerebral vascular malformation, accounting for 55% of all such lesions. The exact etiology remains uncertain but may relate to arrested development of medullary veins likely occurring late in the first trimester and early in the second trimester of gestation. Instead of the normal parallel appearance of the medullary veins as they drain into subependymal or superficial cortical veins, a disorganized network of dilated medullary veins converges in a "caput medusa" appearance and drains into an enlarged venous channel that subsequently drains superficially to cortical veins or sinuses, or deeply to subependymal veins of the lateral ventricle and then into the galenic system. It is important to note that normal cerebral tissue intervenes between the dilated veins. The brain parenchyma surrounding a venous angioma is typically normal, although occasional gliosis, seen as mild T2W hyperintensity, may be present. DVAs are found most commonly in the frontal lobes, followed by the parietal and temporal lobes. Infratentorial DVAs occur most commonly in the cerebellum. These can drain to the fourth ventricle and then to the pontomesencephalic vein, or to the precentral cerebellar vein and into the galenic system.

More than 99% of developmental venous malformations are asymptomatic; however, rarely, these lesions may hemorrhage. Hemorrhagic complications are usually secondary to coexisting cavernous malformations. Rare hemorrhage related specifically to the DVA is most common with cerebellar lesions. DVA thrombosis may lead to venous ischemic infarction, parenchymal hemorrhage, venous congestive edema, or subarachnoid hemorrhage. Patients may present with headache, seizure, or focal neurologic symptoms. Asymptomatic (essentially all) DVAs are not treated because they represent a compensatory venous drainage route for the normal brain. Sacrifice of these lesions could result in venous infarction of the normal brain that they drain.

REFERENCES

Assadsangabi R, Mohan S, Nabavizadeh SA. Clinical manifestations and imaging findings of thrombosis of developmental venous anomalies. *Clin Radiol.* 2018;73(11):985.e7-985.e12. doi:10.1016/j.crad.2018.06.022.

Iv M, Fischbein NJ, Zaharchuk G. Association of developmental venous anomalies with perfusion abnormalities on arterial spin labeling and bolus perfusion-weighted imaging. *J Neuroimaging.* 2015;25(2):243-250.

Jung HN, Kim ST, Cha J, et al. Diffusion and perfusion MRI findings of the signal-intensity abnormalities of brain associated with developmental venous anomaly. *AJNR Am J Neuroradiol.* 2014;35(8):1539-1542.

Neuroradiology: THE REQUISITES. 4th ed. pp 145-146.

REFERENCES

Kucharczyk W, Bishop JE, Plewes DB, Keller MA, George S. Detection of pituitary microadenomas: comparison of dynamic keyhole fast spin-echo, unenhanced, and conventional contrast-enhanced MR imaging. *AJR Am J Roentgenol.* 1994;163(3):671-679.

Lee HB, Kim ST, Kim HJ, et al. Usefulness of the dynamic gadolinium-enhanced magnetic resonance imaging with simultaneous acquisition of coronal and sagittal planes for detection of pituitary microadenomas. *Eur Radiol.* 2012;22(3):514-518.

Sano T, Rayhan N, Yamada S. [Pathology of pituitary incidentaloma]. *Nihon Rinsho.* 2004;62(5):940-945. [Japanese].

Neuroradiology: THE REQUISITES. 4th ed. pp 352-354.

CASE 26

Pituitary Microadenoma

1. **C.** Subcentimeter hypoenhancing lesion in the right lateral pituitary gland in keeping with a microadenoma.
2. **D.** During the dynamic contrast-enhanced MRI, gadolinium washes into the gland from the infundibulum located superiorly, then into the central gland, gradually spreading to more peripheral portions. Note that the lateral portions of the gland opacify last and should not be mistaken for small adenomas.
3. **A.** Pituitary apoplexy is a clinical syndrome manifested by the acute onset of headache, nausea and vomiting, visual disturbance, cranial neuropathies, or a change in mental status. It is most commonly associated with hemorrhage within an adenoma, although it has been described with nonhemorrhagic pituitary necrosis (infarction). Note that most pituitary hemorrhages are asymptomatic.
4. **A.** Bromocriptine treatment (a dopamine agonist) is used to treat prolactinomas.

Comment

Pituitary adenomas are slow-growing, benign epithelial neoplasms arising from the anterior lobe of the gland. They are typically demarcated with a "pseudocapsule" that separates them from the normal gland. Pituitary adenomas larger than 10 mm are referred to as macroadenomas, and those less than 10 mm in diameter are referred to as microadenomas. Many adenomas are incidental findings, are asymptomatic, and can be seen in up to 10% of MRI scans.

The clinical presentation of pituitary adenomas depends on their size, the presence of hormone secretion resulting in endocrine hyperfunction, and the presence of extension beyond the sella (leading to visual symptoms or cranial nerve palsies related to compression). In vivo, approximately 75% of pituitary adenomas are hormonally active (however, in autopsy series, nonsecreting adenomas are much more common).

The most common clinically significant secreting adenoma is the prolactinoma (which arises from the prolactin-secreting cells [lactotrophs]). In women, the most common clinical presentation is irregular menses, galactorrhea, and infertility. In men, impotence may be present. Hormonally active pituitary adenomas arising from somatotrophs, the growth hormone-secreting cells, cause acromegaly in adults and gigantism in children.

MRI is the mainstay of imaging requiring dedicated thin-section pituitary sequences. Contrast-enhanced MRIs have a sensitivity of 90%. Dynamic contrast-enhanced imaging improves diagnostic accuracy and demonstrates a rounded region of delayed enhancement compared to the rest of the gland. These lesions are usually hyperintense on T2. Inferior petrosal sinus sampling is reserved for patients who are suspected of having a pituitary source, especially in the case of Cushing disease and lateralize the microadenoma, to aid in surgical exploration.

CASE 27

Cavernous Malformation (Cavernous Hemangioma, Occult Cerebrovascular Malformation)

1. **B.** The presence of a complete circumferential hemosiderin ring and the absence of edema are typical of uncomplicated cavernous malformations.
2. **B.** Methemoglobin.
3. **D.** SWI is found to be exquisitely sensitive in the detection of intravascular venous deoxygenated blood as well as extravascular blood products as in CMs. It is a high-spatial-resolution, 3D gradient-echo technique that makes use of the phase information to accentuate and measure the susceptibility difference between tissues. In addition, hemosiderin and calcification can be differentiated on the filtered phase images of SWI as they affect the phase in opposite directions.
4. **D.** Patients with a familial multiple cavernous malformation syndrome with mutations in one of the three genes: KRIT1, CCM2, or PDCD10. This patient has a CCM 2 mutation (see the following comments).

Comment

Cavernous malformations, also referred to as cavernomas, cavernous hemangiomas, and angiographically occult cerebrovascular malformations, represent a sinusoidal network of blood vessels without intervening in normal brain parenchyma. Frequently, gliosis is also present. On an unenhanced CT, CMs may be mildly hyperdense as a result of the pooling of blood in the sinusoids. They may also be associated with focal calcification. On MR imaging, CMs are recognized by their characteristic "popcorn" appearance, representing blood products of different ages. Typically, cavernomas have a central region of high signal intensity on unenhanced T1W and T2W images, representing methemoglobin, surrounded by a complete rim of hemosiderin that is hypointense on T2W and SWI (as in this case). In the absence of recent hemorrhage, there should be no surrounding edema. Angiographically, CMs are usually occult. Unlike other occult vascular malformations, such as capillary telangiectasias and venous angiomas, these patients may present clinically with seizures or symptoms related to mass effect in cases in which there has been recent hemorrhage.

CMs may be present in as much as 5% of the population. The majority of CMs are located superficially in the cerebrum and are often closely associated with the adjacent subarachnoid space. They may occur deep within the cerebral hemispheres, although this is less common. CMs occur less frequently in the infratentorial compartment. The most common brainstem location is the pons. Symptoms may be related to lesion location or acute hemorrhage. In the cerebrum, the most common presentation is seizures. In the infratentorial compartment, neurologic deficits may occur on the basis of acute hemorrhage, thrombosis, or progressive enlargement of a CM related to recurrent hemorrhage.

Familial CM has an autosomal dominant pattern of inheritance and should have one or more of the following: (1) five or more CMs, (2) one CM and at least one other family member with one or more CM, (3) mutations in one of the three genes: KRIT1, CCM2 (as in this case), or PDCD10.

REFERENCES

Cauley KA, Andrews T, Gonyea JV, Filippi CG. Magentic resonance diffusion tensor imaging and tractography of intracranial cavernous malformations: preliminary observations and characterization of the hemosiderin rim. *J Neurosurg.* 2010;112(4):814-823.

Ginat DT, Meyers SP. Intracranial lesions with high signal intensity on T1-weighted MR images: differential diagnosis. *Radiographics.* 2012; 32(2):499-516.

Hegde AN, Mohan S, Lim CC. CNS cavernous haemangioma: "popcorn" in the brain and spinal cord. *Clin Radiol.* 2012;67(4):380-388. doi:10.1016/j.crad.2011.10.013.

Razek AA, Castillo M. Imaging lesions of the cavernous sinus. *AJNR Am J Neuroradiol.* 2009;30(3):444-452.

Neuroradiology: THE REQUISITES. 4th ed. pp 145-146.

CASE 28

Dandy–Walker Malformation

1. **D.** The differential diagnosis of posterior fossa cystic includes arachnoid cyst, Dandy–Walker malformation, and giant cisterna magna.
2. **B.** Dandy–Walker malformation other CNS abnormalities can be seen, including cortical dysplasia, polymicrogyria, subependymal grey matter heterotopia, dysgenesis of the corpus callosum, lipoma of the corpus callosum, holoprosencephaly, schizencephaly, and occipital encephalocele.
3. **B.** Dandy–Walker malformation.
4. **D.** Dandy–Walker malformation is the most common posterior fossa malformation. It is characterized by the classic triad of: (1) hypoplasia of the vermis, (2) cystic dilatation of the fourth ventricle extending posteriorly, and (3) enlarged posterior fossa with torcular-lambdoid inversion.

Comment

The Dandy–Walker complex (which includes Dandy–Walker malformation and its variants) is a congenital anomaly believed to be related to an in utero insult to the fourth ventricle leading to complete or partial outflow obstruction of CSF. As a result, there is cyst-like dilation of the fourth ventricle, which protrudes up between the cerebellar hemispheres to prevent their fusion, and there is an incomplete formation of all or part of the inferior vermis. The spectrum of Dandy–Walker variant depends on the time in utero at which the insult occurs, as well as the severity of the insult (the degree of fourth ventricular outflow obstruction). Dandy–Walker malformations are associated with hydrocephalus in approximately 75% of cases that usually develop in the postnatal period. Dandy–Walker malformations may be associated with atresia of the foramen of Magendie and, possibly, the foramen of Luschka. In addition, 70% of patients have associated supratentorial anomalies, including dysgenesis of the corpus callosum, migrational anomalies, encephaloceles, etc.

This case demonstrates characteristic MR findings of a Dandy–Walker malformation including a large retrocerebellar cyst (A, B), enlargement of the posterior fossa with osseous remodeling, abnormally high position of the straight sinus, torcular herophili, and tentorium, and torcular-lambdoid inversion. The radiologic hallmark of Dandy–Walker malformation is a communication of the retrocerebellar cyst with the fourth ventricle, which is readily appreciated on the sagittal MR image (A).

Macrocephaly is the most common manifestation, and in 80% of cases, the diagnosis is made by the first year of life. Despite severe cerebellar abnormalities, cerebellar signs are not common.

A mega cisterna magna consists of an enlarged posterior fossa secondary to an enlarged cisterna magna, but with a normal cerebellar vermis and fourth ventricle. Retrocerebellar arachnoid cysts of developmental origin are clinically important. They displace the fourth ventricle and cerebellum anteriorly and show a significant mass effect. Differentiation of posterior fossa arachnoid cyst from Dandy–Walker malformation is essential as surgical therapy differs between the two entities.

REFERENCES

Bosemani T, Orman G, Boltshauser E, Tekes A, Huisman TA, Poretti A. Congenital abnormalities of the posterior fossa. *Radiographics.* 2015;35(1):200-220.

Wong AM, Bilaniuk LT, Zimmerman RA, Liu PL. Prenatal MR imaging of Dandy-Walker complex: midline sagittal area analysis. *Eur J Radiol.* 2012;81(1):26-30.

Neuroradiology: THE REQUISITES. 4th ed. pp 279, 280-281.

CASE 29

Tuberous Sclerosis (Bourneville's Disease)

1. **C.** The most likely diagnosis is tuberous sclerosis which classically presents with Vogt triad seizures, mental retardation, and adenoma sebaceum. Other clinical signs include skin lesions (ash-leaf spots, shagreen patches, and subungual fibromas).
2. **D.** Subependymal giant cell astrocytomas (SEGAs) are benign tumors (WHO grade I) seen exclusively in patients with tuberous sclerosis.
3. **B.** Subependymal hamartomas. The vast majority are associated with calcification and have a variable signal and enhancement. The most useful feature in distinguishing them from SEGA is serial growth.
4. **D.** The kidneys may have hamartomas (angiomyolipomas), cysts, and rarely, renal cell carcinoma; rhabdomyomas may occur along the ventricular septum in the heart; the lungs may be affected by lymphangioleiomyomatosis (LAM); with pancreatic neuroendocrine tumors; and hepatic angiomyolipoma. A variety of skeletal lesions (bone islands and cysts) and occasionally vascular lesions (aneurysms or stenoses) may also be present.

Comment

Tuberous sclerosis (TS) most commonly occurs as a sporadic mutation with the remainder inherited as an autosomal dominant condition. The mutations have been narrowed down to two tumor suppressor genes, both part of the mTOR pathway. TSC1—encoding hamartin—on chromosome 9q32-34 and TSC2—encoding tuberin—on chromosome 16p13.3. There is a spectrum of clinical signs and symptoms in these patients; however, the imaging manifestations should be sufficient to make the diagnosis in the majority of cases. Seizures, intellectual disability, and adenoma sebaceum are the classic clinical triad (Vogt triad) described in TS; however, the three together are seen in ~ 30% of patients with this diagnosis.

The CNS manifestations of TS are numerous and include subependymal hamartomas, cortical and subcortical tubers, white matter lesions (believed to represent dysplastic white matter or foci of hypomyelination), subependymal giant cell astrocytomas, and ventriculomegaly. Subependymal hamartomas are seen in essentially all patients with TS, and the majority are calcified. Because of the high incidence of calcification, these lesions are easily detected on CT, but they can be difficult to detect on MR imaging. Gradient-echo imaging is best for the detection of these lesions, which are hypointense (as seen in this case).

Cortical tubers are present in approximately 50% of these patients, and approximately half are calcified. Cortical tubers are hyperintense on T2-weighted images and are frequently bilateral and symmetric. They affect the frontal, parietal, occipital, and temporal lobes in descending order of frequency. Up to 33% of subependymal nodules and 5% of cortical tubers may enhance.

REFERENCES

Ertan G, Arulrajah S, Tekes A, et al. Cerebellar abnormality in children and young adults with tuberous sclerosis complex: MR and diffusion weighted imaging findings. *J Neuroradiol*. 2010;37(4):231-238.

Gama HP, da Rocha AJ, Valerio RM, et al. Hippocampal abnormalities in an MR imaging series of patients with tuberous sclerosis. *AJNR Am J Neuroradiol*. 2010;31(6):1059-1068.

Wong AM, Wang HS, Schwartz ES, et al. Cerebral diffusion tensor MR tractography in tuberous sclerosis complex: correlation with neurologic severity and tract-based spatial statistical analysis. *AJNR Am J Neuroradiol*. 2013;34(9):1829-1835.

Neuroradiology: THE REQUISITES. 4th ed. pp 294-296, 487.

CASE 30

Porencephalic Cyst

1. **A.** Porencephalic cyst is a cystic lesion in the brain due to an encephalomalacic insult, lined by white matter, and communicates with the ventricles and/or the subarachnoid space.
2. **D.** Schizencephalic cleft extends from the ependymal surface to the pia mater, and the two layers meet in the cleft: the so-called pial-ependymal seam. The gray matter that lines the cleft is abnormal, usually representing polymicrogyria.
3. **B.** White matter that is frequently gliotic.
4. **E.** All of the mentioned entities can result in porencephalic cysts.

Comment

Porencephalic cysts occur in regions of the encephalomalacic brain. Insults that occur in utero after the development of the brain, postnatally, or in childhood, such as hemorrhage, infarction, trauma, or infection (especially viral agents, such as herpes and cytomegalovirus) involving the cerebral cortex and underlying subcortical white matter, typically predispose to this entity. Porencephalic cyst often communicates with the ventricles and/or subarachnoid spaces. Transmission of CSF pulsations from the ventricles into the cyst or development of adhesions within the cyst, resulting in a ball-valve mechanism, leads to ventricular and cystic enlargement, which may result in remodeling or expansion of the inner table of the calvarium, as is seen with large superficial arachnoid cysts. On imaging, these cysts typically appear isointense to CSF on all pulse sequences, and may also be multiloculated, as seen in this case.

Another entity that extends from the superficial surface of the cerebrum to the ventricular margin is open-lip schizencephaly, which may resemble a porencephalic cyst on a quick initial observation. Schizencephaly is a developmental migrational abnormality (unlike a porencephalic cyst, which is the destruction of a normally developed brain). Schizencephaly can be distinguished from porencephaly in that the schizencephalic CSF cleft is lined by gray matter, usually polymicrogyric, whereas the porencephalic cyst is lined by white matter, usually gliotic.

REFERENCES

Barkovich AJ, Norman D. MR imaging of schizencephaly. *AJR Am J Roentgenol*. 1988;150(6):1391-1396. doi:10.2214/ajr.150.6.1391.

Yang DN, Townsend JC, Ilsen PF, Bright DC, Welton TH. Traumatic porencephalic cyst of the brain. *J Am Optom Assoc*. 1997;68(8):519-526.

Neuroradiology: THE REQUISITES. 4th ed. pp 278-280.

CASE 31

Hemangioblastoma (VHL)

1. **B.** Hemangioblastoma.
2. **D.** Subacute stroke is the most common "space-occupying lesion," "mass" in adults. The most common cerebellar neoplasm in an adult is a metastasis, whereas the most common primary cerebellar neoplasm is a hemangioblastoma.
3. **C.** The presence of enhancement in the cyst wall is common in pilocytic astrocytomas but unusual in hemangioblastomas. In addition, the presence of flow voids also favors the diagnosis of hemangioblastoma. Pilocytic astrocytomas tend to occur in children, whereas isolated cerebellar hemangioblastomas usually present in young adults.
4. **D.** von Hippel–Lindau disease. Notice the left enucleation from the prior retinal angioma and a history of multiple prior tumors in different organs. This is due to mutations in the VHL tumor suppressor gene on chromosome 3.

Comment

Cerebellar hemangioblastomas are benign neoplasms that represent the most common primary infratentorial neoplasm in adults. They are more common in men, and presentation is typically during adulthood (except when associated with von Hippel–Lindau disease, where presentation may occur in late adolescence). Patients may present with headache, nausea and vomiting, ataxia, and vertigo. Although these neoplasms typically have a vascular nidus, subarachnoid hemorrhage is an uncommon presentation. More than 80% of posterior fossa hemangioblastomas occur in the cerebellum. They may also occur in the spinal cord or medulla (in the region of the area postrema). Cerebral hemangioblastomas are unusual, representing fewer than 2% of all hemangioblastomas, and are usually indicative of von Hippel–Lindau disease (posterior fossa tumors are also usually present in this neurocutaneous syndrome).

There are two characteristic imaging appearances of cerebellar hemangioblastomas. The first is that of a solid and cystic mass (>50% of cases). In most cases, there is no enhancement around the cyst wall, as seen in this case. The solid vascular mural nodule associated with the cyst avidly enhances, and the nodule usually abuts the pial surface, as in this case. Alternatively, hemangioblastomas may present as poorly demarcated, avidly enhancing masses typically associated with numerous vascular flow voids (up to 40% of cases) not seen in this case. Approximately 20% of patients also present with polycythemia due to erythropoietin production.

In addition to a large left cerebellar hemangioblastoma, notice enucleation of the left eye from prior retinal angioma, and flattening of the right optic nerve head from raised intracranial pressure and hydrocephalus.

Management is typically surgical resection, which is considered curative. Recurrence may occur if there has been incomplete resection of the solid vascular nidus.

REFERENCES

Bladowska J, Zimny A, Guzinski M, et al. Usefulness of perfusion weighted magnetic resonance imaging with signal-intensity curves analysis in the differential diagnosis of sellar and parasellar tumors: preliminary report. *Eur J Radiol*. 2013;82(8):1292-1298.

Ho VB, Smirniotopoulos JG, Murphy FM, Rushing EJ. Radiologic-pathologic correlation: hemangioblastoma. *AJNR Am J Neuroradiol.* 1992;13(5):1343-1352.
Neuroradiology: THE REQUISITES. 4th ed. pp 70-72.

CASE 32

Normal-Pressure Hydrocephalus

1. **B.** Communicating hydrocephalus. The combination of ventriculomegaly, Sylvian fissure widening, and crowding at the vertex has been termed disproportionately enlarged subarachnoid space hydrocephalus (DESH), reflecting disproportionality between the superior and inferior CSF spaces and is characteristic of normal-pressure hydrocephalus. Note also how the callosal angle (which is measured at the level of the posterior commissure) appears narrowed.
2. **D.** Normal callosal angle is between 100 and 120°. In patients with idiopathic normal-pressure hydrocephalus (iNPH), it is lower, between 50 and 80°, as seen in this case. All other options are correct as well.
3. **B.** Disproportionately enlarged subarachnoid space hydrocephalus (DESH) is a recently described pattern of communicating hydrocephalus characterized by crowding of the sulci superiorly near the vertex (as in this case, Figure 32.2) accompanied by enlargement of Sylvian fissures and a prominent feature of idiopathic normal pressure hydrocephalus (iNPH). External hydrocephalus is seen in children younger than 2 years of age and results from decreased resorption of CSF at the arachnoid villi. Imaging typically shows an enlargement of the cerebral sulci (especially in the frontal region and along the interhemispheric fissure).
4. **E.** All of these factors indicate a favorable response to CSF shunting.

Comment

Normal-pressure hydrocephalus, a form of communicating hydrocephalus, is characterized by normal mean CSF pressure. In NPH, the lateral and third ventricles are enlarged in comparison with the fourth ventricle. Distention of the lateral ventricles may result in thinning and elevation of the corpus callosum, whereas enlargement of the third ventricle may result in dilation of the infundibular and optic recesses, which may be displaced inferiorly. Patients typically have accentuation of the flow void in the aqueduct of Sylvius on spin-echo images, which is no longer considered a useful sign, as most modern higher field strength scanners demonstrate an aqueductal flow void even in normal subjects. The exact etiology of NPH remains controversial.

Some patients with NPH have marked improvement in their symptoms after shunting. Response to shunting is most favorable when ataxia is the predominant symptom, the patient has had symptoms for only a short time (usually less than 6 months), the patient has a known history of intracranial hemorrhage or infection, MR imaging shows a prominent CSF flow void in the aqueduct (less useful, see above), and there is a relative absence of deep periventricular white matter ischemic changes. Lumbar puncture with the removal of 40 mL or more of CSF and subsequent temporary improvement of clinical symptoms also indicates a patient who may have a favorable response to shunting.

There are no MR imaging findings that have been reliably shown to predict the outcome of shunt surgery in patients with NPH with mixed results from CSF flow studies. The major diagnostic challenge is to differentiate NPH from cerebral atrophy, and callosal angle has been found useful in making this distinction (see above). The decision to perform shunt surgery should be based largely on clinical findings and MR imaging studies that indicate that brain atrophy is not responsible for ventriculomegaly.

REFERENCES

Ivkovic M, Liu B, Ahmed F, et al. Differential diagnosis of normal pressure hydrocephalus by MRI mean diffusivity histogram analysis. *AJNR Am J Neuroradiol.* 2013;34(6):1168-1174.
Stadlbauer A, Salomonowitz E, Brenneis C, et al. Magnetic resonance velocity mapping of 3D cerebrospinal fluid flow dynamics in hydrocephalus: preliminary results. *Eur Radiol.* 2012;22(1):232-242.
Neuroradiology: THE REQUISITES. 4th ed. pp 234-238.

CASE 33

Lipoma Associated with Corpus Callosum

1. **C.** Lipoma of the corpus callosum. Notice the fat-containing lesion in the interhemispheric fissure closely related to the corpus callosum. This is the most common location for an intracranial lipoma.
2. **A.** Approximately 50% of patients present with seizures.
3. **D.** All of these are helpful in confirming the fatty nature of an intracranial mass. Chemical shift artifact on T2W images (which results in hypointensity at the periphery of the lesion along the frequency encoding direction, although the contralateral edge is hyperintense). Another approach is to perform a quick fat-suppressed T1W sequence, such as a fast multiplanar spoiled gradient echo, to assess the loss of signal with the application of fat suppression. Lastly, remember to suppress chemical shift artifacts; all commercial DWI sequences utilize some sort of fat suppression method.

Comment

A widely accepted theory for the development of intracranial lipomas is that they arise from abnormal persistence or differentiation of embryologic meninx primitiva (a mesodermal derivative of the neural crest). The meninx primitiva encases the CNS, and its inner lining is resorbed to allow the formation of the subarachnoid spaces. Intracranial lipomas are not neoplasms, but rather disorders of the development of subarachnoid spaces. Because lipomas are believed to develop from the inner layer of the meninx primitiva that forms the subarachnoid space, pericallosal arteries in interhemispheric lipomas and cranial nerves in cerebellopontine angle lipomas, respectively, often course through the lesions.

Intracranial lipomas most often occur in the interhemispheric fissure (up to 50%), followed by the quadrigeminal cistern (25%), the suprasellar cistern (15%), and the cerebellopontine cistern (10%). They are frequently associated with underdevelopment or dysgenesis of the adjacent brain tissue. Lipomas along the posterior corpus callosum are usually "curvilinear," thin, "ribbon-like," elongated and along the corpus callosum margin, measure <1 cm in thickness, and are more posteriorly situated, with only mild hypoplasia of the corpus callosum, as seen in this case.

Lipomas along the anterior corpus callosum are more common: the "tubulonodular" type; these are rounded, usually measure >2 cm in thickness, and are associated with extensive callosal and often fronto-facial anomalies. These are often "tumefactive" (mass-like in configuration) and are associated with partial agenesis of the corpus callosum.

Lipomas in the quadrigeminal cistern may be associated with underdevelopment of the inferior colliculus.

REFERENCES

Karakas E, Dogan MS, Cullu N, et al. Intracranial lipomas: clinical and imaging findings. *Clin Ter*. 2014;165(2):134-138.

Mehemed TM, Yamamoto A, Okada T, et al. Fat-water interface on susceptibility-weighted imaging and gradient-echo imaging: comparison of phantoms to intracranial lipomas. *AJR Am J Roentgenol*. 2013; 201(4):902-907.

Neuroradiology: THE REQUISITES. 4th ed. pp 55-56.

CASE 34

Fenestration of the Basilar Artery

1. **A.** Basilar artery fenestration. It is the most common intracranial arterial fenestration.
2. **A.** There is an increased incidence of basilar artery aneurysm formation at the site of fenestration, presumably due to abnormal flow dynamics, reported in ~ 7% of fenestrations.
3. **A.** The anterior inferior cerebellar artery (AICA) frequently insinuates itself into the internal auditory canal.
4. **B.** Ruptured aneurysms of the posterior inferior cerebellar artery (PICA) frequently have a tendency to present with fourth ventricular hemorrhage.

Comment

Fenestration of a cerebral artery is defined as a division of the vessel lumen that results in two separate vascular channels that are frequently not equal in size. Each of the channels is lined by endothelium. Pathologic evaluation of basilar artery fenestrations shows that the vascular channels may or may not share a common adventitial layer. Histologically, there are short segmental regions at both the proximal and distal ends of the fenestration in which there are defects in the media, similar to bifurcations of cerebral arteries.

Fenestrations are more common in the posterior circulation, reported in up to 0.6% of cerebral angiograms. In comparison, the angiographic incidence of fenestrations in the anterior circulation has been reported in up to 0.2% of cases. On postmortem examination, fenestrations in the posterior and anterior circulation have been reported in 6% to 7% of cases. The discrepancy between pathologic and angiographic incidence is likely due to the increased sensitivity at pathology. The basilar artery is formed by the early fusion of bilateral longitudinal neural arteries. Fenestrations occur along regions where there is a failure of complete fusion of the medial aspects of these longitudinal arteries. Aneurysms may arise from a fenestration; however, when considering all fenestrations (anterior and posterior circulation), the incidence is approximately 3%, which is not significantly different from the incidence of aneurysms arising at the circle of Willis. Aneurysms arising from fenestrations of the posterior circulation may occur more frequently (in up to 7% of cases). Aneurysms arise most commonly at the proximal end of the fenestration.

The vertebral arteries are formed by the fusion of primitive cervical segmental arteries and basivertebral anastomotic vessels. Extracranial duplications of a vertebral artery are most likely related to a failure of regression of the cervical segmental arteries, whereas intracranial duplications likely arise as a result of persistence of basivertebral anastomoses.

REFERENCES

Tanaka S, Tokimura H, Makiuchi T, et al. Clinical presentation and treatment of aneurysms associated with basilar artery fenestration. *J Clin Neurosci*. 2012;19(3):394-401.

Uchino A, Saito N, Okada Y, et al. Fenestrations of the intracranial vertebobasilar system diagnosed by MR angiography. *Neuroradiology*. 2012;54(5):445-450.

Neuroradiology: THE REQUISITES. 4th ed. pp 33-34.

CASE 35

Acute Sinusitis

1. **D.** Acute left maxillary sinusitis. Notice the fluid level in the left maxillary sinus (Figures 35.1 and 35.2) with opacified bilateral ostiomeatal units, also notice a small fluid level in the right concha bullosa (Figure 35.3).
2. **A.** Most cases are related to antecedent upper respiratory tract infection. Mucosal edema results in mucosal apposition. These factors lead to the obstruction of normal sinus drainage, retained sinus secretions, and bacterial overgrowth with infection.
3. **E.** All of these can be manifestations of COVID-19. There is no information yet on whether COVID-19 causes sinusitis.
4. **D.** All of the above are true regarding concha bullosa.

Comment

It is estimated that more than 30 million people in the United States are diagnosed with sinus inflammatory disease annually; more than half of these result in doctor visits. Approximately 0.5% of viral upper respiratory tract infections are complicated by sinusitis. Although many patients are treated for sinusitis based on clinical presentation, CT imaging has increasingly become a part of the standard workup for these patients.

The radiologist should comment on the location of the disease within the sinonasal cavity (mucosal thickening, air–fluid levels in specific parts of the sinuses), affected mucous circulatory passageways (such as the infundibulum of the ostiomeatal complex), and the presence (or absence) of the osseous structures confining the paranasal sinuses, such as the cribriform plate and medial orbital walls. The location of sinusitis is more significant in the production of symptoms than the extent of the disease. Opacification of the infundibulum of the ostiomeatal complex is one of the best predictors for the development of maxillary sinusitis, with a positive predictive value of approximately 80%, whereas opacification of the middle meatus has greater than 90% specificity in predicting maxillary and ethmoid sinusitis. Obstruction of the sphenoethmoidal recess occurs in fewer than 10% of cases and may result in inflammation involving the sphenoid sinus and posterior ethmoid air cells.

In cases of acute sinusitis, an air–fluid level or sinus opacification is present in approximately 50% of cases. These acute changes may be superimposed on chronic changes, including mucosal thickening, neo-osteogenesis, polyposis, and retention cysts. Sinusitis is a clinical diagnosis with supporting radiologic findings. The presence of sinus changes, including air–fluid levels, does not always equate sinusitis.

REFERENCES

Cornelius RS, Martin J, Wippold FJ II, et al. ACR appropriateness criteria sinonasal disease. *J Am Coll Radiol*. 2013;10(4):241-246. doi:10.1016/j.jacr.2013.01.001.

Groppo ER, El-Sayed IH, Aiken AH, et al. Computed tomography and magnetic resonance imaging characteristics of acute invasive fungal sinusitis. *Arch Otolaryngol Head Neck Surg*. 2011;137(10):1005-1010.

Neuroradiology: THE REQUISITES. 4th ed. pp 419-423.

CASE 36

Fahr Disease (Familial Cerebrovascular Ferrocalcinosis, Primary Familial Brain Calcification is now the preferred term)

1. **J.** Basal ganglia calcification is commonly encountered on CT scans of the brain. It is considered a normal incidental and

physiologic finding in elderly patients but should be considered pathologic in persons younger than the age of 40 years unless proven otherwise. There are many causes of calcification, some of which are mentioned here.

2. **D.** Cytomegalovirus. It is the most common TORCH infection, and periventricular calcification is considered one of the most common features.
3. **B.** Bilateral globus pallidus is typically affected by pallidal necrosis.
4. **C.** Bilaterally symmetric calcification within the basal ganglia, thalami, dentate nuclei, and white matter, with subsequent atrophy.

Comment

This case shows bilateral symmetric calcification within the basal ganglia (Figure 36.1) (including the caudate and lentiform nuclei) and dentate nuclei of the cerebellum (Figure 36.5) in a patient with a long-standing history of depression and anxiety. Mineral deposition is frequently noted to be hypointense on T1 (Figure 36.3) and T2 (Figure 36.2) weighted images with susceptibility on the SWI sequence (Figures 36.4 and 36.5). Fahr disease represents a relatively uncommon spectrum of neurologic disorders characterized by extensive abnormal calcium deposition in characteristic locations, such as the bilateral basal ganglia, with associated cell loss and atrophy. This condition has been referred to as idiopathic basal ganglia calcification. Variable neurologic manifestations, including movement disorders such as athetosis (slow, involuntary movements) and chorea, dementia, and psychological impairment, occur. Calcification may also be seen in the dentate nuclei (as in this case), as well as within the white matter, including the centrum semiovale, corona radiata, and subcortical white matter.

Familial patterns of Fahr disease have been commonly noted in the literature. Transmission may be an autosomal recessive trait or may occur in large affected families as an autosomal dominant inheritance pattern.

The differential diagnosis of calcification within the deep gray matter of the cerebral hemispheres, particularly the basal ganglia, is extensive. Probably the most common cause is idiopathic. Calcification in the globus pallidus bilaterally may be noted as a normal finding, representing senescent calcification that occurs with advancing age. A variety of endocrine disorders, including abnormalities in phosphate and calcium metabolism, may result in calcification in these locations. Hypoparathyroidism has not infrequently been identified. Symptomatic patients may respond to correction of serum calcium phosphate abnormalities.

Another common cause of calcium deposition is in the postinflammatory setting. Specifically, calcification may be seen in infections, such as in utero cytomegalovirus exposure, tuberculosis, and cysticercosis, although in these instances, the pattern of calcification is not similar to that seen in Fahr disease. In recent years, calcification within the basal ganglia has been described in patients with in utero HIV infection. Some experts believe that Fahr disease in general may be the result of in utero infections.

REFERENCES

Livingston JH, Stivaros S, Warren D, Crow YJ. Intracranial calcification in childhood: a review of aetiologies and recognizable phenotypes. *Dev Med Child Neurol.* 2014;56(7):612-626. doi:10.1111/dmcn.12359.
Toscano M, Canevelli N, Giacomelli E, et al. Transcranial sonography of basal ganglia calcifications in Fahr disease. *J Ultrasound Med.* 2011; 30(7):1032-1033.
Neuroradiology: THE REQUISITES. 4th ed. p 251.

CASE 37

Sturge–Weber Syndrome (Encephalotrigeminal Angiomatosis)

1. **D.** Sturge–Weber syndrome. Notice gyriform calcification on lateral scout (Figure 37.1), confirmed on the axial bone (Figure 37.2) and soft tissue windows (Figure 37.3) with s usceptibility on GRE (Figure 37.4). The facial skin lesion represents a port-wine stain.
2. **A.** Port wine stain (nevus flammeus), which typically occurs in the trigeminal nerve distribution; the ophthalmic division (cranial nerve V1) is most common.
3. **A.** Unlike most phakomatoses, Sturge–Weber syndrome occurs sporadically and has a relatively equal predilection in both men and women.

Comment

The pathogenesis of Sturge–Weber syndrome is uncertain; however, it is believed to result from persistence of the primitive vascular plexus as a result of a failure of development of the normal cortical venous drainage in affected areas of the brain. A pial vascular malformation develops, which is characterized pathologically by thin-walled, dilated capillaries and venules. The pial angiomatous malformation is usually ipsilateral to the facial port-wine nevus and most commonly affects the posterior cerebral hemisphere (most frequently the occipital lobe, followed by the parietal and temporal lobes), as seen in this case.

In patients older than 2 years of age, plain film radiographs or CT may show "tram-track" calcifications, representing cortical calcification; see scout topogram (Figure 37.1). Enhanced MR imaging shows the extent of the angiomatous malformation because there is an enhancement of the pia in regions involved with the vascular abnormality (Figure 37.5). Collateral venous drainage is manifested by an increase in both the size and number of medullary and subependymal veins. There is also compensatory hypertrophy of the ipsilateral choroid plexus from increased flow (Figure 37.5), and frequently, the internal cerebral veins are enlarged. The involved brain may have abnormal T2W hyperintensity within the white matter related to gliosis and demyelination, cortical enhancement related to anoxic injury, and atrophy, as seen in this case. Secondary calvarial changes include compensatory hypertrophy of the diploic space and enlargement of the ipsilateral paranasal sinuses and mastoid air cells. This case shows many of these abnormalities, including the extent of the pial vascular malformation, leptomeningeal angiomatosis, and ipsilateral enlargement of the choroid plexus.

The finding of decreased *N*-acetylaspartate on proton MR spectroscopy has been observed in affected regions, suggesting neuronal dysfunction or loss. MR perfusion imaging allows evaluation of the time course of bolus arrival and clearance that may provide information about abnormalities due to either the arterial or venous phase. A marked delay of venous clearance of contrast has been observed in areas of leptomeningeal angiomatous involvement. Venous stasis may be distinguished from hypoperfusion, which shows both delayed arrival and clearance of contrast.

REFERENCES

Miao Y, Juhasz C, Wu J, et al. Clinical correlates of white matter blood flow perfusion changes in Sturge-Weber syndrome: a dynamic MR perfusion-weighted imaging study. *AJNR Am J Neuroradiol.* 2011; 32(7):1280-1285.
Wu J, Tarabishy B, Hu J, et al. Cortical calcification in Sturge-Weber Syndrome on MRI-SWI: relation to brain perfusion status and seizure severity. *J Magn Reson Imaging.* 2011;34(4):791-798.
Neuroradiology: THE REQUISITES. 4th ed. pp 296-297.

CASE 38

Pilocytic Astrocytoma of the Optic Pathway—Neurofibromatosis Type 1

1. **B.** Optic pathway gliomas are relatively uncommon tumors with a variable clinical course and are usually seen in the setting of neurofibromatosis type 1.
2. **E.** The bilateral basal ganglia, brain stem, cerebellar peduncles, and dentate nuclei.
3. **B.** Most optic pathway gliomas are pilocytic astrocytomas (WHO grade I tumors). These may appear smooth, fusiform, eccentric, or lobulated and can demonstrate varying degrees of cystic change and enhancement.
4. **C.** The RASopathies are a clinically defined group of genetic syndromes caused by germline mutations in genes encoding components or regulators of the Ras/mitogen-activated protein kinase (MAPK) pathway. These disorders include NF1, Noonan syndrome, Noonan syndrome with multiple lentigines, capillary malformation-arteriovenous malformation syndrome, Costello syndrome, cardio-facio-cutaneous syndrome, and Legius syndrome. Note that the available option, NF2, also an autosomal dominant disorder, affects the NF2 gene on chromosome 22, which encodes merlin (or schwannomin), a tumor suppressor that is not known to affect the Ras/MAPK pathway.

Comment

Neurofibromatosis type 1 (von Recklinghausen's disease) is an autosomal dominant disorder caused by a mutation to the NF1 gene on chromosome 17, which encodes for "neurofibromin," a negative regulator of Ras, which when dysfunctional results in increased signaling of the Ras/MAPK pathway. NF1 can be diagnosed when two or more of the following criteria are present: a first-degree relative with neurofibromatosis type 1, one plexiform neurofibroma or two or more neurofibromas, six or more café-au-lait spots, two or more Lisch nodules (iris hamartomas), axillary or inguinal freckling, optic pathway glioma, and a characteristic bone abnormality (dysplasia of the greater wing of the sphenoid, overgrowth of a digit or limb, pseudarthrosis, lateral thoracic meningocele, or dural ectasia with vertebral dysplasia).

The most common CNS tumor in NF1 is a low-grade optic nerve pilocytic glioma, reported in 15% to 28% of patients. Growth along the optic tract, the lateral geniculate, and the optic radiations may occur. MR imaging is the study of choice for assessing the extent of these tumors, typically when there is posterior extension along the optic tracts and radiations, with variable enhancement. In this case, bilateral optic nerves and the optic chiasm are enlarged, with extension along the posterior optic pathways. Low-grade astrocytic tumors in other locations, such as the brain stem, are also seen with increased incidence in NF1. Neoplasms seen with increased incidence in NF1 include pheochromocytoma, malignant peripheral nerve sheath tumor (MPNST) ~10% of patients, medullary thyroid carcinoma, leukemia, and Wilms' tumor.

NF1 is associated with nonneoplastic focal areas of signal abnormality on T2W sequences within the basal ganglia, thalamus, cerebellar peduncles, dentate nuclei, brain stem, and white matter and may be present in up to 60% of patients, especially in the pediatric age group. Pathology studies have characterized these as spongiform myelinopathy or myelin vacuolar change with no inflammatory reaction and no demyelination.

REFERENCES

Oystreck DT, Morales J, Chaudhry I, et al. Visual loss in orbitofacial neurofibromatosis type 1. *Ophthalmology.* 2012;119(10):2168-2173.
Rauen KA. The RASopathies. *Annu Rev Genomics Hum Genet.* 2013;14: 355-369. doi:10.1146/annurev-genom-091212-153523.
Neuroradiology: THE REQUISITES. 4th ed. pp 64-65, 291-293.

CASE 39

Reversible Posterior Leukoencephalopathy

1. **B.** Imaging findings are consistent with posterior reversible encephalopathy syndrome (PRES).
2. **B.** In patients with PRES, vasogenic edema is seen within the occipital and parietal regions (posterior circulation). "Reversible cerebral edema" is a combination of vasogenic and cytotoxic edema and is seen with seizure-related changes.
3. **D.** Severity of PRES is classified on the basis of the extent of vasogenic edema, mass effect, signs of herniation, and involvement of the cerebellum, brain stem, or basal ganglia.
   Mild: Cortical/subcortical white matter signal-intensity alterations without the involvement of periventricular white matter and without mass effect, or involvement of none or only one of the following: cerebellum, brain stem, or basal ganglia.
   Moderate: Edema involving the cortex and subcortical white matter without the involvement of the periventricular white matter, with mild mass effect but without midline shift/herniation, or involvement of two of the following: cerebellum, brain stem, or basal ganglia.
   Severe: Edema extending from the cortex to the periventricular white matter or the presence of midline shift/herniation, or involvement of all three of the following: cerebellum, brain stem, and basal ganglia. CT shows low attenuation in areas of involvement, whereas T2W images show increased signal intensity within the cortex and subcortical white matter that is frequently bilateral and symmetric. The occipital and parietal lobes are most often affected.
4. **A.** Hypertensive microangiopathy is characterized by central microhemorrhages affecting the basal ganglia, brain stem, and cerebellum and is best seen on susceptibility-weighted imaging (SWI). Note: microhemorrhages secondary to amyloid angiopathy are peripherally distributed in a more lobar-type distribution.

Comment

The images show foci of increased signal intensity within the subcortical white matter (and cortex) that is predominantly in the occipital lobes; however, regions of signal alteration are also present in the parietal and frontal lobes (Figures 39.2–39.4). This case shows many typical imaging manifestations of posterior reversible encephalopathy syndrome (PRES). The posterior circulation is more sensitive to changes in accelerated hypertension. This may be related to a difference in sympathetic innervation (sparse innervation by sympathetic nerves). One theory is that the normal autoregulatory control of the cerebral vasculature that allows continuous perfusion over a range of blood pressures is exceeded. This may result in engorgement of the distal cerebral vessels, with hyperperfusion and breakdown of the blood–brain barrier. Signal abnormalities represent vasogenic edema with facilitated diffusion (Figure 39.5), as seen in this case. Usual clinical presentation with elevated blood pressure is associated with progressive neurologic symptoms, including changes in mental status, headache, blurred vision, seizures, and focal neurologic deficits. Both the symptoms and the radiologic findings may be reversible with treatment of elevated blood pressure.

In addition to foci of abnormal signal intensity at the gray–white matter interface in the occipital and parietal lobes, the frontal and temporal lobes may be affected, as well as the deep gray nuclei, brain stem (Figure 39.3), and cerebellum. Enhancement in regions of signal abnormality may be observed. Acute hemorrhage may be present, although this is less common.

Similarly, potentially reversible changes may occur with the use of intravenous drugs, such as cocaine; in patients treated with chemotherapeutic agents (cytosine arabinoside, methotrexate, cisplatin, tacrolimus); in those undergoing radiation therapy; and in patients with eclampsia.

REFERENCES

Covarrubias DJ, Luetmer PH, Campeau NG. Posterior reversible encephalopathy syndrome: prognostic utility of quantitative diffusion-weighted MR images. *AJNR Am J Neuroradiol.* 2002;23(6):1038-1048.

Fitzgerald RT, Wright SM, Samant RS, et al. Elevation of serum lactate dehydrogenase at posterior reversible encephalopathy syndrome onset in chemotherapy-treated cancer patients. *J Clin Neurosci.* 2014;14:111-118.

Junewar V, Verma R, Sankhwar PL, et al. Neuroimaging features and predictors of outcome in eclamptic encephalopathy: a prospective observational study. *Am J Neuroradiol.* 2014;35(9):1728-1734.

Kastrup O, Schlamann M, Moenninghoff C, et al. Posterior reversible encephalopathy syndrome: the spectrum of MR imaging patterns. *Clin Neuroradiol.* 2015;25(2):161-171.

Neuroradiology: THE REQUISITES. 4th ed. pp 220-221.

CASE 40

Wernicke Encephalopathy

1. **D.** Emergently administer thiamine (vitamin B1). There is a signal abnormality in the paraventricular thalami, mammillary bodies, periaqueductal gray, and dorsal medulla (Figures 40.1–40.5), consistent with the diagnosis of Wernicke encephalopathy.

2. **D.** Enhancement of mammillary bodies is considered pathognomonic of Wernicke encephalopathy (Figure 40.6).

3. **D.** Wernicke encephalopathy is commonly associated with prolonged alcohol use but can also be seen with malignancy, total parenteral nutrition, abdominal surgery, hyperemesis gravidarum, hemodialysis, or any situation that predisposes to a chronically malnourished state. Signal-intensity alterations of atypical locations include the cerebral cortex (23%), ninth cranial nerve nuclei (23%), corpus callosum (5%), basal ganglia (5%), and cerebellum (14%). More recent studies have shown no significant differences between alcoholic and non-alcoholic patients.

4. **D.** Besides Wernicke encephalopathy, the differential diagnosis of symmetric lesions of the medial thalami includes the artery of Percheron infarction, deep cerebral vein thrombosis, variant Creutzfeldt–Jakob disease, West Nile virus meningoencephalitis, etc.

Comment

This case shows many of the imaging findings seen in Wernicke encephalopathy including signal intensity and enhancement in the mammillary bodies with FLAIR hyperintensity in the paraventricular thalami. Wernicke encephalopathy is best assessed with MR imaging, which is more sensitive than CT in evaluating the small structures involved in this entity. Abnormal T2W and FLAIR hyperintensity is seen in the mammillary bodies (in essentially all patients) and may also be seen in the hypothalamus, periaqueductal gray matter, medial thalami, and dorsal medulla. Imaging findings are often bilateral and symmetric. In the acute setting, there may be mild swelling associated with the signal alteration, and enhancement has also been reported, as seen in this case. Resolution of the signal alterations after treatment with thiamine has been reported. In the late stages, atrophy (particularly of the mammillary bodies) may be the main finding.

Wernicke encephalopathy is related to thiamine deficiency and is found most commonly in chronic alcoholism; however, this vitamin deficiency may also be present in other conditions that result in chronic malnutrition, such as anorexia nervosa, prolonged infectious or febrile conditions, hyperemesis gravidarum, etc. It has also been reported in association with long-term parenteral therapy. Wernicke encephalopathy clinically manifests with the triad of acute confusion, ataxia, and ophthalmoplegia. It can evolve into the chronic form of thiamine deficiency known as Korsakoff psychosis, characterized by, memory loss and confabulation, together referred to as Wernicke–Korsakoff syndrome.

REFERENCES

Elefante A, Puoti G, Senese R, et al. Non-alcoholic acute Wernicke's encephalopathy: role of MRI in non typical cases. *Eur J Radiol.* 2012;81(12):4099-4104.

Ha ND, Weon YC, Jang JC, et al. Spectrum of MR imaging findings in Wernicke encephalopathy: are atypical areas of involvement only present in nonalcoholic patients? *AJNR Am J Neuroradiol.* 2012;33(7):1398-1402.

Hegde AN, Mohan S, Lath N, Lim CC. Differential diagnosis for bilateral abnormalities of the basal ganglia and thalamus. *Radiographics.* 2011;31(1):5-30.

Zuccoli G, Siddiqui N, Cravo I, et al. Neuroimaging findings in alcohol-related encephalopathies. *AJR Am J Roentgenol.* 2010;195(6):1378-1384.

Neuroradiology: THE REQUISITES. 4th ed. p 223.

CASE 41

Osmotic Demyelination Syndrome

1. **C.** Osmotic demyelination syndrome. Signal abnormality in the central pons with peripheral sparing (Figure 41.1). Symmetric signal abnormality in bilateral middle cerebellar peduncles (Figure 41.2). The patient's metabolic status, in this case, indicated elevated serum osmolarity with low normal sodium levels. All of these factors culminated in osmotic demyelination, with no abrupt changes in serum sodium. This case represents the ataxic form of central pontine myelinolysis with bilateral middle cerebellar peduncular lesions, which are clinically relevant to gait disturbances and instability.

2. **E.** Pseudobulbar palsy is a clinical syndrome of dysarthria, dysphagia, a hyperactive gag reflex, and labile emotional responses, resulting from brainstem lesions.

3. **A.** Osmotic demyelination is most commonly seen in alcoholics and in chronically debilitated and malnourished patients after rapid correction of hyponatremia.

4. **D.** Hyperintensity in bilateral globus pallidi represents manganese deposition from underlying chronic liver dysfunction.

Comment

Osmotic demyelination may be seen in underlying systemic processes that have a predilection for electrolyte abnormalities. It is most commonly seen in alcoholics and in chronically debilitated and malnourished patients after rapid correction of hyponatremia. It is not the low serum level but rather the rapidity with which it is corrected that is believed to be responsible for this disorder. Overzealous correction of serum sodium levels may be followed by acute or subacute clinical deterioration, including changes in mental status, coma, quadriparesis, extrapyramidal signs, and if unrecognized, death. This process not uncommonly involves extrapontine structures, such as the midbrain, thalamus, deep periventricular white matter, and cerebellum. Pathologically, demyelination is noted without a significant inflammatory response, with relative sparing of axons. There is an associated reactive astrocytosis.

The earliest change is seen on DWI with restriction in the lower pons. Note that "central pontine myelinolysis" is an older term that has now been replaced. Eventual T2 hyperintensity is seen with sparing of the peripheral parts of the pons, and the corticospinal tracts are usually spared as well, giving rise to a "trident sign" which is reminiscent in this case. Usually, osmotic demyelination is not associated with enhancement or significant mass effect.

When osmotic demyelination is localized only to the pons, the imaging diagnosis is usually easy. However, if there is pontine and extrapontine involvement or involvement only in extrapontine structures, the differential diagnosis is somewhat broad, including other demyelinating disorders, encephalitis, and ischemia.

REFERENCES

Alleman AM. Osmotic demyelination syndrome: central pontine myelinolysis and extrapontine myelinolysis. *Semin Ultrasound CT MR.* 2014; 35(2):153-159.
Kim J, Song T, Park S, Choi IS. Cerebellar peduncular myelinolysis in a patient receiving hemodialysis. *J Neurol Sci.* 2007;253(1-2):66-68.
Lim CC. Neuroimaging in post-infectious demyelination and nutritional disorders of the central nervous system. *Neuroimaging Clin N Am.* 2011;21(4):843-858.
Neuroradiology: THE REQUISITES. 4th ed. p 222.

CASE 42

Colloid Cyst of the Third Ventricle

1. **D.** Colloid cyst. Well-defined hyperdense lesion on an unenhanced CT (Figure 42.1), attached to the anterosuperior portion of the third ventricle, hyperintense on T1 (Figures 42.2 and 42.5) and isointense to the brain on T2-weighted images (Figure 42.3) with faint peripheral rim enhancement (Figure 42.6). Note that there is no susceptibility on SWI (Figure 42.4).
2. **D.** Anterior commissure
3. **B.** The classic location of a colloid cyst is the anterosuperior portion of the third ventricle.
4. **C.** Nearly half of all patients with symptomatic colloid cysts present with obstructive hydrocephalus, which has a 3.1% risk of death. Endoscopic, stereotactic resection of the colloid cyst was performed in this symptomatic patient.

Comment

Colloid cysts are benign masses typically located in the superior aspect of the anterior third ventricle between the columns of the fornices. They are lined by a single layer of epithelium and represent the most common type of neuroepithelial cyst (the origin of these cysts has been debated). Many of these lesions are incidental findings in patients being evaluated for other reasons. Alternatively, signs and symptoms of hydrocephalus (headache, nausea, vomiting) that may be positional in nature may occur intermittently due to the obstruction of the foramen of Monro. These benign masses, even if an incidental finding, are usually treated because their mobility with changes in head position put the patient at risk for acute obstructive hydrocephalus. Management options include stereotactic aspiration, surgical resection, and shunting, or a combination of these treatments.

These cystic masses are usually radiologically characteristic, allowing them to be distinguished from other mass lesions in this location that are typically more solid, including those related to the choroid plexus (the occasional choroid plexus papilloma), craniopharyngiomas, gliomas, and occasionally meningiomas. A thick, mucoid material as well as a variety of other products, including old blood, CSF, other proteins, and paramagnetic ions, such as magnesium, are found within colloid cysts. The location of these cysts and their contents give them a characteristic radiologic appearance, including variable density and intensity characteristics on CT and MR imaging, respectively. Depending on the

specific contents within an individual cyst, on an unenhanced CT, these lesions may range from isodense (low protein concentration) to extremely hyperdense (high protein concentration) to the CSF and brain tissue. Colloid cysts also vary extensively in their signal characteristics on T1W and T2W MR imaging, ranging from very hyperintense to isointense or hypointense on unenhanced T1W images. The signal characteristics will depend on the protein concentration, viscosity, water content, and cross-linking of glycoproteins. A thin wall is usually seen that commonly enhances after contrast administration. With the exception of this mild, thin, peripheral enhancement of the epithelial lining, these lesions should not demonstrate solid or central enhancement.

REFERENCES

Armao D, Castillo M, Chen H, Kwock L. Colloid cyst of the third ventricle: imaging-pathologic correlation. *AJNR Am J Neuroradiol.* 2000;21(8):1470-1477.
Bender B, Honegger JB, Beschorner R, et al. MR imaging findings in colloid cysts of the sellar region: comparison with colloid cysts of the third ventricle and Rathke's cleft cysts. *Acad Radiol.* 2013;20(11):1457-1465.
Sener RN. Colloid cyst: diffusion MR imaging findings. *J Neuroimaging.* 2007;17(2):181-183.
Yadav YR, Yadav N, Parihar V, Kher Y, Ratre S. Management of colloid cyst of third ventricle. *Turk Neurosurg.* 2015;25(3):362-371. doi:10.5137/1019-5149.JTN.11086-14.1.
Neuroradiology: THE REQUISITES. 4th ed. pp 80-81.

CASE 43

Juvenile Pilocytic Astrocytoma

1. **D.** Pilocytic Astrocytoma. Left parietal cystic mass (Figures 43.1) with enhancing nodule (Figure 43.4) which demonstrates mild reduced diffusion (Figure 43.3), as well as mild elevation of relative cerebral blood volume (Figure 43.5). Usually, juvenile pilocytic astrocytomas present before the age of 20 years, and hemangioblastomas present after the age of 20 years. Abnormal vessels or flow voids are associated with the enhancing nodule in hemangioblastoma.
2. **E.** All of these tumors can present with a cystic mass with eccentric enhancing mural nodule.
3. **D.** The most common location of a pilocytic astrocytoma is the cerebellum, with the optic pathway being the next most common, particularly in patients with neurofibromatosis type 1, as seen in Patient 2.
4. **A.** Neurofibromatosis type 1.

Comment

Astrocytomas are the most common intracranial tumors in children, accounting for up to 50% of such neoplasms. Approximately two-thirds are located in the posterior fossa. Cerebellar astrocytomas and medulloblastomas are the most common infratentorial neoplasms in children. Approximately 80% of all cerebellar astrocytomas in children are of the pilocytic variety. Most patients with pilocytic astrocytomas have normal karyotypes; however, long-arm deletions of chromosome 17 have been associated with them as well.

Pilocytic astrocytoma, as well as pleomorphic xanthoastrocytomas, frequently have BRAF alterations (present in ~70% of cases). Patient 2 had a BRAF V600E mutation. Note that, unlike adult low-grade tumors, these tumors frequently lack IDH mutations and TP53 mutations. Pilocytic astrocytomas represent one of the more benign forms of glial neoplasms and are classified as World Health Organization grade 1 tumors with a good prognosis. Surgical resection is considered curative. Histologically, tightly packed, piloid (elongated hair-like projections) arise from tumor cells. Eosinophilic granular bodies and Rosenthal fibers (astrocytic processes) are also present.

On imaging, ~ 70% of these tumors had a large cystic component with avidly enhancing mural nodule, as seen in Patient 1. There is a variable enhancement of the cyst wall. Note that no clear enhancement was seen in the cyst wall in Patient 1. In a small minority, these tumors can be more heterogeneous with mixed solid and cystic components, or can be completely solid, as seen in Patient 2. Hemorrhage is uncommon, but calcification may be seen in up to 20% of patients, as seen in Patient 2.

REFERENCES

Mandiwanza T, Kaliaperumal C, Khalil A, et al. Suprasellar pilocytic astrocytoma: one national centre's experience. *Childs Nerv Syst.* 2014; 30(7):1243-1248.

Paixao Becker A, de Oliveria RS, Saggioro FP, et al. In pursuit of prognostic factors in children with pilocytic astrocytomas. *Childs Nerv Syst.* 2010;26(1):19-28.

Neuroradiology: THE REQUISITES. 4th ed. p 57.

CASE 44

Orbital Cellulitis and Abscess

1. **C.** Preseptal orbital cellulitis is limited to the soft tissues anterior to the orbital septum and is often managed with oral antibiotics. It is commonly caused by contiguous spread of infection from adjacent structures such as the face, tooth, and eyelid or by direct inoculation from local trauma or insect bites.
2. **D.** Orbital cellulitis is a postseptal soft-tissue infection with a threat to vision, typically resulting from the extension of a paranasal sinus (most commonly the ethmoid air cells). It generally requires hospital admission with the administration of intravenous antibiotics and close monitoring of the patient's vision.
3. **C.** Orbital cellulitis and abscess on an axial CT image of the orbits reveals right proptosis with globe deformity ("guitar pick" sign) and periorbital edema with small pockets of fluid collection in the extraconal spaces, displacing the right medial and lateral rectus muscles.
4. **D.** OCS is a serious ophthalmologic emergency and may result in ischemia of the optic nerve causing vision loss. Posttraumatic retrobulbar hemorrhage is the most common cause of OCS. It can also be seen after infection, inflammation, tension pneumo-orbitus, or orbital/sinus surgeries. Symptoms include decreased visual acuity, and evidence of increased intraorbital pressure. Note: OCS is a clinical diagnosis, and emergent canthotomy and orbital decompression are needed because only 60–100 minutes of elevated pressure can cause permanent vision loss. On imaging, OCS will manifest as severe proptosis with tenting of the posterior globe and stretching of the optic nerve, as seen in this case.

Comment

It is important to distinguish orbital cellulitis, which is a medical emergency from preseptal cellulitis. There are many superficial similarities between the two diseases, including lid edema and redness, and pronounced pain on palpation. However, orbital cellulitis manifests with proptosis and extraocular muscle restriction, whereas preseptal cellulitis does not. Also, patients with orbital cellulitis have fever and frequently have decreased vision. Proptosis develops due to intraorbital or postseptal abscess. Ophthalmoplegia results from toxic myopathy and soft tissue edema. Visual loss may occur due to increased intraorbital pressure from

abscess and inflammation compressing the optic nerve. There typically will be a precipitating factor, such as sinusitis, penetrating lid trauma, odontogenic infection, or facial trauma. The patient may be systemically ill and have a fever. Orbital cellulitis results from microbial infection with subsequent inflammation of the postseptal orbital tissues. Common organisms include *Staphylococcus aureus*, *Streptococcus pyogenes*, *Streptococcus pneumoniae*, and *Haemophilus influenzae* in children. There is significant potential morbidity and even mortality as a postseptal lid infection can spread through a valveless venous system, leading to cavernous sinus thrombosis, meningitis, and brain abscess.

Often, the degree of proptosis in orbital cellulitis cannot be readily appreciated due to the extreme lid edema. For this reason, CT or MR imaging may be useful not only to identify orbital abscesses but also to ascertain precipitating sinus involvement and to exclude intracranial extension. Management involves immediate hospitalization with inpatient parenteral antibiotic therapy.

REFERENCES

Capps EF, Kinsella JJ, Gupta M, et al. Emergency imaging assessment of acute, nontraumatic conditions of the head and neck. *Radiographics.* 2010;30(5):1335-1352.

Pinto A, Brunese L, Danielle S, et al. Role of computed tomography in the assessment of intraorbital foreign bodies. *Semin Ultrasound CT MR.* 2012;33(5):392-395.

Sepahdari AR, AAkalu VK, Kapur R, et al. MRI of orbital cellulitis and orbital abscess: the role of diffusion-weighted imaging. *AJR Am J Roentgenol.* 2009;193(3):244-250.

Neuroradiology: THE REQUISITES. 4th ed. pp 338-339.

CASE 45

Bilateral Subacute Subdural Hematomas

1. **D.** Bilateral subacute subdural hematomas.
2. **D.** Bilateral subacute subdural hematomas can be difficult to detect on CT. If MRI is unavailable, all of these findings can be helpful in its identification.
3. **C.** Hyperintense on T1W (methemoglobin) and T2W imaging.

Comment

The appearance of blood products on CT and MRI is dependent on several factors. Acute hematomas on CT are hyperdense, typically >50–60 HU. Rarely, acute blood products may be isodense with the adjacent cerebral cortex in patients with anticoagulation, coagulopathies, or severe anemia when the hemoglobin is below 8 g/dL. As the clot ages and protein degradation occurs, the density of the blood clot starts to drop. In the subacute stage (10–14 days), the density drops to 35–40 HU and becomes isodense to the adjacent cortex, making identification difficult.

The appearance of blood products on MR imaging is dependent on several factors, most importantly, the structure of hemoglobin at the time of imaging. Oxyhemoglobin (oxygen bound to the iron of hemoglobin) is diamagnetic because it effectively has no unpaired electrons. Upon giving up its oxygen, deoxyhemoglobin is formed and hemoglobin undergoes a small but significant structural change such that water molecules in the vicinity of deoxyhemoglobin are unable to bind to the iron. Deoxyhemoglobin has four unpaired electrons and may be oxidized to methemoglobin. Methemoglobin has five unpaired electrons, and water molecules are able to bind to the iron atom.

Susceptibility effects, proton–electron dipole–dipole interactions, and other factors contribute to the variable signal characteristics of blood products on MR imaging. When placed in a magnetic field, certain substances may induce an additional smaller magnetic field that may add to the externally applied field. This phenomenon may be seen with paramagnetic substances (deoxyhemoglobin and methemoglobin). Alternatively, other substances, when placed in a magnetic field, may induce magnetic fields that subtract from the externally applied field (seen with diamagnetic materials, such as oxyhemoglobin). Susceptibility effects of blood products depend on the proportionality constant between the strength of the applied magnetic field and the induced magnetic field.

Methemoglobin induces a local magnetic field significantly greater than that of a proton. Therefore, if a proton gets close enough to this field, a spin transition may occur. To have a proton–electron dipole–dipole interaction, water must bind to heme. Even though the number of heme molecules is small relative to that of water, the exchange rate of water molecules is quite rapid compared with the repetition time; hence, many water molecules are bound to heme during MR imaging. Proton–electron dipole–dipole interactions result in the shortening of T1 and T2.

REFERENCES

Bradley Jr WG. MR appearance of hemorrhage in the brain. *Radiology*. 1993;189(1):15-26. doi:10.1148/radiology.189.1.8372185.
Tosaka M, Sato N, Fujimaki H, et al. Diffuse pachymeningeal hyperintensity and subdural effusion/hematoma detected by fluid-attenuated inversion recovery MR imaging in patients with spontaneous intracranial hypotension. *AJNR Am J Neuroradiol*. 2008;29(6):1164-1170.
Neuroradiology: THE REQUISITES. 4th ed. pp 154-157.

CASE 46

Herpes Simplex Encephalitis—Type 1

1. **B.** The pattern of imaging findings is typical for herpes simplex encephalitis with bilateral asymmetrical involvement of the limbic system, medial and anterior atemporal lobes, insular cortices, and inferolateral frontal lobes.
2. **D.** Note that the basal ganglia structures are typically spared, an important imaging feature that helps to distinguish herpes encephalitis from middle cerebral artery infarction.
3. **A.** 80% of all neonatal simplex encephalitides is related to HSV-2.
4. **D.** Cingulate gyrus. It is a belt-shaped gyrus that drapes the corpus callosum and is a component of the limbic system.

Comment

Adult herpes encephalitis infection is usually due to HSV-1 in ~90% of cases, whereas 80% of all neonatal simplex encephalitis is related to HSV-2. In adults, there is no particular age, sex, or seasonal predilection. HSV-1 causes necrotizing encephalitis in adults. The clinical presentation varies, ranging from headache, fever, and seizures to coma. Imaging evaluation frequently shows hypodensity with loss of gray–white matter differentiation in the temporal lobes and insular cortex on CT. Hemorrhage may also be present. The CT appearance may simulate an infarction or a primary glial neoplasm. MR imaging findings in the acute stages of encephalitis show hyperintensity on T2 and FLAIR within the involved brain regions (usually the temporal lobes and inferomedial frontal lobes). There is frequently a local mass effect, which manifests as gyral expansion and sulcal effacement. Although bilateral disease is typical, herpes encephalitis usually involves the temporal lobes, insula, inferior frontal lobes, and cingulate gyrus (note the arrow on Figures 46.5) in an asymmetric pattern, as seen in this case. A proposed explanation for this pattern of involvement is the presence of the latent virus within the gasserian ganglion in Meckel's cave. Reactivated virus may spread along the trigeminal nerve fibers, with subsequent spread

along the meninges around the temporal lobes and the undersurface of the frontal lobes. Meningoencephalitis commonly results. Diagnosis is established with CSF herpes simplex virus polymerase chain reaction testing, although the combination of the clinical presentation, CSF pleocytosis and elevated protein, and typical imaging is usually highly suggestive. Cortical gyriform enhancement is often present and may be associated with meningeal enhancement, as seen in this case (Figures 46.4 and 46.6).

A good outcome from herpes simplex encephalitis relies on an early diagnosis, which is of course dependent on considering herpes as a diagnosis! Remember, bilateral temporal lobe lesions in a sick patient should be considered herpes encephalitis unless proven otherwise. Delay in therapy (acyclovir) or untreated herpes is associated with a high mortality rate (50%–75%), with little chance of full neurologic recovery.

REFERENCES

Grydeland H, Walhovd KB, Westlye LT, et al. Amnesia following herpes simplex encephalitis: diffusion-tensor imaging uncovers reduced integrity of normal-appearing white matter. *Radiology*. 2010;257(3):774-781.
Noguchi T, Yoshiura T, Hiwatashi A, et al. CT and MRI findings of human herpesvirus 6-associated encephalopathy: comparison with findings of herpes simplex virus encephalitis. *AJR Am J Roentgenol*. 2010;194(3):754-760.
Neuroradiology: THE REQUISITES. 4th ed. pp 184-186.

CASE 47

Global Anoxic Brain Injury

1. **C.** Diffuse hypodensity in the brain parenchyma with loss of gray–white matter differentiation (Figure 47.1), with T2/FLAIR hyperintense signal in superficial cortical as well as deep gray matter nuclei (Figures 47.2 and 47.3) with reduced diffusion (Figures 47.4 and 47.5).
2. **E.** The "insular ribbon sign" represents the loss of the definition of the insular cortex, aka the "insular ribbon," and is considered an early CT sign of MCA infarction.
3. **D.** All of these are radiographic signs of brain death.

Comment

Global hypoxic-ischemic injury is typically related to decreased perfusion; less commonly, it may be related to a disturbance in blood oxygenation. Postanoxic encephalopathy typically occurs after a period in which a diffuse episode of cerebral hypoperfusion has occurred.

In the acute setting of global hypoxic-ischemic injury, an unenhanced CT may show global loss of gray–white matter differentiation, diffuse gray matter hypodensity, and sulcal effacement, as seen in this case. On MR imaging, T2W hyperintensity may be seen in the highly metabolic areas of the brain involving hippocampi and superficial and deep gray matter. Note that diffusion-weighted imaging (DWI) is the earliest imaging modality to become positive with low ADC values, usually within the first few hours after a hypoxic-ischemic event due to cytotoxic edema. Note that there is thalamic involvement in anoxic brain injury which helps to differentiate from hypoglycemia which can have similar imaging findings. DWI abnormalities usually pseudonormalize by the end of the first week.

Imaging in the subacute phase may demonstrate cortical laminar necrosis, which is commonly of gyriform high signal intensity on unenhanced T1W images. These T1 hyperintensities usually become evident after two weeks. Note that the T1 hyperintense signal of cortical laminar necrosis does not represent hemorrhage or calcification. It is believed to be caused by the accumulation of denatured proteins in dying cells and/or lipid-laden macrophages.

REFERENCES

Muttikkal TJ, Wintermark M. MRI patterns of global hypoxic-ischemis injury in adults. *J Neuroradiol.* 2013;40(3):164-171.

Pollock JM, Whitlow CT, Deibler AR, et al. Anoxic injury-associated cerebral hyperfusion identified with arterial spin-labeled MR imaging. *AJNR Am J Neuroradiol.* 2008;29(7):1302-1307.

Neuroradiology: THE REQUISITES. 4th ed. pp 115-116.

CASE 48

Chiari II Malformation with Associated Anomalies

1. **B.** This case illustrates several classic imaging findings of a Chiari II malformation including small posterior fossa with inferior descent of the brain stem and cerebellar tonsils, tectal beaking, heart-shaped cerebellum, callosal dysgenesis, fenestrated falx (Figures 48.1), a prior history of spina bifida/lumbar myelomeningocele and tethered cord (Figures 48.5–48.7).
2. **C.** The banana sign is seen on axial ultrasound images through the posterior fossa of fetuses with Chiari II malformation. It is secondary to cerebellar wrapping around the brain stem secondary to a small posterior fossa and inferior descent of the posterior fossa contents.
3. **C.** Tethered cord syndrome is a stretch-induced functional neurological disorder caused by fixation (tethering) of the caudal spinal cord. In these cases, most commonly, the conus medullaris terminates in a low position below the lower border of the L2 vertebral body.
4. **B.** Chiari III malformation is an extremely rare anomaly characterized by a low occipital and high cervical encephalocele. Extreme cerebellar hypoplasia is seen with Chiari III malformation.

Comment

Chiari malformations typically occur during the first 3 to 4 weeks of gestational life and are dorsal induction–neural tube defects. Chiari II malformations are the most common symptomatic form. This case illustrates several findings of Chiari II malformations, which are reviewed later. In Chiari II malformations, the vermis, cerebellar tonsils, and medulla herniate through the foramen magnum and upper cervical canal. The cerebellar hemispheres wrap around the brain stem (banana sign), the cerebellar vermis herniates up through the tentorial incisura ("towering cerebellum"), and the tectum is "beaked." The fourth ventricle is elongated and displaced inferiorly. Chiari II malformations are associated with a spectrum of supratentorial anomalies, including dysgenesis of the corpus callosum (most commonly splenial anomalies), as illustrated in this case. Heterotopias and/or sulcation abnormalities are also seen. Myelomeningoceles are seen in virtually all Chiari II malformations, and more than 50% of cases are associated with syringohydromyelia, also seen in this case.

In Chiari I malformations, there is herniation of the cerebellar tonsils, which are pointed (peg-like) in configuration into the cervical spinal canal. The remainder of the cerebellum, brain stem, and fourth ventricle are normal in location. Syringohydromyelia is frequently seen in Chiari I malformations; myelomeningoceles are not.

Chiari III malformations have the same findings as Chiari II malformations but also include herniation of the posterior fossa contents into a high cervical or occipital encephalocele. There is no associated lumbosacral myelomeningocele.

REFERENCES

Ando K, Ishikura R, Ogawa M, et al. MRI tight posterior fossa sign for prenatal diagnosis of Chiari type II malformation. *Neuroradiology.* 2007;49(12):1033-1039.

Mignone Philpott C, Shannon P, Chitayat D, et al. Diffusion-weighted imaging of the cerebellum in the fetus with Chiari II malformation. *AJNR Am J Neuroradiol.* 2013;34(8):1656-1660.

Ou X, Glasier CM, Snow JH. Diffusion tensor imaging evaluation of white matter in adolescents with myelomeningocele and Chiari II malformation. *Pediatr Radiol.* 2011;41(11):1407-1415.

Neuroradiology: THE REQUISITES. 4th ed. pp 283-288.

CASE 49

Infiltrating Astrocytoma—Low Grade

1. **A.** Imaging findings are most consistent with an infiltrating low-grade astrocytoma.
2. **A.** Among lower-grade gliomas (WHO grades 2 and 3), the T2-FLAIR mismatch sign represents a very specific imaging biomarker for the IDH-mutant, 1p/19q non-codeleted molecular subtype.
3. **A.** Detection of 2-hydroxyglutarate on MRS has excellent diagnostic performance in the prediction of IDH mutant gliomas, with a pooled sensitivity of 95% and a pooled specificity of 91%.
4. **D.** cIMPACT-NOW (the Consortium to Inform Molecular and Practical Approaches to CNS Tumor Taxonomy) was established to make practical recommendations on the basis of recent molecular advances in the field of CNS tumor classification. All of these are proposed changes by the working committee as considerations for inclusion in future CNS tumor classifications.

Comment

The WHO classification of CNS tumors is the most widely accepted system for the classification of CNS tumors. The 2016 update included molecular and genetic parameters into the diagnostic schema for the first time. The upcoming fifth edition will incorporate some important changes to diffuse gliomas and glioblastoma as outlined in recent cIMPACT recommendations.

Diffuse low-grade gliomas, also referred to as low-grade infiltrative astrocytomas, are designated as WHO II, typically seen in young adults with a mean age of 35 years with seizures as the most common initial presenting symptom.

According to the 2016 update of the WHO classification of CNS tumors, diffuse astrocytomas are subdivided into two molecular groups based on IDH mutational status (IDH mutated vs. IDH wildtype). If IDH is shown to be mutated, then 1p19q status is determined. IDH mutated and 1p19q co-deleted tumors are classified as oligodendrogliomas.

On imaging, these IDH mutant low-grade astrocytomas frequently demonstrate the "T2-FLAIR mismatch sign" which is considered highly specific for diffuse astrocytoma (IDH-mutant, 1p/19q-non-codeleted molecular status), as seen in this case, which on pathology turned out to be a grade II astrocytoma, positive for IDH1 mutation.

REFERENCES

Louis DN, Wesseling P, Aldape K, et al. cIMPACT-NOW update 6: new entity and diagnostic principle recommendations of the cIMPACT-Utrecht meeting on future CNS tumor classification and grading. *Brain Pathol.* 2020;30(4):844-856. doi:10.1111/bpa.12832.

Patel SH, Poisson LM, Brat DJ, et al. T2-FLAIR mismatch, an imaging biomarker for IDH and 1p/19q status in lower-grade gliomas: a TCGA/TCIA Project. *Clin Cancer Res.* 2017;23(20):6078-6085.

Suh CH, Kim HS, Jung SC, Choi CG, Kim SJ. 2-Hydroxyglutarate MR spectroscopy for prediction of isocitrate dehydrogenase mutant glioma: a systemic review and meta-analysis using individual patient data. *Neuro Oncol.* 2018;20(12):1573-1583.
Neuroradiology: THE REQUISITES. 4th ed. pp 57-59.

CASE 50

Intraventricular Hemorrhage

1. **B.** Intraventricular hemorrhage with early hydrocephalus from a ruptured 3.4 mm × 3.6 mm right posterior inferior cerebellar artery (PICA) origin aneurysm.
2. **A.** Rupture of a posterior inferior cerebellar artery aneurysm usually presents with fourth ventricular hemorrhage.
3. **C.** Thalamic hemorrhages are often hypertensive in etiology. All others are commonly seen in patients with a closed-head injury.
4. **D.** Left anterior inferior cerebellar artery (AICA). Remember, 99% of AICAs arise from the basilar artery (lower third).

Comment

This case shows intraventricular hemorrhage in bilateral lateral, third, and fourth ventricles, with early acute hydrocephalus. Intraventricular hemorrhage is common in the setting of closed-head injury, occurring in 2% to 40% of patients, depending on the severity of injury. Traumatic intraventricular hemorrhage is most commonly associated with diffuse axonal injury, particularly of the corpus callosum, and may also be seen with injury to the septum pellucidum due to tearing of small subependymal veins.

Nontraumatic causes of intraventricular hemorrhage include rupture of large parenchymal hematomas, as is seen with hypertension or amyloid angiopathy in the elderly. In patients with primary intraventricular hemorrhage, in the absence of other findings to suggest a cause, vascular abnormalities, such as choroidal arteriovenous malformations, must be excluded, and CT angiography, MR imaging, or MR angiography or conventional angiography is usually indicated for further evaluation. Ruptured aneurysms of the posterior inferior cerebellar artery (PICA) usually present with intraventricular hemorrhage, although the hemorrhage is usually located preferentially in the fourth ventricle. Isolated intraventricular hemorrhage in the absence of a parenchymal bleed is unusual. In this case, CT angiography as well as conventional angiography shows a 3.4 mm × 3.6 mm aneurysm arising from the origin of the right PICA, which was successfully treated with coil embolization.

REFERENCES

Phan CM, Yoo AJ, Hirsch JA, et al. Differentiation of hemorrhage from iodinated contrast in different intracranial compartments using dual-energy head CT. *AJNR Am J Neuroradiol.* 2012;33(6):1088-1094.
Romanova AL, Nemeth AJ, Berman MD, et al. Magnetic resonance imaging versus computed tomography for identification and quantification of intraventricular hemorrhage. *J Stroke Cerebrovasc Dis.* 2014;23(8): 2036-2040.
Neuroradiology: THE REQUISITES. 4th ed. pp 123-131.

Fair Game

CASE 51

Idiopathic Orbital Inflammation (Orbital Pseudotumor)

1. **A.** Thyroid-associated orbitopathy is the most common cause of proptosis in adults and is most frequently associated with Graves' disease.
2. **D.** Patients with idiopathic orbital inflammation typically present with rapid onset, of usually unilateral (90%), painful proptosis and diplopia with a rapid response to corticosteroids. Note: periorbital edema is typically present, and therefore it does not help distinguish from infection.
3. **A.** The superior ophthalmic vein.
4. **A.** Cavernous venous malformations of the orbit, also known as cavernous hemangiomas, are the most common vascular lesions of the orbit in adults.

Comment

Idiopathic orbital inflammation, also known as nonspecific orbital inflammation (orbital pseudotumor), is a nonspecific inflammatory disorder of an unknown etiology that involves the contents of the orbit. Clinical presentations include proptosis, pain, and diplopia. This disorder is usually unilateral, but may be bilateral in ~10% of patients. An orbital pseudotumor should be considered a diagnosis of exclusion, with evaluation directed at eliminating other causes of orbital disease. Underlying systemic disorders should be considered, including sarcoid, lymphoma, connective tissue disease, Wegener's granulomatosis, and autoimmune disorders. In the early stages of orbital pseudotumor, histologic features are characterized by inflammation and edema, with an abundance of lymphocytes, plasma cells, and giant cells. In the late stages of the disease, fibrosis may be abundant. Orbital pseudotumor may present with a spectrum of manifestations, including myositis (as seen in this case), dacryoadenitis (lacrimal gland involvement), periscleritis (uveal and scleral thickening), or retrobulbar soft tissue abnormality. In myositis, pseudotumor may involve one or more muscles, and unlike thyroid ophthalmopathy, it often involves the tendinous insertion of the muscle as well as the muscle bellies. When idiopathic orbital inflammation primarily involves the cavernous sinus and the orbital apex, it is referred to as Tolosa–Hunt syndrome. Ophthalmoplegia is secondary to the involvement of cranial nerves III through VI in the cavernous sinus.

Because idiopathic orbital inflammation radiologically may appear similar to a variety of disease processes, patient history is important (rapidity of onset and pain). Importantly, there is usually a dramatic response to corticosteroids that may be useful in confirming the diagnosis. A small percentage of patients do not respond to steroids and may require radiation or chemotherapy.

REFERENCES

Ginat DT, Bokhari A, Bhatt S, Dogra V. Inflammatory pseudotumors of the head and neck in pathology-proven cases. *J Neuroradiol.* 2012;39(2):110-115.

Sepahdari AR, Aakalu VK, Setabutr P, et al. Indeterminate orbital masses: restricted diffusion at MR imaging with echo-planar diffusion-weighted imaging predicts malignancy. *Radiology.* 2010;256(2):554-564.

Neuroradiology: THE REQUISITES. 4th ed. pp 324-329.

CASE 52

Fibrous Dysplasia

1. **C.** Cutaneous pigmentation (café-au-lait spots). This patient has McCune–Albright syndrome (MAS) which is a genetic disorder characterized by endocrinopathies (precocious puberty), polyostotic fibrous dysplasia, and cutaneous pigmentation (coast of Maine—"café au lait" spots).
2. **D.** Elevated serum alkaline phosphatase levels and elevated levels of urine hydroxyproline are found in patients with actively growing fibrous dysplasia lesions. Remember, these abnormalities are not specific to fibrous dysplasia! In addition, increased tracer uptake was observed in Tc99 bone scans.
3. **C.** Note that MRI is usually more confusing in patients with fibrous dysplasia that has marked variability and heterogeneity, and the appearance of these bone lesions is often misdiagnosed as a more aggressive lesion with heterogeneous areas of contrast enhancement.
4. **D.** All of the above.

Comment

Fibrous dysplasia (FD) is a nonhereditary developmental disorder of the bone forming mesenchyme in which osteoblasts do not undergo normal differentiation and maturation. Medullary bone is replaced with fibrous tissue. Trabeculae of woven bone contain fluid-filled cysts embedded in a collagenous fibrous matrix. The etiology is unknown. FD may be monostotic (a solitary lesion) or polyostotic (lesions in multiple bones or multiple lesions in one bone). The majority (approximately 75%) of cases are monostotic. Polyostotic fibrous dysplasia more commonly involves the skull and facial bones, pelvis, spine, and shoulder. Polyostotic disease is more commonly unilateral in distribution. Common areas of calvarial involvement include the ethmoid, maxillary, frontal, and sphenoid bones. Involvement of these bones may result in orbital abnormalities such as proptosis, visual disturbances, and displacement of the globe. Involvement of the temporal bone may result in hearing loss or vestibular dysfunction. Although Paget's disease may occur in these same locations of the calvaria, unlike FD, concomitant involvement of the facial bones is less common.

Cutaneous pigmentation is the most common extraskeletal manifestation of FD. It occurs in more than 50% of cases of the polyostotic form. Cutaneous pigmentation is ipsilateral to the side of bony lesions, a feature that differentiates this disease from pigmentation in neurofibromatosis. The pigmented macules, or café-au-lait spots, are related to increased amounts of melanin in the basal cells of the epidermis. They tend to be arranged in a linear or segmental pattern near the midline of the body, usually overlying the lower lumbar spine, sacrum, upper back, neck, and shoulders.

This patient has features typical of FD. There is a "ground glass" appearance of the involved clivus, occipital bones, left temporal bone, and multiple maxillofacial bones. There is relative preservation of the cortex and expansion of involved bones that maintain their normal configuration.

REFERENCES

Chong VF, Khoo JB, Fan YF. Fibrous dysplasia involving the base of the skull. *AJR Am J Roentgenol.* 2002;178:717-720.

Lisle DA, Monsour PA, Maskiell CD. Imaging of craniofacial fibrous dysplasia. *J Med Imaging Radiat Oncol.* 2008;52(4):325-332.

Neuroradiology: THE REQUISITES. 4th ed. pp 432-434.

CASE 53

Retinoblastoma

1. **F.** Retinoblastoma, persistent hyperplastic primary vitreous, toxocara endophthalmitis, Coats' disease (congenital retinal telangiectasia), and retrolental fibroplasia.
2. **D.** Leukocoria, also known as the loss of red reflex. On eye examination, when a light source is directed to the eye through the iris, the retina appears red. In children with leukocoria, the retina abnormally appears white.
3. **B.** The third eye refers to a pineoblastoma of the pineal gland.
4. **B.** They are bilateral in 30% to 40% of patients.

Comment

Retinoblastoma represents the most common intraocular tumor in childhood. The typical clinical presentation is leukocoria, an abnormal pupillary reflex characterized by a "white" pupil. Other common clinical presentations include strabismus, decreased visual acuity, and eye pain (which may be related to glaucoma). The majority of retinoblastomas (98%) present before 3 years of age. Retinoblastomas most commonly represent isolated sporadic tumors; however, they may be heritable in an autosomal dominant pattern. Up to 30% to 40% of patients with retinoblastoma have bilateral tumors; familial disease should be considered in these cases.

Because the radiologic hallmark of retinoblastoma is the presence of intraocular calcification before the age of 3 years, CT remains the best imaging modality for the detection of retinoblastoma, as seen in this case (A). CT is also important in assessing the other eye for small calcifications. MR imaging is not as sensitive in detecting calcification. Not all retinoblastomas (particularly small ones) have calcification, so the absence of calcification does not exclude the possibility of retinoblastoma. MR imaging plays an important role in assessing these patients because retinoblastoma may spread along the nerves and vessels to the retrobulbar orbit, and there may be subarachnoid seeding. Both modes of transmission may result in intracranial dissemination of the disease. Therefore, patients with retinoblastoma should be evaluated with MR imaging to determine the extent of the disease.

Diffusion-weighted imaging (DWI) is particularly helpful as these tumors demonstrate reduced diffusion with low ADC values, which provides a good contrast to the high intensity of the vitreous on the ADC maps. DWI is also valuable in evaluating the response to eye-preservation treatment. A small percentage (<5%) of patients with bilateral retinoblastomas may also have a pineoblastoma of the pineal gland ("third eye").

REFERENCES

de Graaf P, Pouwels PJ, Rodjan F, et al. Single-shot turbo spin-echo diffusion-weighted imaging for retinoblastoma: initial experience. *AJNR Am J Neuroradiol*. 2012;33(1):110-118. doi:10.3174/ajnr.A2729.

Jansen RW, de Bloeme CM, Brisse HJ, et al. MR imaging features to differentiate retinoblastoma from Coats' disease and persistent fetal vasculature. *Cancers (Basel)*. 2020;12(12):3592.

Neuroradiology: THE REQUISITES. 4th ed. pp 318-319.

CASE 54

Perivascular Spaces (Virchow–Robin Spaces)

1. **A.** Imaging findings are consistent with perivascular spaces.
2. **B.** Tumefactive perivascular spaces can mimic cystic neoplasms, but usually have no edema and no enhancement. The only exception is the "anterior temporal pole perivascular space," which can have surrounding edema.
3. **C.** A variety of low-grade cystic neoplasms can mimic the appearance of dilated PVSs. Pilocytic astrocytomas, gangliogliomas, and pleomorphic xanthoastrocytomas (PXA) are easily distinguished from enlarged PVSs, as they generally contain areas of solid enhancement with variable surrounding edema. Dysembryoplastic neuroepithelial tumors (DNETs) and multinodular and vacuolating neuronal tumors (MVNTs) could be mistaken for dilated PVSs. DNETs are benign, slow-growing WHO grade I tumors classically seen in temporal lobes and present with seizures, with a characteristic "bubbly" cystic appearance and 30% may have minimal enhancement. MVNT is a more recently described entity characterized by clustered "bubbly" subcortical tumors that are not suppressed on FLAIR with no enhancement.
4. **B.** Cryptococcus (especially in immunocompromised patients).

Comment

This case illustrates the typical appearance of perivascular spaces (PVSs) previously known as Virchow–Robin spaces. PVSs are divided into three subtypes based on location: Type I appear along lenticulostriates entering the basal ganglia through the anterior-perforated substance. Type II are found along the path of perforating medullary arteries as they enter cortical gray matter over the high convexities. Type III appear in the midbrain.

Diagnostic considerations for PVSs, particularly along the basal ganglia, include chronic lacunar infarcts (which typically have a surrounding rim of gliosis on FLAIR); however, other developmental cysts, cystic neoplasms, and occasionally chronic infections could potentially share many of the same imaging features. Dilated PVSs can usually be distinguished from a lacunar infarct on the basis of typical imaging findings. Lacunar infarcts tend to occur in the upper half of the putamen, whereas PVSs occur along the inferior half. In addition, whereas PVSs are usually isointense to CSF on all pulse sequences, lacunar infarcts usually have a thin hyperintense rim on T2-weighted and FLAIR images, representing gliosis. Dilated PVSs are not associated with edema or enhancement, have a characteristic location along the anterior commissure, and are frequently bilateral and symmetric.

PVSs are extensions of the subarachnoid space that follow the perforating vessels at the base of the brain into the basal ganglia. Virchow–Robin spaces may range from 1 to 15 mm in size, although occasionally they can be larger, as seen in this case. They tend to enlarge with age and in the presence of hypertension. This makes sense because most vessels (including those along the PVSs) become more ectatic under both of these circumstances. In addition, just as the subarachnoid spaces become more prominent with age in that the PVSs are extensions of the subarachnoid space, it makes sense that they enlarge in a similar manner. Given the extension of the PVSs from the subarachnoid space into the brain, they are a conduit for the spread of a variety of inflammatory and neoplastic processes (e.g., Cryptococcus, neurosarcoidosis, intravascular lymphoma, carcinomatosis, etc.).

REFERENCES

Eluvathingal Mittikkal TJ, Raghavan P. Spontaneous regression and recurrence of a tumefactive perivascular space. *Neuroradiol J*. 2014;27(2):195-202.

Hernandez Mdel C, Piper RJ, Wang X, et al. Towards the automatic computational assessment of enlarged perivascular spaces on brain magnetic resonance images: a systematic review. *J Magn Reson Imaging*. 2013;38(4):774-785.

Rudie JD, Rauschecker AM, Nabavizadeh SA, Mohan S. Neuroimaging of dilated perivascular spaces: from benign and pathologic causes to mimics. *J Neuroimaging*. 2018;28(2):139-149. doi:10.1111/jon.12493.

Salzman KL, Osborn AG, House P, et al. Giant tumefactive perivascular spaces. *AJNR Am J Neuroradiol*. 2005;26(2):298-305.

Neuroradiology: THE REQUISITES. 4th ed. p 214.

CASE 55

Agenesis of the Corpus Callosum

1. **A.** Colpocephaly. Note that the asymmetric prominence of the occipital horns of the lateral ventricles, secondary to agenesis of the corpus callosum, gives a characteristic "racing car appearance" on axial images (Figure 55.1) and a "Texas longhorn" appearance on coronal images (Figure 55.3). Other features as seen in this case are elevated and slightly prominent third ventricle and small frontal horns. This baby was born at 36 weeks of gestation, and was large for gestational age, with respiratory distress syndrome of newborn, agenesis of the corpus callosum, and neonatal hypoglycemia.
2. **C.** Isolated dysgenesis of the corpus callosum is often asymptomatic. Note that the clinical picture in patients with agenesis is dictated by other abnormalities that are frequently associated.
3. **D.** The corpus callosum forms from the front (genu) to back (splenium) with the rostrum formed at the last. Also remember, in partial dysgenesis of the corpus callosum, the anterior portion of the corpus callosum (except the rostrum) is typically spared.
4. **E.** Lipomas, migrational abnormalities, Dandy–Walker syndrome, Chiari malformations, and holoprosencephaly, to name just a few!

Comment

Axons arising from the right and left cerebral hemispheres grow into the lamina reuniens (the dorsal aspect of the lamina terminalis), giving rise to the corpus callosum (and the hippocampal commissures). The corpus callosum develops between the 11th and 20th gestational weeks in an organized manner, with the formation of the anterior genu first followed in order by the anterior body, posterior body, splenium, and rostrum. Given this pattern of development, in partial dysgenesis of the corpus callosum, the anterior portion is formed and partial dysgenesis affects the posterior portions (posterior body, splenium) and rostrum. In cases in which the splenium is very small or is not visualized, partial dysgenesis of the corpus callosum can be readily distinguished from an insult to a previously fully developed splenium by checking for the presence of the rostrum. If the rostrum is absent, the splenial abnormality corresponds to partial dysgenesis. However, if the rostrum is present, given that it forms after the splenium, a splenial abnormality must have occurred on the basis of an insult resulting in secondary atrophy or volume loss.

Imaging findings in complete agenesis of the corpus callosum include lack of convergence of the lateral ventricles, which are displaced laterally and oriented in a vertical fashion; a high-riding third ventricle (which may form an interhemispheric cyst); and ex vacuo enlargement of the occipital and temporal horns (colpocephaly) related to deficient white matter. The Probst bundles are the white matter tracts that were destined to cross the corpus callosum. The axons that would usually cross from the right to left in the corpus callosum instead form tracts that run anterior to posterior along the medial walls of the lateral ventricles parallel to the interhemispheric fissure.

REFERENCES

Bayram E, Topcu Y, Yis U, et al. Comparison of cranial magnetic resonance imaging findings and clinical features in patients with corpus callosum abnormalities. *Neuropediatrics.* 2014;45(1):30-35.

Cignini P, D'Emidio L, Padula F, et al. The role of ultrasonography in the diagnosis of fetal isolated complete agenesis of the corpus callosum: a long-term prospective study. *J Matern Fetal Neonatal Med.* 2010;23(12):1504-1509.

Neuroradiology: THE REQUISITES. 4th ed. pp 265-270.

CASE 56

Calvarial Metastases—Lung Carcinoma

1. **C.** Imaging findings are consistent with multiple calvarial metastases.
2. **F.** All of these primary cancers can present with blastic osseous metastases.
3. **E.** All of these primary cancers can present with lytic osseous metastases.
4. **D.** DWI is a more sensitive sequence for identifying focal skull metastases for breast and lung malignancies and, compared with conventional MR imaging, provides improved detection of these lesions. Note that DWI is insensitive for detecting skull metastases from prostate carcinoma.

Comment

This case shows multiple calvarial lytic metastases in a patient with lung carcinoma. Primary tumors that commonly metastasize to the skull are breast, lung, melanoma, prostate and thyroid cancer (usually follicular). Prostate carcinoma is the most common cause of blastic metastases in men. Other carcinomas that may present with blastic metastases include breast carcinoma and, less commonly, Hodgkin's lymphoma, and mucinous carcinomas of the lung, colon, transitional cell carcinoma (TCC), carcinoid, medulloblastoma, and neuroblastoma. On the other hand, lytic metastases, which are more common than sclerotic metastases, are seen with non-small-cell lung cancer (as in this case), thyroid cancer, renal cell cancer, melanoma, etc.

In older patients, blastic or mixed metastases (blastic and lytic) can be mistaken for the "cotton-wool" appearance of diffuse calvarial Paget's disease. On close examination of a CT scan, these can often be distinguished. In addition to having regions of sclerosis or lysis, Paget's disease is usually associated with thickening of the diploic space, as well as cortical thickening. In contrast, metastatic disease (as in this case) is typically not associated with significant bone expansion, and instead causes cortical destruction (Figure 56.2) with transcalvarial soft tissue (Figures 56.1–56.8) and intracranial dural enhancement (Figure 56.8).

When there is a question about the diagnosis, particularly in a patient without a known systemic malignancy, a bone scan may be performed. In most instances, both pagetoid bone and metastatic disease will be "hot"; however, the reason to perform the bone scan is not to assess the skull, but rather to assess the remainder of the skeleton for evidence of additional foci of metastatic disease. Paget's disease is not infrequently polyostotic (involving multiple sites); however, plain radiographs of additional pagetoid lesions detected on bone scans usually have a characteristic appearance.

Bone metastases are usually hypointense on T1-weighted images (normal intradiploic fat is hyperintense on T1) and hyperintense on DWI with a low ADC value due to the restriction of water and generally enhance after contrast administration, as seen in this case. Note that DWI provides improved detection of all types of skull metastasis over conventional MR imaging by 20% for breast cancer and 36% for lung cancer. DWI is also more useful for detecting focal metastases, especially in areas with complex anatomy and multiple different normal signal intensities, such as the supraorbital region and the skull base. DWI is not helpful relative to conventional MR imaging for detecting skull metastases when the primary lesion is prostate carcinoma or when the skull metastases are diffuse.

REFERENCES

Kotecha R, Angelov L, Barnett GH, et al. Calvarial and skull base metastases: expanding the clinical utility of Gamma Knife surgery. *J Neurosurg.* 2014;121:91-101.

Nemeth AJ, Henson JW, Mullins ME, Gonzalez RG, Schaefer PW. Improved detection of skull metastasis with diffusion-weighted MR imaging. *AJNR Am J Neuroradiol.* 2007;28(6):1088-1092.

Pinker K, Stadlbauer A, Bogner W, et al. Molecular imaging of cancer: MR spectroscopy and beyond. *Eur J Radiol.* 2012;81(3):566-577.

Neuroradiology: THE REQUISITES. 4th ed. pp 72-74, 432-433, 438.

CASE 57

Giant Aneurysm—Left Superior Cerebellar Artery

1. **C.** Giant, partially thrombosed aneurysm of the left superior cerebellar artery, incorporating the tip of the basilar artery as well as the P1 segment of the left posterior cerebral artery. The patent lumen measures >2.5 cm. Although angiography will adequately assess the patent lumen, it cannot evaluate the true size of these aneurysms because the thrombosed portions are not visualized, as seen in this case (Figures 57.1–57.4).
2. **C.** Painful ophthalmoplegia.
3. **C.** An aneurysm with a maximal diameter larger than 2.5 cm.
4. **D.** All of these include the middle cerebral artery, cavernous internal carotid artery, and tip of the basilar artery.

Comment

Giant intracranial aneurysms are those that exceed 25 mm in the greatest dimension and make up ~ 5% of all intracranial aneurysms. These typically manifest during the fifth to seventh decades of life with a female predominance. Common predisposing factors include advanced age, hypertension, tobacco use, arteriovenous malformations, connective tissue disorders (including Ehlers–Danlos syndrome, Marfan syndrome, and autosomal dominant polycystic renal disease), and vasculitis. Fibromuscular dysplasia (FMD) is an arterial disease of an unknown etiology and can also be rarely associated with giant intracranial aneurysms, as seen in this case (arrow in Figure 57.6).

Giant aneurysms may present with subarachnoid hemorrhage or symptoms caused by mass effect (nausea, vomiting, focal neurologic deficits) related to aneurysm size or intraparenchymal rupture or hematoma.

A thrombus may form within large aneurysms and may be a source of distal emboli. Unenhanced CT may show the giant aneurysm as a hyperdense mass (Figure 57.1). At its periphery, there may be heterogeneous density related to the presence of thrombus. On MR imaging, giant aneurysms have a characteristic appearance, as seen in this case. Findings include signal void consistent with the flow in the patent lumen, phase artifacts related to flow, and heterogeneous signal intensity representing thrombi of varying ages.

Recent investigations with CT angiography in the setting of subarachnoid hemorrhage have shown detection rates for all aneurysms as high as 96%. False-negative findings may be related to the CT angiography technique, aneurysm size (especially those < 3 mm), and aneurysm location. Advantages of CT angiography include its rapidity, noninvasiveness, ability to provide information about potential neuroangiographic intervention, and ability to provide preoperative information about the relationship of an aneurysm to adjacent bony landmarks. Catheter angiography is still the most commonly used technique and remains the accepted gold standard.

Management of giant intracranial aneurysms is challenging due to their complex anatomy. Optimal therapy requires careful planning with consideration of aneurysm size, shape, neck dimensions, relation to adjacent neural structures and branch artery origins, among other factors. Endovascular management (including embolization with or without stent or balloon assistance) may be used alone (as was done in this case), in combination with surgical techniques. When feasible, clipping is usually the preferred neurosurgical technique.

REFERENCES

Kalani MY, Zabramski JM, Hu YC, Spetzler RF. Extracranial-intracranial bypass and vessel occlusion for the treatment of unclippable giant middle cerebral artery aneurysms. *Neurosurgery.* 2013;72(3):428-435.

Labeyrie MA, Lenck S, Bresson D, et al. Parent artery occlusion in large, giant, or fusiform aneurysms of the carotid siphon: clinical and imaging results. *AJNR Am J Neuroradiol.* 2015;36(1):140-145.

Mehta RI, Salamon N, Zipser BD, Mehta RI. Best cases from the AFIP: giant intracranial aneurysm. *Radiographics.* 2010;30(4):1133-1138.

Neuroradiology: THE REQUISITES. 4th ed. pp 142-145.

CASE 58

Vascular Infundibulum—Posterior Communicating Artery (PCOM)

1. **B.** The ophthalmic artery.
2. **A.** The most common location for an infundibulum is the origin of the posterior communicating artery (PCOM) from the supraclinoid internal carotid artery and can be seen in up to 25% of all cerebral angiograms.
3. **D.** An infundibulum should meet the following criteria: (1) it measures 3 mm or smaller; (2) it is triangular or funnel-shaped; and (3) the posterior communicating artery arises from its apex.
4. **B.** Approximately 15%.

Comment

These angiographic images demonstrate the typical appearance of a posterior communicating artery infundibulum, showing its funnel shape as well as the origin of the posterior communicating artery from the apex of the infundibulum. Because the management is dramatically different, angiographic images in anteroposterior, lateral, and oblique projections should be obtained to accurately differentiate an aneurysm from an infundibulum.

CT angiography is increasingly used in the diagnosis and evaluation of intracranial aneurysms. In the acute setting, there are several indications for prompt imaging evaluation, including nontraumatic subarachnoid hemorrhage; acute-onset third nerve palsy that involves the pupil (to exclude a posterior communicating or superior cerebellar artery aneurysm); and in the postoperative setting, to evaluate complications after placement of an aneurysm clip. In approximately 15% of patients with spontaneous subarachnoid hemorrhage, no aneurysm is found on initial angiography. In patients with angiogram-negative acute nontraumatic subarachnoid hemorrhage, follow-up angiography is usually indicated. It is important to remember that all potential sites of aneurysm formation must be assessed with conventional angiography. False-negative interpretations of a CTA can be in the following situations: (1) small aneurysms <3 mm, (2) presence of vasospasm, (3) thrombosed aneurysms, (4) nonsaccular aneurysms (dissecting aneurysms), (5) blister-type aneurysms, and (6) mycotic aneurysms.

In the acute setting, postoperative angiography is often indicated in the evaluation of perioperative ischemic sequelae (which may be due to embolic phenomena, vasospasm, or vascular occlusion). Postoperative or intraoperative angiography on an elective basis may be performed to assess for residual aneurysm after aneurysm clipping.

REFERENCES

Conijn MM, Hendrikse J, Zwanenburg JJ, et al. Perforating arteries originating from the posterior communicating artery: 7.0-Tesla MRI study. *Eur Radiol.* 2009;19(12):2986-2992.

Fischer S, Hopf N, Henkes H. Evolution from an infundibulum of the posterior communicating artery to a saccular aneurysm. *Clin Neuroradiol.* 2011;21(2):87-90.

Shi WY, Li YD, Li MH, et al. Differential diagnosis of infundibular dilation versus a small aneurysm of the internal carotid artery: assessment by three-dimensional rotational angiography with volume rendering. *Neurol Sci.* 2013;34(7):1065-1070.

Neuroradiology: THE REQUISITES. 4th ed. pp 144-145, 358.

CASE 59

Closed-Head Injury—Diffuse Axonal Injury

1. **D.** Imaging findings are consistent with grade 3 diffuse axonal injury (DAI), also known as shear injury, with several small regions of susceptibility at the gray–white matter junction, corpus callosum, and in the brainstem (Figures 59.2, 59.4–59.7), surrounded by areas of FLAIR hyperintensity (Figure 59.3).

2. **E.** Demyelinating diseases (multiple sclerosis and/or acute disseminated encephalomyelitis) present with white matter lesions typically involving the callososeptal interface but with no associated susceptibility on GRE/SWI. Note that no lesions were seen in the callososeptal interface in Figure 59.1.

3. **D.** The lobar white matter, the corpus callosum (most commonly the splenium, but also the undersurface of the posterior body), and the dorsolateral aspect of the upper brainstem (midbrain and pons).

4. **B.** DAI is difficult to diagnose on CT as the findings can be very subtle. All others are correct.

   DAI lesions are more common in the posterior and splenial regions of the corpus callosum because with a rotational acceleration of the head, shear forces develop across the corpus callosum. Anteriorly, there is less strain because the falx is shorter and allows transient displacement of the frontal lobes across the midline. Posteriorly, the falx is broader and more rigid, preventing motion of the cerebral hemispheres across the midline.

Comment

Diffuse axonal injury (DAI) is the result of shear-strain forces induced by angular rotation or acceleration of the head that result in partial or complete disruption of involved axons. Patients have loss of consciousness and a spectrum of cognitive impairment and neurological dysfunction beginning at the moment of trauma. Symptoms may range from transient loss of consciousness at the time of injury to permanent coma (vegetative state) or death in the most severe diffuse forms. DAI is most commonly seen in patients involved in high-velocity acceleration–deceleration motor vehicle accidents, but it can also be seen in more minor forms of trauma, such as a fall down the stairs and occasionally falls from a standing position. It is characterized by multiple focal lesions in the lobar white matter at the gray–white matter interface, in the corpus callosum, and in cases of severe head trauma, in the dorsolateral brainstem. Shear injuries are typically elliptical in shape, with the long axis parallel to the direction of the involved axons, as seen in this case.

MRI is the most sensitive imaging modality for the detection and evaluation of DAI; in the acute setting, however, the initial imaging study should still be a noncontrast head CT to exclude potentially treatable acute intracranial hemorrhage (subdural and epidural hematomas or large parenchymal hematomas). If there is concern about shear injury, MR imaging should be performed when the patient is stable. Shear injuries, unless hemorrhagic or of substantial size, frequently go undetected on CT. The presence of intraventricular hemorrhage should raise suspicion of injury to the septum pellucidum or corpus callosum. On MRI,

shear injuries are hyperintense on T2W and FLAIR images with susceptibility on SWI or GRE sequences, which are extremely sensitive to paramagnetic blood products, as seen in this case. Nonhemorrhagic lesions will, however, be visible as regions of high FLAIR signal.

DAI can be graded as (1) stage 1 (lobar), with lesions confined to the gray–white matter junction, (2) stage 2 (callosal), with lesions in the corpus callosum (posterior body and splenium), invariably in addition to the lobar white matter, and (3) stage 3 (brainstem), with lesions in the brainstem, in addition to the lobar white matter and corpus callosum.

REFERENCES

Bodanapally UK, Shanmuganathan K, Saksobhavivat N, et al. MR imaging and differentiation of cerebral fat embolism syndrome from diffuse axonal injury: application of diffusion tensor imaging. *Neuroradiology.* 2013;55(6):771-778.

Gentry LR. Imaging of closed head injury. *Radiology.* 1994;191(1):1-17. doi:10.1148/radiology.191.1.8134551.

Mamere AE, Saraiva LA, Matos AL, et al. Evaluation of delayed neuronal and axonal damage secondary to moderate and severe traumatic brain injury using quantitative MR imaging techniques. *AJNR Am J Neuroradiol.* 2009;30(5):947-952.

Rutgers DR, Fillard P, Paradot G, et al. Diffusion tensor imaging characteristics of the corpus callosum in mild, moderate, and severe traumatic brain injury. *AJNR Am J Neuroradiol.* 2008;29(9):1730-1735.

Neuroradiology: THE REQUISITES. 4th ed. pp 162-165.

CASE 60

Cerebral Amyloid Angiopathy (CAA)

1. **F.** All of these conditions can present with multiple small foci of susceptibility on SWI.

2. **C.** In patients with CAA, microhemorrhages are typically seen peripherally and larger hemorrhages are lobar in distribution. In contrast, hypertensive microhemorrhages are located in a more central distribution in the basal ganglia, thalami, pons, and cerebellar hemispheres.

3. **E.** All of the above. This case illustrates several of the imaging findings of CAA in this elderly patient with multiple bilateral lobar cerebral microhemorrhages and superficial siderosis. Notice the lack of microhemorrhages in the deep gray nuclei (Figure 60.3). In addition, CAA can also present with convexity subarachnoid hemorrhage; the presence of they have been incorporated into the Modified Boston Criteria to diagnose CAA without the need for an invasive biopsy. Additional imaging findings include ischemic leukoencephalopathy (Figures 60.1 and 60.2), lacunar infarcts, prominent perivascular spaces as well cerebral atrophy.

4. **B.** Scattered lobar hemorrhages in a patient aged 55 years or older have been incorporated into the Modified Boston Criteria to diagnose CAA without the need for an invasive biopsy. This increases the likelihood of Alzheimer's disease that is associated with cerebral amyloid deposition and accumulation of cerebral amyloid-β (Aβ) in various parts of the CNS.

Comment

Cerebral amyloid angiopathy (CAA) results from the deposition of β-pleated proteins within the media and adventitia of small- and medium-sized vessels of the superficial layers of the cortex and leptomeninges. Amyloid deposition increases with age and results in loss of elasticity of the walls of involved vessels. On pathological examination, microaneurysms and fibrinoid degeneration are often present. Amyloid stains intensely with Congo red dye (previously referred to as congophilic angiopathy) and demonstrates yellow-green birefringence under polarized light.

On CT and MR imaging, hemorrhages are characteristically lobar in location, and the most commonly occur in the frontal and parietal lobes. Multiple hemorrhages of different ages, as well as multiple simultaneous hemorrhages, are often present. Subarachnoid and subdural blood may be present due to perforation of blood through the pia arachnoid or involvement of superficial blood vessels with amyloid deposition. MR imaging, including GRE and SWI sequences, may be especially useful for demonstrating the full extent of intracranial involvement (as seen in this case). Multiple hypointense foci on GRE/SWI may also be related to multiple cavernomas, prior radiation, hypertensive microhemorrhages, etc. Importantly, there is no association of hypertension with the development of amyloid angiopathy.

REFERENCES

Fountas KN, Tsougos I, Gotsis ED, et al. Temporal pole proton preoperative magnetic resonance spectroscopy in patients undergoing surgery for mesial temporal sclerosis. *Neurosurg Focus.* 2012;32(3):E3.

Howe KL, Dimitri D, Heyn C, et al. Histologically confirmed hippocampul structural features revealed by 3T MR imaging: potential to increase diagnostic specificity of mesial temporal sclerosis. *AJNR Am J Neuroradiol.* 2010;31(9):1682-1689.

Linn J, Halpin A, Demaerel P, et al. Prevalence of superficial siderosis in patients with cerebral amyloid angiopathy. *Neurology.* 2010;74(17):1346-1350.

Neuroradiology: THE REQUISITES. 4th ed. pp 133-134.

CASE 61

Mesial Temporal Sclerosis

1. **C.** Mammillary body. Notice the atrophy of the contralateral (R) mammillary body in this patient with right mesial temporal sclerosis.
2. **C.** Asymmetric atrophy and signal abnormality of the right hippocampus, with distortion of intrinsic architecture (Figures 61.1–61.3). Notice the associated ex vacuo prominence of the right temporal horn, with a small size of the right mammary body and fornix. The constellation of these findings is consistent with mesial temporal sclerosis (MTS).
3. **D.** Fornix. Atrophy of the ipsilateral fornix and mammillary body is seen in patients with long-standing MTS, as seen in this case (Figure 61.4).
4. **D.** MTS is characterized by volume loss of the hippocampus with associated ex vacuo dilation of the adjacent temporal horn which is considered one of the least specific neuroimaging findings. High signal intensity on T2W and FLAIR images in the hippocampus (Figures 61.1–61.3) is present. Note that the administration of IV gadolinium is not necessary for establishing the diagnosis of MTS.

Comment

Temporal lobe epilepsy is the most common epilepsy syndrome in adults. Seizures usually begin in late childhood or adolescence. Virtually all patients have complex partial seizures. In most patients, the epileptogenic focus involves the structures of the mesial temporal lobe. These structures include the hippocampus, amygdala, and parahippocampal gyrus. The histologic substrate in approximately two-thirds of cases is mesial temporal sclerosis (MTS). The hippocampal formation located in the mesial temporal lobe protrudes into the medial temporal horn

and is roofed by the choroidal fissure. It is a complex structure composed of the hippocampus proper, subiculum, dentate gyrus, parahippocampal gyrus, fimbria, and fornix. The hippocampus proper (or cornu ammonis) can be subdivided into four subfields, CA1 to CA4, depending on the appearance of pyramidal neurons. Neuronal loss is accompanied by fibrillary gliosis, leading to hippocampal atrophy. In MTS, gliosis may also affect the amygdala, uncus, and parahippocampal gyrus.

The differential diagnosis for hippocampal sclerosis includes cortical dysplasias and primary brain neoplasm. MTS is usually characterized by high-resolution thin-section coronal FLAIR and T2W and T1W gradient volumetric sequences as illustrated in this case. This case highlights the classic MR imaging appearance of MTS with atrophy of the right hippocampus, ipsilateral dilation of the adjacent temporal horn, and atrophy of the ipsilateral fornix and mammillary body.

Whether MTS is the cause or the result of temporal lobe epilepsy is controversial and so is the relationship of MTS with febrile seizures. It was demonstrated that there was no clear occurrence of increased incidence of MTS in patients even after prolonged febrile seizures.

REFERENCES

Chen YJ, Nabavizadeh SA, Vossough A, Kumar S, Loevner LA, Mohan S. Wallerian Degeneration beyond the corticospinal tracts: conventional and advanced MRI findings. *J Neuroimaging.* 2017;27(3):272-280. doi:10.1111/jon.12404.

Tarkka R, Pääkkö E, Pyhtinen J, Uhari M, Rantala H. Febrile seizures and mesial temporal sclerosis: no association in a long-term follow-up study. *Neurology.* 2003;60(2):215-218.

Neuroradiology: THE REQUISITES. 4th ed. pp 308-310.

CASE 62

Mineral Deposition in the Basal Ganglia on T1W Imaging—Mineralizing Microangiopathy

1. **C.** There is bilaterally symmetric hyperintensity in the basal ganglia and thalami on unenhanced T1W imaging (Figure 62.5), low signal on T2 (Figure 62.1) and FLAIR (Figure 62.2) with susceptibility on GRE (Figure 62.4), findings consistent with mineral deposition, "mineralizing microangiopathy," in this patient with a history of prior cranial radiotherapy.
2. **F.** All of these can be seen as a late complication of cranial irradiation among childhood brain tumor survivors, and many of them can even present with devastating strokes during the follow-up period. Although cranial irradiation remains necessary for the treatment of brain tumors, strategies to prevent and treat its late effects on cerebral vasculature are urgently required.
3. **A.** Neurofibromatosis type 1.
4. **E.** All of these can present with T1 hyperintensity in the basal ganglia.

Comment

Mineralizing microangiopathy, a distinctive histopathologic process involving the microvasculature of the central nervous system (CNS), is usually seen following combined radiation and chemotherapy for the treatment of CNS neoplasms in childhood. CT typically demonstrates calcification within the basal ganglia and subcortical white matter. The areas of calcification may give paradoxically increased signal on T1-weighted MRI due to a surface-relaxation mechanism, and decreased signal on T2-weighted images, as seen in this case. It is important to note that the axial image (Figure 62.5) is a precontrast T1W image, and the bilaterally symmetric high signal intensity in the basal ganglia should not be mistaken for enhancement.

In a large study assessing the risk of damage to cerebral vasculature in long-term survivors of childhood brain tumors after radiotherapy, the incidence of mineralizing microangiopathy was found to be about 30%, with a cumulative prevalence at 20 years of follow-up of 25% (95% CI, 16%–39%). Clinical background is essential to differentiate from other conditions that have a similar appearance on neuroimaging such as Fahr disease and other abnormalities of calcium and phosphate metabolism.

High signal intensity in the basal ganglia on unenhanced T1W images is also described in patients with manganese deposition secondary to chronic liver dysfunction, patients receiving hyperalimentation, and those with portosystemic shunting. Other causes of T1 hyperintensity in the basal ganglia include Wilson's disease, hyperglycemia, and recently described gadolinium deposition.

Neurofibromatosis type 1 (NF1) is the most common neurocutaneous disorder. It is associated with a variety of intracranial lesions, the most common of which are foci of high signal intensity on long TR images within the brain parenchyma. The foci of high signal intensity are seen most commonly in the basal ganglia; however, they are frequently noted in the white matter tracts of the corpus striatum, in the brainstem, and in the cerebellum. The basal ganglia lesions may be hyperintense on unenhanced T1W images. It has been suggested that the pathologic basis of these foci in neurofibromatosis type 1 may be related to hypomyelination, migrational abnormalities, and nonneoplastic hamartomatous changes. A recent study in which pathologic correlation was obtained suggests that at least some of the foci of signal abnormality may be related to vacuolar or spongiotic change.

REFERENCES

Hegde AN, Mohan S, Lath N, Lim CC. Differential diagnosis for bilateral abnormalities of the basal ganglia and thalamus. *Radiographics*. 2011;31(1):5-30.

Remes TM, Suo-Palosaari MH, Koskenkorva PKT, et al. Radiation-induced accelerated aging of the brain vasculature in young adult survivors of childhood brain tumors. *Neurooncol Pract*. 2020;7(4):415-427.

Shanley DJ. Mineralizing microangiopathy: CT and MRI. *Neuroradiology*. 1995;37(4):331-333.

Neuroradiology: THE REQUISITES. 4th ed. pp 84, 223, 291-293.

CASE 63

Basilar Meningitis—Tuberculosis

1. **B.** Diffuse enhancement of the basal cisterns with associated FLAIR hyperintensity, findings consistent with tuberculous meningitis.
2. **D.** All of the above. CNS infections such as tuberculosis, neurosyphilis, pyogenic infections, *Cryptococcus*, other inflammatory conditions such as neurosarcoidosis, leptomeningeal seeding of tumor (carcinomatosis from systemic malignancies or primary brain tumors), lymphoma, and chemical meningitides can all present with basilar meningitis.
3. **A.** The hydrocephalus is usually "communicating" due to blockage of the basal cisterns and arachnoid villi with an inflammatory exudate. Hydrocephalus may also result from mass effect related to a parenchymal lesion, or from entrapment of a ventricle related to ependymitis.
4. **A.** Diffuse leptomeningeal glioneuronal tumor is a recently described CNS tumor (2016 WHO update) presenting with numerous subpial cystic nodular areas and prominent leptomeningeal enhancement, often without an identifiable parenchymal mass, mimicking chronic meningitis.

Comment

There has been an increased incidence of tuberculosis in the United States. The cause of this is multifactorial and is related in part to HIV/AIDS and the emergence of drug-resistant strains of the bacillus. Approximately 5% to 10% of patients with tuberculosis go on to have CNS disease (approximately 5%–20% of patients with AIDS have CNS manifestations). Tuberculous infection in children is usually related to primary infection, whereas in adults, it is usually caused by postprimary infection.

Tuberculous meningitis is the most common presentation of intracranial tuberculosis and usually refers to infection of the leptomeninges. Besides meningitis, CNS tuberculosis has a spectrum of other clinical and radiologic presentations, including cerebritis or encephalitis, abscess formation, and tuberculoma. Intracranial tuberculosis has two related pathologic correlates—meningitis and tuberculoma—which coexist in approximately 10% of cases. Tuberculomas are tubercles that form as a result of cell-mediated immunity. They are walled off by a fibrous capsule and are centrally necrotic, with surrounding lymphocytes and giant cells. Tuberculomas may be dormant for years. They may resolve, cause symptoms related to lesion location (seizure, mass effect), or rupture into the subarachnoid space, causing meningitis to form a gelatinous exudate in the basal cisterns. FLAIR imaging is very sensitive in the detection of subarachnoid and leptomeningeal disease, which manifests as sulcal hyperintensity in the affected areas. Avid enhancement of the involved areas is the rule. Arteritis may be seen in up to one-third of patients with basilar meningitis. This is because the vessels coursing through this inflammatory exudate may become directly involved. Consequences of arteritis include vasospasm and infarction. CNS tuberculosis is usually related to hematogenous dissemination from a systemic source, most commonly, the lung, but also possibly the genitourinary system or gastrointestinal tract.

REFERENCES

Kalita J, Prasad S, Maurya PK, Kumar S, Misra UK. MR angiography in tuberculous meningitis. *Acta Radiol*. 2012;53(3):324-329.

Mohan S, Jain KK, Arabi M, Shah GV. Imaging of meningitis and ventriculitis. *Neuroimaging Clin N Am*. 2012;22(4):557-583.

Oztoprak I, Gumus C, Oztoprak B, Engin A. Contrast medium-enhanced MRI findings and changes over time in stage I tuberculous meningitis. *Clin Radiol*. 2007;62(12):1206-1215.

Pienaar M, Andronikou S, van Toorn R. MRI to demonstrate diagnostic features and complications of TBM not seen with CT. *Childs Nerv Syst*. 2009;25(8):941-947.

Neuroradiology: THE REQUISITES. 4th ed. pp 191-195.

CASE 64

Dural Metastases—Breast Carcinoma

1. **B.** Metastatic disease. CT and MRI show a dural-based mass in the left frontal lobe involving the overlying calvarium with surrounding vasogenic edema and midline shift. Note the additional osseous metastases in the skull and upper cervical spine (Figure 64.1). Also note dural tails on Figure 64.6 which are not specific for meningiomas and can be seen in sarcoidosis, lymphoma, pleomorphic xanthoastrocytomas (PXA), and dural metastases (as in this case). This patient had stage IV breast cancer with metastatic disease to the bone and previously underwent a breast lumpectomy with subsequent chemotherapy and radiation therapy.
2. **A.** Cortical metastases. Tiny cortical metastases may be missed in the absence of intravenous gadolinium contrast.
3. **A.** Breast carcinoma.
4. **B.** Neuroblastoma.

Comment

This case of metastatic breast carcinoma illustrates several findings and imaging patterns of metastatic disease. There is a diffuse enhancement of the dura over the left cerebral convexity with a large left frontal dural-based mass. Notice the additional osseous metastases in the calvarium, skull base, and visualized upper cervical spine.

Dural metastases are usually secondary to hematogenous dissemination of tumors from extracranial systemic tumors but can also occur secondary to retrograde seeding through the vertebral venous plexus (particularly in the spine), as well as lymphatic seeding. Dural metastases may also result from direct extension of adjacent calvarial or skull base bone metastases, as was seen in this case. Breast, lung, and prostate carcinoma as well as melanoma and lymphoma are commonly associated with dural metastases in adults. In children, neuroblastoma and leukemia are most commonly associated with dural metastases. Neuroblastoma may also metastasize to the cranial sutures. In infancy, this may present as widened sutures. Inflammatory processes that may mimic dural metastases include granulomatous infections (tuberculosis, syphilis, and fungal), neurosarcoidosis, Langerhans cell histiocytosis, and Erdheim–Chester disease.

REFERENCES

Cipolla V, Santucci D, Guerrieri D, et al. Correlation between 3T apparent diffusion coefficient values and grading of invasive breast carcinoma. *Eur J Radiol.* 2014;83(12):2144-2150.
Trimboli RM, Veradi N, Cartia F, et al. Breast cancer detection using double reading of unenhanced MRI including T1-weighted, T-2 weighted STIR, and diffusion-weighted imaging: a proof of concept study. *AJR Am J Roentgenol.* 2014;203(3):674-681.
Neuroradiology: THE REQUISITES. 4th ed. pp 47-48.

CASE 65

Rathke's Cleft Cyst

1. **D.** Rathke's cleft cyst. Craniopharyngiomas demonstrate calcification (on CT), an associated soft tissue mass, or areas of solid enhancement. Pituitary apoplexy is an acute clinical syndrome with the presence of blood products on MRI, also see case 26.
2. **A.** The vast majority of Rathke's cleft cysts are asymptomatic and are detected incidentally, as in this case.
3. **B.** Unlike pituitary adenomas, which are more frequently localized in the lateral portion of the gland, large autopsy series have shown that the vast majority of Rathke's cleft cysts are localized in the center of the gland (pars intermedia), aka "pars intermedia cysts."
4. **C.** Eccentric nonenhancing intracystic nodule has been demonstrated in up to 77% of cases and is considered pathognomonic of a Rathke's cleft cyst. It is slightly hyperintense to the surrounding fluid on T1 and hypointense on T2, as seen in this case. On histologic examination, these intracystic nodules appear as mucinous material and as cholesterol and protein on biochemical analysis. The amount of protein in these intracystic nodules influences signal intensity on MRI.

Comment

Rathke's cleft cysts are embryologic remnants of Rathke's pouch, the neuroectoderm that ascends from the oral cavity to the sella to form the anterior pituitary lobe and pars intermedia. In the majority of cases, Rathke's cleft cysts are asymptomatic and are incidentally noted at autopsy or identified on imaging studies performed for other reasons. In a recent series of 1000 autopsy specimens, 11% of the pituitary glands had an incidental Rathke's cleft cyst. These lesions are typically localized within the pituitary sella, although they may also extend into the suprasellar region. In addition, Rathke's cleft cysts may be centered in the suprasellar cistern anterior to the hypothalamic stalk. A single layer of cuboidal or columnar epithelium, which may contain goblet cells, typically lines these cysts.

The contents within the cysts are mucoid, resulting in their typical MR imaging appearance. Most Rathke's cleft cysts are circumscribed and hyperintense on both unenhanced T1W and T2W images. Although this is the most common pattern, cysts may also be hypointense or isointense on either T1W or T2W images, depending on their protein concentration and viscosity. In this case, the cyst is hyperintense on unenhanced T1W imaging and hyperintense on T2W imaging, with an intracystic nodule that is slightly hyperintense on unenhanced T1W images and hypointense on T2W images. These cysts do not enhance (although there may be mild peripheral enhancement), as seen in this case. At surgery, these appear as yellow, waxy solid masses, and the pathologic correlate shows a mucin clump.

Although most Rathke's cleft cysts are incidental findings, symptoms may occur with larger lesions that compress the optic chiasm (resulting in headache and visual disturbances) or pituitary gland (patients may present with diabetes insipidus or hypopituitarism).

REFERENCES

Binning MJ, Gottfried ON, Osborn AG, Couldwell WT. Rathke cleft cyst nodule: a characteristic magnetic resonance image finding. *J Neurosurg.* 2005;103(5):837-840.
Byun WM, Kim OL, Kim D. MR imaging findings of Rathke's cleft cysts: significance of intracystic nodules. *AJNR Am J Neuroradiol.* 2000; 21(3):485-480.
Neuroradiology: THE REQUISITES. 4th ed. pp 271-272, 358-360.

CASE 66

Optic Neuritis (Demyelinating Disease)

1. **D.** Optic neuritis. High signal intensity within the right optic nerve was associated with avid solid enhancement of the optic nerve sheath complex.
2. **B.** Marcus Gunn pupil is the term given to an abnormal pupil showing an aberrant pupillary response and is often used synonymously with a relative afferent pupillary defect (RAPD). The "swinging light test" or Marcus Gunn test is used to detect an RAPD, which means detecting differences between the two eyes in how they respond to a light shone in one eye at a time. This test is very useful for detecting unilateral or asymmetrical disease of the retina or optic nerve.
   Argyll Robertson pupil (ARP): bilateral small irregular pupils that do not react to light but constrict to accommodation and are classically seen in late neurosyphilis. Pseudo-Argyll Robertson pupil: when this is seen in nonsyphilitic conditions, e.g., diabetes mellitus, midbrain lesions, stroke, etc.
3. **D.** Contrast enhancement on fat-suppressed, T1W images is seen in more than 94.5% of patients with acute optic neuritis due to blood–brain barrier breakdown (as in this case).

Comment

A wide spectrum of disease processes may be associated with optic neuritis, most commonly, demyelinating disease followed by idiopathic disease. Approximately 50% of patients with optic neuritis have multiple sclerosis, and approximately 15% of patients with multiple sclerosis have optic neuritis as their initial clinical presentation. Typical optic neuritis (as is encountered in multiple sclerosis) is a unilateral and short segment. In contrast, in the setting of neuromyelitis optica (NMO) and anti-MOG, encephalomyelitis involvement is usually bilateral and longitudinally extensive, which mirrors the pattern of involvement in the spinal cord.

In older patients, vasculopathies and ischemia are more common causes of optic neuritis. Other potential etiologies include toxins, prior radiation, human immunodeficiency virus (HIV), and other systemic viral infections such as varicella or herpes.

Patients presenting with optic neuritis can be assessed using high-resolution, fat-suppressed, fast spin-echo T2W, STIR and enhanced T1W images, as in this case. Imaging in the coronal plane is particularly useful. Imaging may demonstrate increased T2W signal intensity within the nerve itself, and postcontrast images may demonstrate enhancement of the nerve in more than 90% of patients due to blood–brain barrier breakdown (as in this case). Note that the normal optic nerve does not enhance, but the optic nerve sheath may mildly enhance due to the pial vascular network.

In cases of clinically diagnosed optic neuritis, MR imaging of the brain is especially useful and is recommended because it may help to establish the diagnosis of demyelinating disease. In patients with their first episode of optic neuritis, up to 65% have asymptomatic cerebral white matter lesions on brain MRI.

REFERENCES

Hickman SJ, Wheeler-Kingshott CA, Jones SJ, et al. Optic nerve diffusion measurement from diffusion-weighted imaging in optic neuritis. *AJNR Am J Neuroradiol.* 2005;26(4):951-956.
Kupersmith MJ, Alban T, Zeiffer B, Lefton D. Contrast-enhanced MRI in acute optic neuritis: relationship to visual performance. *Brain.* 2002;125(Pt 4):812-822. doi:10.1093/brain/awf087.
McKinney AM, Lohman BD, Sarikaya B, et al. Accuracy of routine fat-suppressed FLAIR and diffusion-weighted images in detecting clinically evident acute optic neuritis. *Acta Radiol.* 2013;54(4):455-461.
Neuroradiology: THE REQUISITES. 4th ed. pp 212-213, 326-328.

CASE 67

Toxoplasmosis Infection in Acquired Immunodeficiency Syndrome

1. **B.** In immunocompromised patients where neuroimaging shows multiple lesions, whether serologic results are negative or positive, antitoxoplasmosis therapy should be initiated. Open biopsy with decompression is reserved for extremely sick patients with impending herniation.
2. **C.** Toxoplasmosis is rare in immunocompetent patients.
3. **A.** Thallium-201 SPECT will demonstrate minimal or no uptake in cerebral toxoplasmosis as opposed to primary CNS lymphoma.
4. **C.** Congenital cerebral toxoplasmosis presents with multiple calcifications in the basal ganglia and cortex as well as hydrocephalus. In severe cases, there may be microcephaly.

Comment

Cerebral toxoplasmosis is caused by the intracellular protozoan *Toxoplasma gondii.* Toxoplasma encephalitis is most commonly seen in immunocompromised patients with impaired cellular immunity, especially in the setting of HIV/AIDS. Other immunodeficient conditions associated with increased infection include following organ transplantation, long-term steroid therapy or chemotherapy, and impaired immunity from an underlying malignancy. In the setting of HIV/AIDS, radiologic differentiation

between toxoplasmosis and lymphoma can be difficult. Both entities may have multiple lesions, and both may have solid or ring enhancement. Toxoplasmosis has a predilection for the basal ganglia and the corticomedullary junction. T2 signal intensity of the lesions is variable, from hyperintense to isointense, or may show concentric alternating zone of hypo/hyper/isointense signal, "concentric target sign." Lesions may be hemorrhagic, as shown in this case.

Diffusion-weighted imaging with apparent diffusion coefficient (ADC) maps has been used to distinguish these two lesions. Toxoplasmosis lesions have demonstrated significantly greater diffusion than lymphoma, with increased diffusion relative to that in normal white matter, in contrast to the restricted diffusion seen within pyogenic abscesses. Increased diffusion in toxoplasmosis lesions has been postulated to reflect relatively decreased viscosity within the central cores of the lesions, perhaps due to an impaired cellular immune response related to the immunocompromised state of these patients. The core of the lesion, in this case, demonstrates primarily facilitated diffusion. These lesions often demonstrate ring or nodular enhancement, with infolding of the cyst wall also referred to as "eccentric target sign" on postcontrast images. Recent investigations with perfusion MR imaging have shown decreased relative cerebral blood volumes in toxoplasmosis lesions (attributed to the avascularity of abscesses) compared with increased blood volumes in lymphoma (attributed to increased vascularity in regions of metabolically active tumors).

Findings favoring lymphoma are hyperdense masses on an unenhanced CT, ependymal spread on enhanced MR imaging (rare in toxoplasmosis), and a periventricular distribution. Distinguishing these two disease processes is important because they are treated differently. Primary lymphoma responds to radiation therapy; however, the benefit of radiation therapy is diminished when treatment is delayed, as may happen in patients first treated empirically for toxoplasmosis. Thallium-201 SPECT can be effective (sensitive and specific) in distinguishing lymphoma (takes up thallium) from toxoplasmosis (normally does not take up thallium). Positron emission tomography has been shown to be useful in the accurate differentiation of hypometabolic toxoplasmosis lesions versus metabolically active lymphoma.

REFERENCES

Evaluation and management of intracranial mass lesions in AIDS. Report of the Quality Standards Subcommittee of the American Academy of Neurology. *Neurology.* 1998;50(1):21-26. doi:10.1212/WNL.50.1.21.
Kumar GG, Mahadevan A, Guruprasad AS, et al. Eccentric target sign in cerebral toxoplasmosis: neuropathological correlate to the imaging feature. *J Magn Reson Imaging.* 2010;31(6):1469-1472.
Mahadevan A, Ramalingaiah AH, Parthasarathy S, et al. Neuropathological correlate of the "concentric target sign" in MRI of HIV-associated cerebral toxoplasmosis. *J Magn Reson Imaging.* 2013;38(2):488-495.
Neuroradiology: THE REQUISITES. 4th ed. pp 199-200.

CASE 68

Neurocysticercosis

1. **C.** Cysticercosis. However, these lesions can mimic a spectrum of infectious and inflammatory processes (e.g., septic emboli, bacterial abscesses) as well as metastatic disease.
2. **A.** The most common parasitic infection of the CNS is cysticercosis. Other less frequent infections are toxoplasmosis, echinococcosis, and schistosomiasis.
3. **B.** Seizures are seen in 30% to 90% of symptomatic patients. Symptoms are dependent on the stage of infestation, as well

as the sites of parasitic CNS involvement. Patients remain frequently asymptomatic in the initial stages of cerebral infection and the mature cystic phase of infection, when the larvae are alive. Patients may become symptomatic as the larvae die because the larvae incite a significant inflammatory reaction. Headache, vertigo, and vomiting are seen in patients with "Bruns syndrome" with an obstructing intraventricular lesion.

4. **C.** Fourth ventricle.

Comment

Cysticercosis is the most common parasitic infection of the CNS. It usually involves the intracranial compartment, and it may rarely involve the spinal cord. Cysticercosis is endemic to Central and South America, parts of Asia, Mexico, Africa, and India. The pork tapeworm (*Taenia solium*) is the causative agent. Humans may become the definitive host (the parasite sexually reproduces) by eating inadequately cooked pork that harbors the larvae of the pork tapeworm (cysticerci). These larvae develop into tapeworms in the small intestine that release eggs that pass into the stool. If humans ingest food or water contaminated by these ova, they may serve as an intermediate host. In the stomach, the ova release oncospheres (primary larvae), which enter the bloodstream through the gastrointestinal mucosa. These primary larvae may deposit within muscle and subcutaneous tissue, although they have a propensity to infect the CNS. There are multiple patterns of neurocysticercosis, including the parenchymal pattern (the larvae penetrate directly into the brain), the intraventricular pattern (which involves the ependyma or choroid plexus), and the subarachnoid pattern (involves the meninges). In mixed neurocysticercosis, there is involvement of the parenchyma, ventricles, or subarachnoid spaces. Patients with parenchymal involvement may present with seizures and neurologic signs (e.g., confusion, dementia, paresis, paresthesias, visual disturbances). Intraventricular involvement may be symptomatic if there is obstructive hydrocephalus, and meningeal involvement may result in communicating hydrocephalus.

There is a spectrum of radiologic appearances, depending on the stage of the disease; however, imaging findings are frequently characteristic. In the initial stage of cerebral infection, the larvae result in small, edematous lesions that are hypodense on CT and hyperintense on T2W images. The cysticerci then develop into cysts that range in size from millimeters to centimeters and contain a scolex. There may be mild surrounding edema in the brain. As the cysts die, there is an intense inflammatory reaction in the adjacent brain parenchyma that may result in prominent edema and mass effect. It is at this time that patients may be most symptomatic, presenting with seizures or focal neurologic signs. After years of infestation, the cysts finally collapse and often calcify (as seen in this patient). Rim enhancement has been described in as many as 38% of calcified lesions, also seen in this patient who was a pig farmer in Burma. He had long-standing seizures and developed right-sided mesial temporal sclerosis (not shown).

REFERENCES

Gupta RK, Awasthi R, Garg RK, et al. T1-weighted dynamic contrast-enhanced MR evaluation of different stages of neurocysticercosis and its relationship with serum MMP-9 expression. *AJNR Am J Neuroradiol.* 2012;35(4):997-1003.

Lucato LT, Guedes MS, Sato JR, et al. The role of conventional MR imaging sequences in the evaluation of neurocysticercosis: impact on characterization of the scolex and lesion burden. *AJNR Am J Neuroradiol.* 2007;28(8):1501-1504.

Neuroradiology: THE REQUISITES. 4th ed. pp 198-201.

CASE 69

Paget's Disease—Osteodystrophica Deformans (Osteitis Deformans)

1. **A.** Osteoporosis circumscripta. Osteolysis is most commonly seen in the frontal or occipital region.
2. **C.** Paget's disease is a disease of middle-aged and elderly persons, whereas fibrous dysplasia is typically seen in children and young adults. In contrast to fibrous dysplasia, extensive involvement of the facial bones is uncommon in Paget's disease. Paget's disease causes cortical thickening, compared with fibrous dysplasia, in which the cortex is relatively spared.
3. **G.** All of these are known complications of Paget's disease.

Comment

In Paget's disease, there is a malfunction in the normal process of bone remodeling. When an area of bone is destroyed, the new bone replacing it is soft and porous. Bone affected with Paget's disease also has increased vascularity. The cause of Paget's disease is unknown; however, a viral etiology (paramyxovirus) is postulated. Paget's disease is more common in men than in women, and it usually presents after the age of 40 years. It is often an incidental finding detected on radiographs obtained for other reasons, as seen in this case. Patients may be symptomatic, depending on the distribution of the disease. Involvement of the calvarium may present with enlarging head size. Involvement of the skull base, resulting in platybasia, may lead to neurologic symptoms (weakness and paralysis). Hearing loss may result if there is fixation of the ossicles. Compression of the eighth cranial nerve due to overgrowth of bone may cause sensorineural hearing loss. There is usually relative sparing of the otic capsule. Paget's disease has multiple stages, including an initial osteolytic phase characterized by osteoclastic activity with resorption of normal bone. This phase is followed by excessive and sporadic new bone formation as a result of osteoblastic activity. Eventually, Paget's disease enters its inactive stage.

Neoplastic involvement within the pagetoid bone is not uncommon and includes sarcomatous degeneration, giant cell tumors, superimposed hematologic neoplasms (myeloma, lymphoma), and metastatic disease. Giant cell tumors are typically confined to the skull and less often to the facial bones. It is speculated that the increased blood flow within the pagetoid bone may make it more susceptible to deposition of metastases. Clinically, the development of neoplastic disease in the pagetoid bone should be suspected if there is increased pain or an associated soft tissue mass.

The differential diagnosis of Paget's disease of the skull includes other sclerotic bone lesions, hyperostosis frontalis, fibrous dysplasia, and metastatic disease. In the elderly, metastatic disease may have the cotton-wool appearance of Paget's disease (prostate cancer in men and breast cancer in women).

REFERENCES

Libicher M, Kasperk C, Daniels M, et al. Dynamic contrast-enhanced MRI in Paget's disease of bone—correlation of regional microcirculation and bone turnover. *Eur Radiol.* 2008;18(5):1005-1011.

Scutellari PN, Giorgi A, De Sario V, Campanati P. Correlation of multimodality imaging in Paget's disease of bone. *Radiol Med.* 2005;110:603-615.

Neuroradiology: THE REQUISITES. 4th ed. pp 403, 584.

CASE 70

Carbon Monoxide Poisoning

1. **B.** Globus pallidus. Note the sparing of the putamina, a classic finding of carbon monoxide poisoning.

2. **C.** The most common cause is carbon monoxide poisoning. Other toxic exposures that can cause bilateral pallidal abnormalities include cyanide and manganese (hyperalimentation).
3. **D.** All of these conditions can present with bilateral pallidal abnormalities.
4. **D.** Excitotoxic brain injury is a final common pathway of many toxic and metabolic disorders where there is an excessive release of glutamate in the synaptic cleft which can lead to cell swelling and subsequent death (i.e., cytotoxic edema) in the event of ischemia and cell failure with disruption of glutamate reuptake. If the reuptake of glutamate is maintained, cell swelling and death may not occur; instead, intramyelinic edema occurs. Intramyelinic edema is a reversible non-neurotoxic edema characterized by restricted diffusion. The periventricular white matter and the splenium, which are known to have a higher metabolism, are especially susceptible to these changes, as seen in this case.

Comment

Injury to the brain with a particular predilection for the basal ganglia may be seen in a variety of toxic exposures, neurodegenerative processes, and metabolic disorders. Because the globus pallidus is sensitive to hypoxia, its bilateral symmetric necrotic involvement is the hallmark of carbon monoxide poisoning. In addition to the globus pallidi, less common sites that may be involved are the hippocampi, caudate nuclei, putamina, thalami, cerebellum, corpus callosum, and cerebral cortex. The second most commonly affected site is the cerebral white matter (up to one-third of patients), which can show delayed leukoencephalopathy in the subacute phase of carbon monoxide poisoning.

Carbon monoxide is a colorless and odorless gas and binds hemoglobin ~250 times stronger than O_2 causing hypoxic/anoxic brain injury. It presents with abnormal hypodensity on CT or T2W hyperintensity on MR imaging within the bilateral globus pallidi, which may enhance in the subacute phase, as seen in this case (Figure 70.5). Although carbon monoxide toxicity has a characteristic imaging appearance, the diagnosis is usually established by the clinical circumstances in which the patient is found. The diagnosis of carbon monoxide toxicity is confirmed by the identification of carboxyhemoglobin in the blood.

Patients with carbon monoxide poisoning may experience sudden neurologic deterioration and coma approximately 2 to 3 weeks after the initial injury. Imaging often shows accompanying toxic leukoencephalopathy, which relates to cerebral white matter alterations that are potentially reversible if rapidly and correctly recognized. It presents with bilateral symmetric confluent areas of restricted diffusion involving the periventricular white matter (Figures 70.7 and 70.8) with sparing the basal ganglia (Figures 70.3 and 70.4). Subsequent normalization of findings is related to intramyelinic edema, as described earlier. On delayed imaging performed months to years after carbon monoxide injury, T2W hypointensity in the deep gray matter, especially the putamen, may be present and is likely due to mineralization.

REFERENCES

Beppu T, Nishimoto H, Fujiwara S, et al. 1H-magnetic resonance spectroscopy indicates damage to cerebral white matter in the subacute phase after CO poisoning. *J Neurol Neurosurg Psychiatry*. 2011;82(8):869-875.
de Oliveira AM, Paulino MV, Vieira APF, et al. Imaging patterns of toxic and metabolic brain disorders. *Radiographics*. 2019;39(6):1672-1695.
Hegde AN, Mohan S, Lath N, Lim CC. Differential diagnosis for bilateral abnormalities of the basal ganglia and thalamus. *Radiographics*. 2011;31(1):5-30.
Lin WC, Lu CH, Lee YC, et al. White matter damage in carbon monoxide poisoning intoxication assessed in vivo using diffusion tensor MR imaging. *AJNR Am J Neuroradiol*. 2009;30(6):1248-1255.
Neuroradiology: THE REQUISITES. 4th ed. pp 116, 219-220.

CASE 71

Wallerian Degeneration

1. **D.** Restricted diffusion along the left corticospinal tract in this neonate with acute right MCA territory infarction reflects acute Wallerian degeneration (WD).
2. **D.** In the spinal cord, WD is seen in the dorsal column cranial to the site of injury and in lateral corticospinal tracts below the level of injury. The length of the involved segment is proportional to the number of axons that are damaged. Therefore, the length is more in the cervical region, where the axons are more tightly packed as compared to the thoracolumbar region.
3. **B.** Ipsilateral atrophy of the corticospinal tract is seen in the chronic stages.
4. **F.** In addition to the corticospinal tract where the occurrence of WD is most common, all of these are additional neural tracts that can demonstrate WD. Besides cerebral infarction, other causes of WD include trauma, necrosis, focal demyelination, or hemorrhage.

Comment

Wallerian degeneration (WD) is a secondary manifestation of brain injury from a spectrum of causes. Secondary antegrade degenerative changes of axons and their myelin sheaths occur along the distal axonal segment as a result of an injury to the proximal axon or neuronal cell body. Among the causes of degeneration of the corticospinal tract pathways, the most common is cerebral infarction, as seen in this neonate. Other injuries and neurodegenerative processes (e.g., amyotrophic lateral sclerosis) may result in WD. It may occur as a result of trauma, hemorrhage, white matter disease, including demyelination, or neoplasia and its treatment (radiation injury). Histologically, WD represents several stages of progressive axonal degradation, ultimately resulting in gliosis and volume loss.

MRI is superior to CT in detecting WD, especially in the acute stages. CT may show the later changes in atrophy of the involved corticospinal pathways within the brainstem, but it does not show the earlier changes. On MRI, signal alteration on T2W or T1W images may be seen as early as 4 weeks after an injury (some studies have shown these changes even earlier), and in the late stages (weeks to months), signal alteration and atrophy are invariably present. In the late stages, T2W hyperintensity is accompanied by hypointensity on corresponding T1W images. More recent work has shown that diffusion-weighted imaging (DWI) and corresponding apparent diffusion coefficient (ADC) maps may reflect the changes of acute WD within a week, manifesting as restricted diffusion (hyperintensity on diffusion-weighted images) and hypointensity on corresponding ADC images (low ADC values), as seen in this case.

REFERENCES

Chen YJ, Nabavizadeh SA, Vossough A, Kumar S, Loevner LA, Mohan S. Wallerian degeneration beyond the corticospinal tracts: conventional and advanced MRI findings. *J Neuroimaging*. 2017;27(3):272-280.
Liu X, Tian W, Kolar B, et al. Hyperintensity on diffusion weighted image alone ipsilateral cortical spinal tract after cerebral ischemic stroke: a diffusion tensor analysis. *Eur J Radiol*. 2012;81(2):292-297.
Mittal P, Gupta R, Mittal A, Mittal K. MRI findings in a case of spinal cord Wallerian degeneration following trauma. *Neurosciences (Riyadh)*. 2016;21(4):372-373.
Puig J, Pedraza S, Blasco G, et al. Wallerian degeneration in the corticospinal tract evaluated by diffusion tensor imaging correlates with motor deficit 30 days after middle cerebral artery ischemic stroke. *AJNR Am J Neuroradiol*. 2010;31(7):1324-1330.
Neuroradiology: THE REQUISITES. 4th ed. pp 223-224.

CASE 72

Thyroid Ophthalmopathy—with Optic Nerve Compression in the Orbital Apex

1. **C.** Thyroid-associated orbitopathy is the most common cause of proptosis in adults.
2. **D.** The lateral rectus muscle. An easy mnemonic to remember the order of extraocular muscle involvement in thyroid-associated orbitopathy is "I'M SLOw." *I*nferior rectus, *M*edial rectus, *S*uperior rectus, *L*ateral rectus, and *O*bliques.
3. **D.** All of these are vascular causes of extraocular muscle enlargement.
4. **C.** Patients with thyroid-associated orbitopathy generally present with dry eyes, puffy eyelids, bulging eyes, diplopia, visual/field loss, and/or ocular pressure. Pain with eye movement is uncommon.

Comment

Thyroid-associated orbitopathy is more common in women by a ratio of 4:1 and is frequently asymptomatic; however, when present, it may be seen in euthyroid or hyperthyroid states. Clinical signs and symptoms may include proptosis, lid retraction, decreased ocular range of motion, visual loss resulting from compression of the optic nerve in the orbital apex, and corneal exposure caused by eyelid retraction. Pain is uncommon. The most common cause of unilateral or bilateral exophthalmos in adults is thyroid-associated orbitopathy. The incidence of bilateral disease may be as high as 90% of cases. Most patients evaluated with CT or MR imaging carry a known diagnosis of thyroid ophthalmopathy, and the role of imaging is to assess for the presence of optic nerve compression in the orbital apex by enlarged muscles, as in these cases. When there is compromised vision in patients who do not respond to medical therapy, orbital decompression by removal of the osseous walls around the orbital apex may be necessary.

MRI may also be useful in evaluating patients with thyroid-associated orbitopathy without laboratory or clinical evidence of thyroid disease. The most common patterns of extraocular muscle involvement are enlargement of all of the extraocular muscles or of the inferior and medial rectus muscles only. Isolated involvement of the lateral rectus muscle is unusual, and when present, it should raise suspicion for a different disease process, such as myositis or pseudotumor. Characteristically, in thyroid ophthalmopathy, there is an enlargement of the muscle bellies, with sparing of the tendinous insertions. In the late stages of the disease, fibrosis resulting in contraction of the muscle bellies may be evident, and there may be fatty replacement of the muscles.

REFERENCES

Parmar H, Ibrahim M. Extrathyroidal manifestations of thyroid disease: thyroid ophthalmopathy. *Neuroimaging Clin N Am.* 2008;18(3):527-536.
Tortora F, Cirillo M, Ferrara M, et al. Disease activity in Graves' ophthalmopathy: diagnosis with orbital MR imaging and correlation with clinical score. *Neuroradiol J.* 2013;26(5):555-564.
Neuroradiology: THE REQUISITES. 4th ed. pp 334-335.

CASE 73

Frontal Sinus Mucoceles

1. **C.** Mucocele. There is opacification of the left frontal sinus with osseous expansion (Figure 73.2) and breakthrough into the superior orbit with a mild displacement of the superior rectus muscle and globe (Figure 73.6).
2. **A.** Two-thirds of all mucoceles occur in the frontal sinus which is most prone to developing mucoceles, followed by ethmoid air cells, whereas the maxillary and sphenoid sinuses are rarely involved.
3. **C.** The signal characteristics of mucoceles on MRI depend on the protein concentration, water content, viscosity, and cross-linking of glycoproteins. They are often hyperintense on both T1W and T2W images, as seen in this case (Figures 73.4 and 73.6).
4. **D.** Air-filled cavities, secretions with increased viscosity/protein concentration or binding of different metals, can appear as a signal void on MRI. In the paranasal sinuses, low signal on T1 and T2 (signal-void) appearance is frequently attributed to fungal rhinosinusitis, giving rise to a pseudo-pneumatized sinus leading to diagnostic errors. In the course of the disease, fungal rhinosinusitis tends to desiccate, and accumulate macromolecular proteins, iron, calcium, magnesium, manganese, and other heavy metals, all contributing to a progressive reduction in signal intensity. This patient underwent FESS with pathology demonstrating sinonasal mucosa with chronic inflammation and fragments of bone. No fungal forms were identified.

Comment

This case shows an expansile lesion in the left frontal sinuses (in this patient with a history of chronic, recurrent sinus infections, and prior sinus surgeries). The material within the expansile frontal sinus is isodense on an unenhanced CT, consistent with mucoid material, and corresponding MR images show the material to be hyperintense on T1W (very common) and heterogeneous and hypointense on T2W images.

Mucoceles develop from obstruction of the sinus ostia or septated compartments of a sinus and represent mucoid secretions encased by mucus-secreting epithelium (sinus mucosa). In more than 90% of cases, mucoceles occur in the frontal sinuses or the ethmoid air cells (the anterior is more common than the posterior) and are least common in the sphenoid and maxillary sinuses. Patients frequently have a history of chronic sinusitis, trauma, or sinus surgery. When symptomatic, mucoceles present with signs and symptoms related to mass effect, including frontal bossing, headache, and orbital pain. Orbital extension, as in this case, may result in proptosis and diplopia. Secondary infection (mucopyocele) and direct extension into the anterior cranial fossa are not infrequent complications. Extension into the anterior cranial fossa or orbit is more likely if there is an associated fracture of an involved sinus wall. Alternatively, as a mucocele expands, it may directly erode a sinus wall, allowing for extrasinus extension. Advances in endoscopic sinus surgery have led to the acceptance of simple drainage procedures, even for some seemingly very complicated mucoceles.

In the radiologic evaluation of mucoceles, CT best demonstrates the osseous changes of the sinus walls, which may be remodeled and expanded, thinned, and with large mucoceles, partially dehiscent. However, MRI best detects the interface of the mucocele with the intraorbital and intracranial structures. When necessary, enhanced MRI is useful in distinguishing a mucocele (which shows thin peripheral enhancement) from a neoplasm (which typically shows solid enhancement).

REFERENCES

Aghakhanyan G, Lupi G, Frihia F, et al. Delayed post-traumatic fronto-ethmoidal sinus mucocele evaluated with short and long TE ME spectroscopy. *Neuroradiol J.* 2013;26(6):693-698.
Batra PS, Manes RP, Ryan MW, Marple BF. Prospective evaluation of intraoperative computed tomography imaging for endoscopic sinonasal and skull-base surgery. *Int Forum Allergy Rhinol.* 2011;1(6):481-487.
Neuroradiology: THE REQUISITES. 4th ed. pp 339-341, 427-429.

CASE 74

Vein of Galen Malformation (VOGM)

1. **D.** There is a marked enlargement of the vein of Galen with peripheral calcification (Figure 74.1), which connects posteriorly to the dilated straight sinus into dilated bilateral transverse and sigmoid sinuses, in keeping with a vein of Galen malformation. The internal cerebral veins are also dilated (Figure 74.4). The partially visualized vertebral arteries are dilated, probably feeding the vein of Galen malformation (Figure 74.3). Mild prominence of the ventricles and sulci.

2. **C.** The presentation varies with age and the type of malformation. In the neonatal period, presentation often results in high-output cardiac failure, although low-flow aneurysms may remain undetected. In infants, presentation is with macrocephaly, hydrocephalus while in a child, presentation is usually with developmental delay, hydrocephalus, and/or seizures.

3. **D.** The arrow in Figure 74.4 denotes the straight sinus. The falcine sinus, on the other hand, is present at birth in 2%–5% of individuals, usually arises from the vein of Galen or the anterior part of the straight sinus, and drains into the superior sagittal sinus. Persistent falcine sinus is the most common venous anomaly associated with the vein of Galen malformation in children, particularly if the straight sinus is absent, thrombosed, or rudimentary. In this situation, the aneurysmally enlarged median prosencephalic vein (MPV) drains into the falcine sinus.

4. **C.** Management of VOG malformations has evolved from bilateral internal carotid artery ligation to the present-day preferred endovascular strategies. Generally, treatment is postponed until the child is 5–6 months of age. Microsurgical obliteration employing occipital-transtentorial and infratentorial supracerebellar approaches has also been described. Radiosurgery has not been used widely due to its latent period. CSF diversion before the obliteration of the malformation can lead to subdural or intraventricular bleeding and also causes reversal of blood flow in the medullary veins, leading to brain hypoperfusion. Therefore, if necessary, shunts are usually performed after the completion of embolization.

Comment

Vein of Galen malformations (VOGM) are rare intracranial vascular anomalies, constituting 30% of all neurovascular abnormalities in children, and 1% of all pediatric congenital anomalies. Abnormal embryonic development causes arterial shunting into the median prosencephalic vein (MPV) of Markowski, which, although a precursor of the vein of Galen (VOG), is a separate entity, making the term VOGM a misnomer, probably better termed as median prosencephalic arteriovenous fistulas.

The CT appearance of a vein of Galen aneurysm in an infant is a characteristic sign. In unenhanced images, the vein of Galen appears as a hyperdense, demarcated mass at the level of the posterior third ventricle and diencephalon. After intravenous contrast administration, there is marked homogeneous enhancement of the malformation. MR imaging not only confirms the presence of flow within this abnormality but also better delineates both the arterial and venous anatomy. In combination with MR angiography, MR imaging may show large choroidal arteriovenous fistulas or the presence of a parenchymal AVM. Increasingly, the diagnosis of VOGM is being made antenatally with third-trimester antenatal ultrasound.

Early in embryologic development, the deep brain structures and diencephalon are drained by the MPV. As the internal cerebral veins begin to develop, this vein slowly regresses. A caudal remnant of the MPV becomes the normal vein of Galen. In patients with VOGM related to either a parenchymal AVM or a direct arteriovenous fistula between the choroidal vessels, a persistent MPV may occur. Because this provides diencephalic venous drainage, the straight sinus may not form (arrow in Figure 74.4). Instead, a falcine sinus is frequently noted. VOGM resulting from direct arteriovenous fistulas is frequently associated with venous obstruction and venous hypertension. High-output heart failure in newborns and hydrocephalus due to obstruction of the aqueduct of Sylvius by the enlarged vein of Galen with macrocephaly are common clinical scenarios in infants.

Treatment of these malformations is catheter angiography and endovascular embolization (both venous and arterial embolization) of the shunt. Several embolization procedures may be necessary to completely obliterate the vascular shunts and communications. This is often done as a staged procedure over a several-month period before the child is a toddler.

REFERENCES

Hassan T, Timofeev EV, Ezura M, et al. Hemodynamic analysis of an adult vein of Galen aneurysm malformation by use of 3D image-based computational fluid dynamics. *AJNR Am J Neuroradiol*. 2003;24(6):1075-1082.

Suazo L, Putman C, Vilchez C, Stoeter P. Unexpected silent infarctions after embolization of cerebral arteriovenous malformations and fistulas. A diffusion-weighted magnetic resonance imaging study. *Interv Neuroradiol*. 2013;19(2):209-214.

Neuroradiology: THE REQUISITES. 4th ed. pp 146-148.

CASE 75

Craniosynostosis—Metopic Suture

1. **B.** Premature closure of sutures that appear closed or nearly closed. This finding is abnormal for age, and the appearance suggests craniosynostosis. CT scan is recommended as the next step in evaluation.

2. **B.** Dolichocephaly, also known as scaphocephaly, is the most common form of craniosynostosis and accounts for approximately 50% of all cases. It is defined as premature closure of the sagittal suture resulting in impediment to the lateral growth of the skull while anteroposterior growth continues, producing a narrow, elongated, "boat-shaped" skull.

3. **A.** The sagittal suture is the most common suture to close prematurely. The next most common suture is coronal in ~20% of cases followed by metopic and lambdoid sutures.

4. **B.** Trigonocephaly refers to the triangular appearance of the frontal skull created by the premature fusion of the metopic suture (metopic craniosynostosis). It accounts for ~ 5% of all craniosynostosis cases.

Comment

Craniostenosis, or craniosynostosis, refers to the premature closure of one or more of the cranial sutures. Isolated premature closure of the sagittal suture is most common, occurring in more than 50% of cases of craniosynostosis. Unilateral or bilateral premature closure of coronal sutures is the next most common, followed by premature closure of the metopic suture. The lambdoid suture undergoes premature closure in ~1% of cases of craniosynostosis. Depending on the sutures involved, there are characteristic deformities of the skull and orbit. Premature closure of the sagittal suture results in a head that has limited growth in the transverse dimension. This results in dolichocephaly (scaphocephaly), in which there is an increase in head size in the anteroposterior dimension.

Plagiocephaly refers to premature closure of a single coronal or lambdoid suture (or, occasionally, a temporosquamous suture). In the majority of cases, plagiocephaly is seen with the closure of a single coronal suture, resulting in elevation of the lesser wing of the sphenoid bone and leading to a "harlequin" appearance of the orbit. Premature closure of both coronal sutures results in brachycephaly. Early fusion of the metopic suture in the frontal region results in trigonocephaly, or simply a "triangular" configuration of the head, as seen in this case. Craniosynostosis is usually an isolated abnormality, although it may be associated with a variety of congenital syndromes. Such conditions include Apert syndrome, which is associated with a "cloverleaf" deformity of the skull resulting from the closure of the coronal, lambdoid, and sagittal sutures. Other syndromes associated with craniostenosis are hypophosphatasia, Crouzon's disease (craniofacial dysostosis), and Treacher Collins syndrome (mandibulofacial dysostosis). Treatment is often with a cranioplasty, as was performed in this case (Figure 75.4 and 75.5).

REFERENCES

Rijken BF, Leemans A, Lucas Y, et al. Diffusion tensor imaging and fiber tractography in children with craniosynostosis syndromes. *AJNR Am J Neuroradiol*. 2015;36(8):1558-1564.
Simanovsky N, Hiller N, Koplewitz B, et al. Effectiveness of ultrasonographic evaluation of the cranial sutures in children with suspected craniosynostosis. *Eur Radiol*. 2009;19(3):687-692.
Neuroradiology: THE REQUISITES. 4th ed. pp 305-306.

CASE 76

Craniopharyngioma—Adamantinomatous Subtype

1. **A.** Suprasellar mass with a solid and a large cystic component representing craniopharyngioma. Notice the solid enhancing nodule measuring 1 cm in the inferior aspect of the mass. The cystic component is T2 (Figure 76.1) and T1 (Figure 76.4) hyperintense and is not suppressed on FLAIR images (Figure 76.2) consistent with proteinaceous material, with smooth thin rim enhancement (Figure 76.5). The mass abuts the posterior aspect of the optic chiasm and causes splaying of the optic tracts with elevation and displacement of the midbrain, mammillary bodies, and hypothalamus. The * on the sagittal image (Figure 76.6) denotes the pituitary gland. The mass is separate from the gland, making a pituitary macroadenoma unlikely.
2. **D.** Craniopharyngiomas are WHO grade I tumors, with a bimodal age distribution. Those in children between the ages of 5 and 10 years are of the adamantinomatous subtype. The second peak occurs later after the fourth decade of life. Adamantinomatous craniopharyngiomas are typically cystic with a lobulated contour. Solid components are present, but often form a relatively minor part of the mass, and demonstrate enhancement, as seen in this case. Calcification is seen in ~90%. On the other hand, papillary craniopharyngiomas tend to be more solid with few smaller cysts. Calcification is rare.
3. **A.** Adamantinomatous craniopharyngiomas are predominantly cystic or cystic and solid, with calcification and enhancement.

Comment

Craniopharyngiomas arise from metaplastic squamous epithelial rests (Rathke's pouch) along the hypophysis or from ectopic embryonic cell rests and are seen in children and adults. Histologically, they are characterized by palisading adamantinomatous epithelium, keratin, and calcification. They account for 1% to 3% of all intracranial neoplasms and 10% to 15% of all supratentorial tumors. There is no gender predilection. The majority of craniopharyngiomas arise within the suprasellar cistern (80%–90%), as in this case; however, they also may arise within the sella turcica and, occasionally, the third ventricle. Clinical

presentation includes visual disturbances related to compression of the optic chiasm, pituitary hypofunction related to compression of the gland or hypothalamus, and symptoms of increased intracranial pressure.

Imaging findings typically include a cystic or a solid and cystic mass lesion. Approximately 80% to 90% of all craniopharyngiomas have a cystic component. Smaller lesions may be purely solid. The majority (90%) of craniopharyngiomas have calcification or regions of avid homogeneous enhancement (in solid portions of the tumor) or peripheral enhancement (around cystic portions). As MRI may not be sensitive in detecting the presence of calcification, CT may be quite useful in establishing the diagnosis of craniopharyngioma. On MRI, the signal characteristics may be quite variable, depending on the contents and viscosity within the cysts. Whereas the cystic portion is frequently hyperintense on T2W and FLAIR imaging, it may be hypointense, isointense, or hyperintense on T1W imaging. High signal intensity on T1W images may be due to high concentrations of protein or methemoglobin "motor oil cysts" (rather than cholesterol or lipid products).

REFERENCES

Cohen M, Bartels U, Branson H, Kulkarni AV, Hamilton J. Trends in treatment and outcomes of pediatric craniopharyngioma. *Neuro Oncol*. 2013;15(6):767-774.
Kim EH, Ahn JY, Kim SH. Technique and outcome of endoscopy-assisted microscopic extended transsphenoidal surgery for suprasellar craniopharyngiomas. *J Neurosurg*. 2011;114(5):1338-1349.
Neuroradiology: THE REQUISITES. 4th ed. pp 358, 363-364, 368.

CASE 77

Subependymal Heterotopia

1. **C.** This infant presented with seizures. Patients with heterotopias most commonly present with seizures and sometimes with developmental delay.
2. **C.** Subependymal heterotopia. Nodules of gray matter are seen immediately deep to the ependyma, distorting the outlines of the ventricles and are most frequently seen in the region of the trigones and occipital horns, as in this case. These nodules follow gray matter on all sequences and do not enhance.
3. **A.** Although the majority of cases are sporadic, some are X-linked recessive (Xq28).
4. **D.** Approximately 90% are calcified on CT with variable enhancement.

Comment

This case illustrates multiple subependymal heterotopias that consist of clusters of disorganized neurons and glial cells that are located in close proximity to the ventricular walls. In subependymal heterotopia, nodules are often bilaterally symmetric along the length of the lateral ventricles, or there may be just a few lesions, as in this case. Heterotopias appear as masses that are isointense to gray matter on all pulse sequences and do not enhance. High signal intensity in the parenchyma surrounding the heterotopia should not occur. The differential diagnosis for subependymal heterotopia is limited, and the diagnosis is usually easily established by the stereotypical imaging appearance. Subependymal nodules in tuberous sclerosis are readily differentiated because they do not follow the signal characteristics of gray matter, and the vast majority are calcified (hypointense on T2W and gradient-echo susceptibility images and mildly hyperintense on unenhanced T1W images). In addition, other sequelae of tuberous sclerosis are commonly present. Metastatic masses are uncommon and typically enhance after contrast administration. Other signs of metastatic disease are frequently present in the intracranial compartment.

Periventricular heterotopia represents failed migration from the germinal region; however, some cases may result from abnormal proliferation of neuroblasts in the periventricular region, failure of regression, or apoptosis of neuroblasts within the germinal matrix. Heterotopia may be associated with a spectrum of other congenital anomalies, including Chiari malformations, ventral induction defects (holoprosencephaly, dysgenesis of the corpus callosum), other migrational abnormalities, and encephaloceles. Some cases have X-linked inheritance, and early antenatal diagnosis is important for appropriate management. In this patient, there is ex vacuo enlargement of the occipital horns of the lateral ventricles (colpocephaly) as a result of underdevelopment of the surrounding deep white matter and dysgenesis of the splenium of the corpus callosum.

REFERENCES

Barkovich AJ. Morphologic characteristics of subcortical heterotopia: MR imaging study. *AJNR Am J Neuroradiol*. 2000;21:290-295.
Donkol RH, Moghazy KM, Abolenin A. Assessment of gray matter heterotopia by magnetic resonance imaging. *World J Radiol*. 2012;4(3):90-96.
Merschhemke M, Mitchell TN, Free SL, et al. Quantitative MRI detects abnormalities in relatives of patients with epilepsy and malformations of cortical development. *Neuroimage*. 2003;18(3):642-649.
Mitchell LA, Simon EM, Filly RA, Barkovich AJ. Antenatal diagnosis of subependymal heterotopia. *AJNR Am J Neuroradiol*. 2000;21(2):296-300.
Neuroradiology: THE REQUISITES. 4th ed. p 274.

CASE 78

Optic Nerve Meningioma

1. **D.** Optic nerve meningioma. There is asymmetric thickening and hyperattenuation of the right optic nerve (Figure 78.1) with thickening and enhancement of the intraorbital and intracanalicular segments of the right optic nerve sheath (Figures 78.4–78.6), consistent with optic nerve meningioma. Note the additional meningiomas. Other entities such as sarcoid, lymphoma, and pseudotumor may result in this "tram-track" enhancement pattern of the optic nerve sheath (enhancing sheath around a filling defect that represents the optic nerve, Figures 78.4 and 78.5).
2. **B.** The vast majority of optic nerve meningiomas are sporadic and are direct extensions from intracranial meningiomas. The classic clinical triad includes painless, slowly progressive vision loss; optic nerve atrophy; and the presence of optociliary shunt vessels, which result after long-term compression of the central retinal vein.
3. **A.** Pneumosinus dilatans. It is characterized by the expansion of a paranasal sinus that contains only air. Pneumosinus dilatans involving the sphenoid sinus are associated with optic nerve meningiomas.

Comment

Optic nerve sheath meningiomas typically present with painless, slowly progressive vision loss. If the lesion goes undetected or misdiagnosed and enlarges, it may present later with proptosis and optic atrophy. These tumors are most commonly present in middle-aged women; however, they may also be present in children with neurofibromatosis type 2 in whom they are also frequently bilateral. Bilateral orbital meningiomas also may rarely occur when they arise from the tuberculum sellae or planum sphenoidale. In this situation, meningiomas normally grow anteriorly along the optic nerves, from the optic canal into the orbit. In every patient with suspected optic meningioma, it is important to assess both eyes and the region of the tuberculum sellae on imaging.

On imaging, "tram-tracking" is the term that has been used to describe both the pattern of enhancement and the pattern of calcification. On CT, 20% to 50% of optic nerve meningiomas have calcification along the nerve sheath. Linear enhancement may be seen on both sides of the optic nerve, as seen in this case. Other findings to assess on CT include secondary bony changes (erosion or hyperostosis) of the optic canal, sphenoid sinus, and planum sphenoidale. There may be enlargement of the optic canal. A major advantage of MRI is its ability to evaluate the optic nerve separately from the surrounding nerve sheath. This is extremely helpful in differentiating lesions arising from the optic nerve itself (optic neuritis, gliomas) from those arising from the nerve sheath (meningiomas, metastases, and granulomatosis disorders). In addition, because of artifacts arising from the bones, MRI is better than CT in evaluating the nerve within the optic canal as well as spread into the intracranial compartment. When performing MRI of the orbits, it is important to use fat suppression so that the full extent of the tumor around the optic nerve can be assessed. Limitations of MRI include its inability to detect small calcifications and artifacts (chemical shift or susceptibility from the aerated paranasal sinuses) in the orbit that may obscure small lesions.

Treatment of optic nerve meningiomas is problematic and depends on the degree of visual impairment and proptosis. In patients with preserved vision and no proptosis, conservative management is preferred with frequent ophthalmologic and imaging follow-ups. Severe proptosis requires surgery but almost invariably results in loss of vision. More recently, stereotactic radiotherapy has been utilized as an alternative approach to surgery.

REFERENCES

Lope LA, Hutcheson KA, Khademian ZP. Magnetic resonance imaging in the analysis of pediatric orbital tumors: utility of diffusion-weighted imaging. *J AAPOS*. 2010;14(3):257-262.
Tailor TD, Gupta D, Dalley RW, et al. Orbital neoplasms in adults: clinical, radiologic, and pathologic review. *Radiographics*. 2013;33(6):1739-1758.
Neuroradiology: THE REQUISITES. 4th ed. pp 327-330.

CASE 79

Venous Sinus Thrombosis

1. **D.** Cerebral venous thrombosis of the left transverse sinus, left sigmoid sinus, left jugular bulb, and proximal left internal jugular vein (not shown), with thrombus extending into the left vein of Labbe (Figure 79.5). Low attenuation with associated cortical expansion in the left inferolateral temporal lobe (Figure 79.1), with findings suggestive of venous ischemia on MRI.
2. **E.** There are several risk factors for cerebral venous sinus thrombosis including dehydration, oral contraceptive pills, pregnancy and postpartum status, steroids, prothrombotic conditions (antiphospholipid antibodies), infections (meningitis and otomastoiditis), trauma (skull fractures involving dural venous sinuses), sepsis, malignancy, etc.
3. **C.** Arachnoid granulations are typical of CSF density on CT and isointense to CSF on MRI, with no contrast enhancement.
4. **C.** The vein of Labbe is also known as the inferior anastomotic vein. It is part of the superficial venous system and is the largest vein on the lateral surface of the brain, connecting the superficial middle cerebral vein to the transverse sinus.

Comment

Cerebral venous thrombosis (dural venous sinus thrombosis, cortical vein thrombosis, and deep cerebral vein thrombosis) and venous infarction are commonly underdiagnosed because of the lack of consideration of these entities. Sinus thrombosis has a spectrum of clinical presentations, including headache and papilledema related to increased intracranial pressure, as well as focal neurologic deficits and seizures in cases complicated by intraparenchymal hemorrhage or venous infarction. Venous thrombosis is associated with a variety of underlying systemic disorders, as discussed earlier. Venous infarctions are frequently hemorrhagic and should be considered in the differential diagnosis of intracerebral hemorrhage in the absence of known risk factors (e.g., trauma, hypertension) and the presence of bilateral or subcortical hemorrhages that are not in a typical arterial vascular distribution.

Diagnosing venous thrombosis has become easier with noninvasive techniques, especially with advanced MRI sequences and CT venography (CTV). On CTV, thrombosis is readily identified as filling defects in the affected venous sinuses, as in this case. CTV is preferred over MRV and has a reported sensitivity of over 95% compared to DSA which remains the gold standard. Remember, filling defects in the venous sinuses should not be confused with arachnoid (Pacchionian) granulations that can be seen in essentially all dural sinuses and are especially common in the superior sagittal sinus and transverse sinus. MRI is superior as it is able to visualize the clot as well as associated parenchymal changes. However, MRI has several pitfalls, e.g., an acute clot is isointense on T1 and hypointense on T2 and thus can mimic a flow void. In addition, hypoplastic venous sinuses and slow flow remain problematic with 2D time of flight (TOF) MR venography (MRV) which is routinely performed in suspected cases. Contrast-enhanced MRV and 3D contrast-enhanced T1 sequences are more sensitive in detecting cerebral venous thrombosis than TOF MRV.

In subacute thrombosis, extracellular methemoglobin within the clot appears hyperintense on both T1W and T2W images. Flow-sensitive time-of-flight gradient echo images often are not helpful because both the methemoglobin in the thrombus and blood flow are hyperintense. In this situation, phase-contrast technique is helpful because it provides suppression of high signal from the hemorrhage such that only flow is shown on these images.

REFERENCES

Bal ZS, Sen S, Yildiz KB, et al. Tuberculous otomastoiditis complicated by sinus vein thrombosis. *Braz J Infect Dis.* 2012;16(6):608-609.
Saindane AM, Mitchell BC, Kang J, et al. Performance of spin-echo and gradient-echo T1-weighted sequences for evaluation of dural venous sinus thrombosis and stenosis. *AJR Am J Roentgenol.* 2013;201(1):162-169.
Neuroradiology: THE REQUISITES. 4th ed. pp 134-137, 386-391.

CASE 80

Osseous Metastases in the Occipital Condyle and C1

1. **C.** Findings are consistent with osseous metastases involving the right occipital condyle and right lateral mass of C1. Notice the normal fatty marrow on the left side.
2. **C.** There is asymmetric extra-osseous soft tissue encroaching into the right hypoglossal canal, as indicated by the arrow in Figure 80.6.
3. **D.** Cranial nerve XII palsy that presents with tongue fasciculations, deviation, and weakness.
4. **E.** All of these are correct regarding occipital condylar fractures that are uncommon injuries usually resulting from high-speed MVC.

Comment

In children, abnormalities of the craniovertebral junction may be congenital (Chiari malformations) or acquired (traumatic, inflammatory, neoplastic). In adults, acquired craniovertebral and occipital condyle lesions may result from trauma (fractures due to axial loading with ipsilateral flexion), inflammatory disorders (such as rheumatoid arthritis), and metabolic disorders (such as Paget's disease and hyperparathyroidism) and may result in basilar invagination. In addition, primary hematologic malignancies and metastatic disease to the craniovertebral junction, and more specifically, the occipital condyles, are not uncommon and are often overlooked. Many primary malignancies such as those arising from the gastrointestinal tract, prostate, breast, and lung may metastasize to the condyles. Spread is most likely hematogenous.

The occipital condyles and pathology affecting them are often missed because they are frequently seen only at the edge of films (the inferior sections of an axial brain MR imaging or CT scan and the lateral sections of a sagittal MR imaging scan).

Most patients present with occipital headaches or neck pain, which may be associated with cranial neuropathies related to the extension of the tumor into the hypoglossal canal as was the case with this patient. Hypoglossal nerve (XII CN) paralysis can result in tongue weakness or fasciculations. Involvement of the jugular foramen will result in neuropathies of cranial nerves IX through XI. Secondary thrombosis of the sigmoid and transverse sinuses may also be present. Sagittal and axial unenhanced non-fat saturated T1W images are most useful in identifying abnormalities of the craniovertebral junction and condyles because the hyperintense fat within the marrow provides an excellent intrinsic "contrast" and replacement of this fat with abnormal hypointense tissue is easily identified. In this case, the right occipital condyle and the lateral mass of C1 are replaced by a metastatic tumor. Lesions are less conspicuous on T2W and enhanced T1W images without fat saturation. The axial diffusion-weighted image shows restricted diffusion (Figure 80.5), with marked hypointensity on the corresponding apparent diffusion coefficient map (not shown), consistent with cellularity.

REFERENCES

Cardoso AC, Fontes RB, Tan LA, et al. Biomechanical effects of the transcondylar approach on the craniovertical junction. *Clin Anat.* 2015;28(5):683-689.
Hanson JA, Deliganis AV, Baxter AB, et al. Radiologic and clinical spectrum of occipital condyle fractures: retrospective review of 107 consecutive fractures in 95 patients. *AJR Am J Roentgenol.* 2002;178(5):1261-1268.
Neuroradiology: THE REQUISITES. 4th ed. pp 27, 72-74, 284.

CASE 81

Moyamoya Disease

1. **G.** In this case, there is multifocal large vessel narrowing and occlusion including the right M1 segment, left supraclinoid ICA, left A1, and left M1 narrowing with retrograde filling of bilateral MCA vascular territories from ACA and PCA collaterals consistent with moyamoya disease. Many other disorders can have similar imaging findings, such as sickle cell disease, neurofibromatosis type-1, atherosclerosis, chronic infections, and radiation therapy.
2. **A.** The term moyamoya disease is reserved for an "idiopathic" condition, which sometimes can be familial (more common in Japan), and leads to characteristic intracranial vascular changes. There are several entities that have been described which mimic the angiographic appearance of moyamoya disease, where the terms "moyamoya pattern," "moyamoya phenomenon," or "moyamoya syndrome" are used.

3. **A.** In children, transient ischemic attacks or ischemic strokes are more common.
4. **B.** In adults, intracranial hemorrhage is probably the most common.

Comment

This case shows multifocal large vessel narrowing and occlusions including right M1 segment, left supraclinoid ICA, left A1, and left M1 segments with retrograde filling of bilateral MCA vascular territories from ACA and PCA collaterals. On arterial spin labeling (ASL), there is decreased delivery of labels to both MCA territories (Figure 81.6), with relative sparing of posterior circulation distributions (not shown). On CTA, notice the near-normal caliber of the right A1 and A2 segments as well as distal ACA branches on the right, though the left ACA is decreased in caliber (Figures 81.1 and 81.2). Mild asymmetry but no clear decreased blood flow in the right basal ganglia, corresponding to acute infarcts (Figure 81.5), suggesting at least some degree of reperfusion.

In these patients, there are collateral vessels arising from the abnormal lenticulostriate, thalamoperforating, leptomeningeal, and dural arteries (transdural branches of the middle meningeal artery) and appear as multiple serpentine tortuous flow voids on T1 and T2 sequences. Pial collaterals appear as the so-called "ivy sign," with sulcal FLAIR hyperintensity in the subarachnoid spaces and contrast enhancement.

Moyamoya refers to slow, progressive occlusive disease of the distal intracranial internal carotid arteries and their proximal branches, including the anterior and middle cerebral arteries. There may also be involvement of the posterior cerebral arteries in up to 50% of cases. Moyamoya disease is predominantly an idiopathic arteriopathy, with fibrocellular proliferation and thickening of the intima resulting in vascular stenoses and occlusions. However, a moyamoya pattern has been associated with a variety of other conditions, including neurofibromatosis type-1, sickle cell disease, radiation therapy, chronic infections, and atherosclerosis. Because of the slowly progressive development of high-grade stenoses or occlusions of the distal internal carotid arteries or its proximal branches, collateral circulation develops through a number of pathways, including leptomeningeal collaterals from the cerebral arteries; parenchymal collaterals through the perforating arteries (particularly the basal ganglia); and transdural collaterals, which most commonly arise from the external carotid artery (ophthalmic and middle meningeal arteries).

Moyamoya disease is more symptomatic when it presents in childhood, typically with transient ischemic attacks and stroke. In adults, the disease is less frequently symptomatic, but when it is, it more commonly presents with intracranial hemorrhage.

REFERENCES

Horie N, Morikawa M, Nozaki A, et al. "Brush Sign" on susceptibility-weighted MR imaging indicated the severity of moyamoya disease. *AJNR Am J Neuroradiol.* 2011;32(9):1697-1702.

Wang R, Yu S, Alger JR, et al. Multi-delay arterial spin labeling perfusion MRI in moyamoya disease – comparison with CT perfusion imaging. *Eur Radiol.* 2014;24(5):1135-1144.

Neuroradiology: THE REQUISITES. 4th ed. pp 118-121.

CASE 82

Spontaneous Intracranial Hypotension

1. **D.** These findings are classic for intracranial hypotension with acquired cerebellar tonsillar ectopia (Figure 82.1, cerebellar tonsils were in the normal position on an earlier MRI scan, not shown), bilateral subdural hygromas (Figure 82.2),

pachymeningeal enhancement (Figure 82.3), and diffuse venous engorgement (Figure 82.4).

2. **D.** Axial and coronal CT myelographic images at the midthoracic level demonstrate accumulation of extrathecal contrast material along the left lateral aspect of the thecal sac indicating the site of CSF leakage. Notice the multiple regions of irregularity of the thecal sac, along the left lateral aspect with a small outpouching without frank contrast extravasation at the T5-6 level (upper arrow, Figure 82.6). An additional outpouching with an apparent extravasation at the left T6-7 level (middle arrow, Figure 82.6), and a larger defect at the left lateral aspect of the thecal sac at T7-8 with adjacent contrast collection (lower arrow, Figure 82.6). An additional small focus of contrast extravasation on the left at T8-9.

3. **E.** Metastatic disease (breast and prostate carcinoma), lymphoma or leukemia, granulomatous disease (tuberculosis, sarcoidosis, Wegener's granulomatosis, Erdheim-Chester disease, lipid granulomatosis), spontaneous intracranial hypotension, and idiopathic hypertrophic pachymeningitis can all present with diffuse dural enhancement.

Comment

This case illustrates classic imaging findings of intracranial hypotension with acquired cerebellar tonsillar ectopia, bilateral subdural hygromas, pachymeningeal enhancement, and venous engorgement. The site of leakage was identified in the midthoracic spine on a CT myelogram which was subsequently treated with a targeted blood patch.

Spontaneous intracranial hypotension is caused by chronic, and often intermittent, leakage of CSF from the subarachnoid space. This leakage of CSF results in low intracranial pressure. Symptomatic patients typically present with headaches that are frequently postural in nature (exacerbated in the upright position, relieved when lying down). Trauma or spontaneous (rupture of perineural/Tarlov's cyst) or iatrogenic (after a lumbar puncture or spine surgery or instrumentation) causes result in CSF leakage, which typically occurs somewhere along the spinal column. Imaging findings may be subtle and nonspecific such that in the absence of providing a history of postural headaches, the diagnosis of intracranial hypotension is frequently overlooked. Imaging findings include sagging of the posterior fossa contents, with low-lying cerebellar tonsils, elongation of the fourth ventricle, bilateral subdural effusions, and diffuse dural enhancement. In addition, prominent dural veins have been reported. Symptoms of intracranial hypotension may resolve spontaneously; however, further workup, including MRI, and if indicated, CT myelography or nuclear scintigraphy, is often necessary to identify the source of the CSF leak. The additional value of decubitus positioning during CT myelography in enhancing the detection of subtle leaks has also been recently reported. If a source can be identified, positioning of an epidural blood patch can be performed and typically results in the resolution of symptoms. Increasingly, prophylactic blood patches are being performed.

REFERENCES

Chazen JL, Talbott JF, Lantos JE, et al. MR myelography for identification of spinal CSF leak in spontaneous intracranial hypotension. *AJNR Am J Neuroradiol.* 2014;35(10):2007-2012.

Kranz PG, Gray L, Taylor JN. CT-guided epidural blood patching of directly observed or potential leak sites for the targeted treatment of spontaneous intracranial hypotension. *AJNR Am J Neuroradiol.* 2011;32(5):832-838.

Shah LM, McLean LA, Heilbrun ME, et al. Intracranial hypotension: improved MRI detection with diagnostic intracranial angles. *AJR Am J Roentgenol.* 2013;200(2):400-407.

Neuroradiology: THE REQUISITES. 4th ed. pp 157-158.

CASE 83
Nonaneurysmal Perimesencephalic Subarachnoid Hemorrhage

1. **A.** This case represents acute subarachnoid hemorrhage localized in the prepontine and perimesencephalic cisterns anterior to the brainstem. CTA is recommended as the next step in the evaluation of perimesencephalic subarachnoid hemorrhage (pmSAH) to investigate for possible aneurysmal causes; remember that 5% of these can be secondary to a vertebrobasilar aneurysm.
2. **D.** Ninety-five percent of cases of perimesencephalic subarachnoid hemorrhage have a normal cerebral angiogram, and the source of bleeding is not identified.
3. **B.** In the vast majority of cases with pmSAH, the etiology is never defined, even after an extensive evaluation. Possible theories regarding its origin include rupture of a perforating artery, and cryptic vascular malformation, such as high cervical spinal dural arteriovenous fistula. However, a venous source for pmSAH is the most accepted explanation, suggested by the limited extension of blood and low rate of subsequent rebleeding, both suggesting a low-pressure bleeding source. It often occurs in the setting of physical exertion, which produces increased intrathoracic pressure, impaired internal jugular venous return, elevated intracranial venous pressure, and leakage of venous blood from susceptible blood vessels.
4. **D.** The arrows are pointing to the posterior inferior cerebellar artery. Remember, the rupture of an aneurysm arising from the origin of the posterior inferior cerebellar artery can present with an isolated fourth ventricular hemorrhage.

Comment

Benign, nonaneurysmal subarachnoid hemorrhage with a distinct radiographic appearance was identified by van Gijn and associates in 1985. Nonaneurysmal perimesencephalic subarachnoid hemorrhage (pmSAH) is an increasingly recognized cause of nontraumatic subarachnoid hemorrhage. These patients typically present in adulthood with an acute headache, as was seen in this patient. Specific criteria for a perimesencephalic pattern of hemorrhage on CT have been described within 72 hours of symptom onset. (1) Hemorrhage is centered anteriorly to the pons and the midbrain, (2) may extend into all perimesencephalic cisterns (interpeduncular, crural, ambient, and quadrigeminal cisterns), foramen magnum, proximal interhemispheric fissure, and Sylvian fissures, and (3) may settle as sediment in the occipital horns of the lateral ventricles and fourth ventricle, but there is no frank intraventricular hemorrhage.

Computed tomography angiography (CTA) or digital subtraction angiography (DSA) is often recommended as the next step in evaluation to exclude an intracranial aneurysm that can be seen in the posterior circulation as a causative factor in ~5% of patients. Subarachnoid hemorrhage in nonaneurysmal bleeds is believed to be related to venous or capillary rupture. In the presence of a characteristic pattern of subarachnoid hemorrhage and negative findings on a high-quality conventional angiogram, follow-up angiography may not be necessary. Patients with this type of subarachnoid hemorrhage generally have an excellent prognosis.

REFERENCES

Brinjikji W, Kallmes DF, White JB, et al. Inter- and intraobserver agreement in CT characterization of nonaneurysmal perimesencephalic subarachnoid hemorrhage. *AJNR Am J Neuroradiol.* 2010;31(6):1103-1105.

Mensing LA, Vergouwen MDI, Laban KG, et al. Perimesencephalic hemorrhage: a review of epidemiology, risk factors, presumed cause, clinical course, and outcome. *Stroke.* 2018;49(6):1363-1370.

Neuroradiology: THE REQUISITES. 4th ed. pp 140-141.

CASE 84
Internal Carotid Artery Dissection

1. **C.** There is a crescent-shaped hyperattenuating area (arrows, Figure 84.3) along the distal left internal carotid artery (ICA), consistent with an intramural hematoma. Axial CT angiography obtained (Figures 84.4–84.6); the intramural wall hematoma (arrowheads) is iso-hypoattenuating relative to the surrounding muscles. Notice the enlargement of the overall vessel diameter and a narrowed eccentric lumen. No acute ischemic injury was seen in the brain.
2. **F.** All of these are risk factors for craniocervical dissections.
3. **A.** In ICA dissections, HS is postganglionic due to the involvement of the pericarotid sympathetic plexus that is compressed by the intramural hematoma. All other options are correct.
4. **A.** In the intracranial ICA, the tunica media and tunica adventitia are only a third as thick as their extracranial counterparts which accounts for the markedly different natural history of intracranial arterial dissections compared to their extracranial counterparts. When a tear occurs, there is little tissue preventing extension into the subarachnoid space, thus accounting for the very high rate of subarachnoid hemorrhage in intracranial dissections.

Comment

This case illustrates the characteristic appearance of a dissection of the internal carotid artery. Noncontrast head CT is usually insensitive for dissection but may demonstrate intracranial infarcts. It can also demonstrate arterial wall hematoma in the distal cervical ICA as a crescent-shaped hyperattenuating focus (Figure 84.3), as was seen in this case. CTA may demonstrate enlargement of the dissected artery (Figure 84.4), with an abnormal contour (Figures 84.5 and 84.6), as well as dissecting pseudoaneurysms. On MR, this intramural hematoma can appear as hyperintense on unenhanced T1W images (methemoglobin), with narrowing of the arterial lumen. MRI combined with MR angiography is sensitive for detecting vascular dissections because they allow evaluation of both the vascular lumen (such as angiography) and the vessel wall and the tissues around the vascular structures. An occluded vessel can usually be differentiated from one that is narrowed but patent using a combination of conventional spin-echo MR imaging and MR angiography. It is important to acquire phase-contrast MR angiography because, with this sequence, the mural hematoma, which has high signal intensity, is nulled. Note, you may be "burned" if only time-of-flight MR angiography is used in which mural hematoma may be mistaken for flow because it remains hyperintense on this sequence.

Vascular dissections (tears in the intima that allow blood to travel in the arterial wall) may result from trauma or neck manipulation (e.g., as provided by chiropractors) and are more common in patients with underlying vascular dysplasias (fibromuscular dysplasia, Marfan syndrome, Ehlers–Danlos syndrome, and cystic medial necrosis). Treatment in uncomplicated cases usually includes anticoagulation therapy and aspirin. It is important to obtain follow-up MR imaging in these patients to assess for recanalization of the vascular lumen or progressive stenosis. In addition, these patients are at an increased risk for the development of pseudoaneurysms, which can be catastrophic if they go undetected and rupture. The most common complication of vascular dissection is thromboembolic disease (transient ischemic attack and stroke), which may occur days to weeks after the dissection.

REFERENCES

Ozdoba C, Sturzenegger M, Schroth G. Internal carotid artery dissection: MR imaging features and clinical-radiologic correlation. *Radiology.* 1996;199(1):191-198.

Provenzale JM, Sarikaya B. Comparison of test performance characteristics of MRI, MR angiography, and CT angiography in the diagnosis of carotid and vertebral artery dissection: a review of the medical literature. *AJR Am J Roentgenol.* 2009;193(4):1167-1174.
Neuroradiology: THE REQUISITES. 4th ed. pp 32, 160-162.

CASE 85

CNS Cryptococcosis

1. **A.** *Cryptococcus neoformans* is the most common fungal infection and the second most common opportunistic infection of the central nervous system.
2. **D.** All of these fungal infections can occur in both immunocompetent and immunocompromised patients.
3. **A.** The most common pattern of CNS cryptococcosis in immunocompromised patients is spread along the perivascular spaces, most commonly involving the basal ganglia.
4. **A.** This likely reflects the inability of these patients to mount significant inflammatory and cell-mediated immune responses.

Comment

This case demonstrates extensive areas of bilateral, mildly expansile T2 prolongation within the basal ganglia (Figure 85.1), with associated patchy foci of abnormal diffusion restriction (Figures 85.2 and 85.3) and contrast enhancement consistent with CNS cryptococcal infection. In addition, there was a lack of FLAIR suppression of cerebral sulci in bilateral cerebral hemispheres with multiple areas of leptomeningeal enhancement, consistent with meningoencephalitis (images not shown).

Focal regions of high signal intensity and enhancement in the basal ganglia represent the spread of infection along the perivascular spaces. In patients with profound immunosuppression, there is a paucity of enhancement which is likely related to the inability to mount an inflammatory reaction, given the immunodeficient state of the patient. The CT and MRI findings are often nonspecific, and the clinician may not be able to distinguish among the various fungal infections, as well as toxoplasmosis and tuberculosis. Lymphoma in the setting of AIDS must also be considered.

Fungal infection in the CNS results in granulomatous changes that may affect the intracranial vasculature, meninges, or brain parenchyma. In patients with CNS cryptococcosis, CT and MRI findings may be normal in up to 40% of cases. Alternatively, a spectrum of imaging findings may occur, including dilated perivascular spaces; parenchymal cryptococcomas (more common in the deep gray matter nuclei than in the cerebral cortex); and less commonly, miliary disease with parenchymal, leptomeningeal, and intraventricular nodules. The diagnosis of CNS cryptococcosis may be established by analysis of the CSF with India ink, detection of cryptococcal antigen, or positive findings on fungal cultures. Treatment is with aggressive antifungal therapy (e.g., intravenous amphotericin B or fluconazole), and if left untreated, it is usually fatal.

REFERENCES

Lu CH, Chen HL, Chang WN, et al. Assessing the chronic neuropsychologic sequelae of human immunodeficiency virus-negative cryptococcal meningitis by using diffusion tensor imaging. *AJNR Am J Neuroradiol.* 2011;32(7):1333-1339.
Sanossian N, Shatzmiller RA, Djabiras C, Liebeskind DS. FLAIR vascular hyperintensity preceding stroke in cryptococcal meningitis. *J Neuroimaging.* 2013;23(1):126-128.
Neuroradiology: THE REQUISITES. 4th ed. pp 196-197.

CASE 86

Subarachnoid Seeding—Leptomeningeal Carcinomatosis

1. **D.** These findings are consistent with leptomeningeal carcinomatosis. There is widespread leptomeningeal enhancement in bilateral internal auditory canals (Figures 86.3 and 86.4), along optic nerves (Figure 86.6), and diffusely along cerebral and cerebellar sulci and cisterns.
2. **B.** There can be several causes of increased leptomeningeal enhancement including carcinomatous meningitis (secondary to a systemic malignancy), CSF subarachnoid seeding from a primary CNS malignancy, inflammatory or granulomatous disease (sarcoidosis, tuberculosis), and infectious meningitis. Melanoma, lung, and breast carcinomas are the most common non-CNS malignancies that seed the subarachnoid space. About 23% of patients with melanoma, 9%–25% of patients with lung cancer, and 5% of patients with breast cancer develop leptomeningeal carcinomatosis. More than 50% of cases have concurrent brain parenchymal lesions, and the most common primary lesion is breast carcinoma of the provided choices.
3. **I.** MRI is superior to CT in the evaluation of suspected meningitis. FLAIR imaging shows CSF space hyperintensity presumably caused by increased protein content (Figures 86.1 and 86.5). Sulcal hyperintensity on the FLAIR sequence has other differential diagnostic considerations, as listed here.
4. **D.** Communicating (with obstruction to CSF absorption) hydrocephalus.

Comment

Leptomeningeal carcinomatosis is a relatively uncommon presentation of metastatic disease to the CNS in patients with extracranial malignancies. Carcinomatous meningitis is reported in approximately 3% to 5% of patients with such malignancies; however, as a treatment for cancer improves and patients live longer, it is likely that the incidence of subarachnoid seeding from systemic malignancies will increase. Patients may present with nonspecific symptoms, including headache and meningeal signs; however, they may also present with cranial neuropathies and symptoms related to communicating hydrocephalus (with obstruction to CSF absorption). Histologic examination of leptomeningeal spread typically shows metastatic cellular infiltrates within the subarachnoid space.

Contrast-enhanced CT is insensitive for the detection of leptomeningeal spread. Contrast-enhanced MRI is the imaging modality of choice for detecting subarachnoid seeding; however, it can be normal in a significant percentage of cases. Lumbar puncture to obtain CSF for cytologic evaluation of malignant cells remains the gold standard for diagnosing carcinomatous meningitis (serial punctures may be necessary).

In this case, enhancement is seen within internal auditory canals bilaterally, with an enhancement of bilateral optic nerves. Notice the flattening and bulging of the optic nerve head (better seen on the right, Figure 86.5), which is suggestive of papilledema secondary to increased intracranial pressure. In hematologic malignancies, such as leukemia and lymphoma, spread usually occurs directly to the leptomeninges. In systemic cancers, such as lung and breast carcinoma, although spread may occur directly to the meninges, frequently, subarachnoid seeding may be the result of the rupture of superficial cerebral parenchymal metastasis into the subarachnoid space. In patients with carcinomatous meningitis, enhancement may be seen along the perivascular spaces within the brain parenchyma and along the ependymal surface of the ventricles. Patients with leptomeningeal carcinomatosis have a poor prognosis with a median overall survival of 2.4 months that can be extended up to 6–10 months with aggressive treatment.

REFERENCES

Francolini M, Sicurella L, Rizzuto N. Leptomeningeal carcinomatosis mimicking Creutzfeldt-Jakob disease: clinical features, laboratory tests, MRI images, EEG findings in an autopsy-proven case. *Neurol Sci.* 2013;34(4):441-444.

Krupa M, Byun K. Leptomeningeal carcinomatosis and bilateral internal auditory canal metastases from ovarian carcinoma. *Radiol Case Rep.* 2017;12(2):386-390.

Mohan S, Jain KK, Arabi M, Shah GV. Imaging of meningitis and ventriculitis. *Neuroimaging Clin N Am.* 2012;22(4):557-583.

Neuroradiology: THE REQUISITES. 4th ed. pp 47-49.

CASE 87

Petrous Apex Cholesterol Granuloma

1. **D.** Large expansile lesion of the right petrous apex with areas of osseous deficiency along the horizontal petrous carotid canal (arrow in Figure 87.1) and the anterior wall of the internal auditory canal (not shown). On MRI, it demonstrates high signal on T2 (Figure 87.2), FLAIR (Figure 87.3), and T1 (Figure 87.5) without associated enhancement (Figure 87.6). Note, no diffusion restriction (Figure 87.4). Imaging findings are consistent with cholesterol granuloma.

2. **A.** On MRI, cholesterol granulomas are typically hyperintense on both T1- and T2-weighted sequences because of the accumulation of blood breakdown products and proteinaceous debris.

3. **A.** The exact mechanisms are not clearly understood. The prevalent hypothesis suggests an initial obstruction to an air cell, leading to negative pressure gradients, and repeated microhemorrhages with gradual expansion and bone remodeling.

4. **A.** Small asymptomatic incidentally discovered cholesterol granulomas can be followed up with serial imaging. However, symptomatic or progressively enlarging lesions should be treated with surgical resection.

Comment

Cholesterol granulomas, also known as blue-domed or chocolate cysts, are the most common primary lesions of the petrous apex. They are believed to be due to chronic obstruction of previously pneumatized petrous air cells, resulting in negative pressure within them. As a result of these negative pressure gradients, there are recurrent microhemorrhages caused by the rupture of small blood vessels. A foreign body reaction involving the mucosal lining of the petrous air cells occurs, with giant cell proliferation and a fibroblastic reaction, as well as deposition of cholesterol crystals within the cyst. These are reportedly more common in the setting of chronic otomastoiditis, with no gender predilection. On CT, these lesions typically have a benign appearance that manifests as an expansile mass lesion with demarcated margins, as in this case involving the right petrous apex. Cholesterol granulomas, when large enough, may be multilobular. There is usually thinning of the cortex with large lesions and areas of osseous dehiscence, as seen in this case. On MRI, cholesterol granulomas are hyperintense on all pulse sequences. In particular, the marked hyperintensity on unenhanced T1W images is classic, distinguishing it from many other lesions, and the presence of hemorrhage–fluid levels within these lesions is highly characteristic. Normal fat may occur in the petrous apex and, because it is hyperintense on both T1W and fast spin-echo T2W imaging, may be mistaken for a cholesterol granuloma. This error can be avoided by obtaining fat-saturated T1W images in which fat will lose signal, but the cholesterol granuloma will continue to glow!

The differential diagnosis of a benign-appearing expansile petrous apex mass includes cholesterol granuloma, mucocele, and cholesteatomas of the petrous apex (aka epidermoid cyst). Mucoceles are frequently unilocular and show peripheral enhancement. The signal characteristics of mucoceles will vary, depending on the protein concentration and viscosity within them, as well as the crosslinking of glycoproteins. Cholesteatomas may have a benign appearance but can have more concerning radiologic findings, such as bone erosion or destruction. They are hypointense on T1, hyperintense on T2, and intermediate in signal on FLAIR with a characteristic restricted diffusion. Less common and more aggressive "cystic-appearing" masses that may involve the petrous apex include hemorrhagic metastases and plasmacytoma and multiple myeloma.

REFERENCES

Chapman PR, Shah R, Curé JK, Bag AK. Petrous apex lesions: pictorial review. *AJR Am J Roentgenol.* 2011;196(suppl 3):WS26-WS37; Quiz S40-S43.

Isaacson K, Kutz Jr JW, Mendelsohn D, et al. CT venography: use in selecting a surgical approach for the treatment of petrous apex cholesterol granulomas. *Otol Neurotol.* 2009;30(3):386-391.

Pietrantonio A, D'Andrea G, Fama I, et al. Usefulness of image guidance in the surgical treatment of petrous apex cholesterol granuloma. *Case Rep Otolaryngol.* 2013;2013:257263.

Neuroradiology: THE REQUISITES. 4th ed. pp 403-404.

CASE 88

Medulloblastoma

1. **B.** There is a heterogeneously enhancing mass (Figures 88.5 and 88.6) measuring approximately 2.6 cm located in the region of the cerebellar vermis and the superior aspect of the fourth ventricle (arrows in Figure 88.8). Notice a few internal cystic foci (Figure 88.1), as well as homogeneously decreased diffusion (Figures 88.3 and 88.4) suggestive of cellularity. On perfusion imaging (Figure 88.7), the mass demonstrates elevated relative cerebral blood volume. The leading diagnostic consideration is medulloblastoma. Ependymomas typically arise in the inferior floor of the fourth ventricle near the obex, whereas medulloblastomas are typically seen related to the roof of the fourth ventricle. Unlike medulloblastomas, ependymomas characteristically extend through the foramina of Magendie and Luschka "plastic tumor."

2. **B.** The 2016 update of the WHO classification of CNS tumors recognizes four distinct molecular subgroups of medulloblastomas: WNT, SHH, Group 3, and Group 4. Location is the key to predict molecular subgroups, and SHH medulloblastomas (second most common and most commonly seen in adults and infants) are most frequently located laterally within the cerebellar hemispheres. In this case, pathology was consistent with a medulloblastoma, non-WNT/non-SHH, most likely a group 3/4, WHO grade IV.

3. **A.** The term "Primitive neuroectodermal tumors" (PNET) has been removed from the 2016 update to the WHO classification of CNS tumors.

4. **B.** In approximately 30% to 40% of patients, there is evidence of CSF seeding at the time of initial diagnosis.

Comment

Medulloblastomas are the most common posterior fossa tumor of childhood, accounting for up to one-third of all pediatric posterior fossa tumors. They occur more commonly in boys than in girls (approximately 2:1) and arise from the superior medullary velum of the fourth ventricle from primitive neuroectoderm. In children, they are typically midline masses associated with the inferior vermis (group 4), but occasionally may present as a lateral cerebellar hemispheric mass, which is generally of the SHH subtype. Importantly, subarachnoid seeding of the leptomeninges is very common at presentation (reported in up to 30%–40% of cases in some series) and portends a poorer prognosis; therefore, patients should have a screening contrast-enhanced MR imaging study of the spine to exclude this type of spread.

On an unenhanced CT, 90% of medulloblastomas are hyperdense relative to the brain parenchyma because of their dense cellularity. They are demarcated masses, and calcification, cystic change, or hemorrhage may be present in up to 10% to 20% of lesions. On MRI, the signal characteristics of medulloblastomas vary considerably on T2W imaging, depending on the presence of hemorrhage and the degree of cellularity. Precisely, 90% of medulloblastomas show avid but heterogeneous contrast enhancement. Typically, they efface the fourth ventricle and present with symptoms of obstructive hydrocephalus.

Accurate preoperative diagnosis is important in pediatric cerebellar tumors because this may affect the surgical approach. Diffusion imaging allows assessment of microscopic water diffusion within tissues, and with neoplasms, this diffusion seems to be primarily based on cellularity. Increasing cellularity leads to increased signal intensity on diffusion imaging and hypointensity on corresponding apparent diffusion coefficient (ADC) maps. Studies have suggested that diffusion imaging and ADC values may be useful in helping to distinguish among histologic types of pediatric brain tumors. Juvenile pilocytic astrocytomas have shown high ADC values. In contrast, medulloblastomas that characteristically are cellular have shown restricted diffusion, as seen in this case. The cellularity of ependymomas is between that of astrocytomas and that of medulloblastomas, and restricted diffusion can be seen in solid components of an anaplastic ependymoma. Taurine peak at 3.4 ppm on MR spectroscopy can sometimes be helpful in group 3 or 4 medulloblastomas.

Besides molecular subgroups, histological features are also important with desmoplastic and nodular histology having a better prognosis than large cell or anaplastic histologic features. Treatment consists of surgical resection, radiation therapy, and chemotherapy, with prognosis influenced by the presence of CSF metastases at the time of initial diagnosis, and expression of the c-erbB-2 (HER2/neu) oncogene (with increased c-erbB-2 expression reflecting increased proliferative activity).

REFERENCES

Perreault S, Ramaswamy V, Achrol AS, et al. MRI surrogates for molecular subgroups of medulloblastoma. *AJNR Am J Neuroradiol.* 2014; 35(7):1263-1269.

Taylor MD, Northcott PA, Korshunov A, et al. Molecular subgroups of medulloblastoma: the current consensus. *Acta Neuropathol.* 2012;123(4):465-472.

Yeom KW, Mobley BC, Lober RM, et al. Distinctive MRI features of pediatric medulloblastoma subtypes. *AJR Am J Roentgenol.* 2013;200(4): 895-903.

Neuroradiology: THE REQUISITES. 4th ed. pp 62-65.

CASE 89

Cavernous Malformation and Developmental Venous Anomaly—Mixed Vascular Malformation

1. **D.** These images show a classic cavernous malformation with an associated developmental venous anomaly (DVA) (Figures 89.6–89.8).
2. **B.** Cavernous malformations are most commonly associated with DVAs in approximately 20% and are then referred to as "mixed vascular malformations."
3. **C.** DVA (previously known as venous angioma) is a congenital vascular malformation that drains normal brain tissue and is recognized as the most common cerebral vascular malformation, accounting for approximately 55% of all such lesions.
4. **B.** Type II is the most common type of cavernous malformation according to the Zabramski classification with a classic "popcorn" appearance, as depicted in this case.

Comment

Cavernous malformations are intracranial vascular malformations that can exist as a single lesion or mixed vascular lesions. The most common mixed form is the coexistence of a cavernous malformation with an associated developmental venous anomaly (DVA). These lesions follow a benign course as individual lesions but have a high risk of hemorrhage when they occur together, which prompts for rapid diagnosis and treatment. MRI is helpful in the detection of individual as well as mixed vascular malformations. Asymptomatic lesions can be managed conservatively, but surgical excision is performed for patients with symptomatic cavernous malformations, and in mixed lesions (when associated with a DVA), the DVA is left untouched due to the potential of devastating venous infarction.

DVAs are typically incidental vascular malformations representing an aberration in venous drainage. Within the venous network is intervening normal brain tissue, and no arterial elements are associated with these lesions. Angiomas are composed of a tuft of enlarged venous channels that drain into a common venous trunk, which then subsequently drains into the deep or superficial venous system. Typically, the lesions are clinically silent, although they may be associated with intracranial hemorrhage. These lesions have a characteristic MR imaging appearance, representing a cluster of veins oriented in a "radial" pattern that drain into a large central vein. There is usually no significant signal abnormality in the adjacent brain parenchyma. Angiographically, the arterial and capillary phases are normal, and there may be opacification of the DVA during the venous phase.

Capillary telangiectasias, on the other hand, represent a cluster of abnormally dilated capillaries with intervening normal brain tissue. They usually represent clinically silent lesions that are detected on imaging studies acquired for unrelated reasons, but remain occult on a conventional angiogram.

This case nicely illustrates a mixed vascular malformation with cavernous malformation and an associated developmental venous anomaly on MRI. Note, a typical type II cavernous malformation (the most common type, according to Zabramski classification) with a classic "popcorn" appearance, with a mixed signal on T1 (Figure 89.5) and T2 (Figure 89.1), a complete low signal rim with blooming on GRE (Figure 89.3), and no appreciable contrast enhancement (Figure 89.6). A DVA is seen along its lateral aspect.

REFERENCES

Chaudhry US, De Bruin DE, Policeni BA. Susceptibility-weighted MR imaging: a better technique in the detection of capillary telangiectasia compared with T2* gradient-echo. *AJNR Am J Neuroradiol.* 2014; 35(12):2302-2305.

El-Koussy M, Schroth G, Gralla J, et al. Susceptibility-weighted MR imaging for diagnosis of capillary telangiectasia of the brain. *AJNR Am J Neuroradiol.* 2012;33(4):715-720.

Idiculla PS, Gurala D, Philipose J, Rajdev K, Patibandla P. Cerebral cavernous malformations, developmental venous anomaly, and its coexistence: a review. *Eur Neurol.* 2020;83(4):360-368.

Pozzati E, Marliani AF, Zucchelli M, et al. The neurovascular triad: mixed cavernous, capillary, and venous malformations of the brainstem. *J Neurosurg.* 2007;107(6):1113-1119.

Neuroradiology: THE REQUISITES. 4th ed. pp 145-146.

CASE 90

Creutzfeldt–Jakob disease (CJD)

1. **D.** Asymmetric increased signal intensity in bilateral deep gray matter of the basal ganglia and thalami with restricted diffusion. There is also asymmetric involvement of the cortices, with greater cortical volume loss than expected for the patient's age. The constellation of findings is consistent with the diagnosis of Creutzfeldt–Jakob disease (CJD).
2. **D.** All of these radiological signs are described in patients with CJD, the most common being the cortical ribbon sign.
3. **D.** The definitive diagnosis of CJD requires a brain biopsy. However, as an alternative, in many institutions, a combination of brain MRI findings as well as CSF 14-3-3 protein and RT-QuIC assays is used to diagnose CJD.
4. **D.** Exponential apparent diffusion coefficient (e-ADC). These are an alternative to the ADC maps where the exponential image removes the T2-shine-through effects from the b-1000 image. The exponential image is simply the b-0 image divided by the conventional DW image. If you do not have an exponential image available, a reasonable alternative is to simply invert the conventional ADC map on your monitor.

Comment

Creutzfeldt–Jakob disease (CJD) is rare and is caused by a prion agent composed of protease-resistant protein that affects the CNS and results in rapid, progressive neurodegeneration. Approximately 1 in every 1 million persons worldwide is infected. It is thought to be caused by a slow virus, an organism devoid of active nucleic acid. The most common clinical presentation is that of rapidly progressive dementia, as was seen in this patient. Other neurologic symptoms include upper motor neuron signs, ataxia, myoclonus, and sensory deficits. The characteristic diagnostic triad of progressive dementia, myoclonic jerks, and periodic sharp-wave electroencephalographic activity is present in approximately 75% of cases. The prognosis is poor, with death usually occurring within 1 year of the onset of symptoms. Histologic evaluation shows neuronal degeneration and gliosis in the gray matter, especially the cortex, but also in the deep gray matter of the corpus striatum and thalami. Spongiform changes are characteristic. Inflammatory changes are usually not present. The disease is best known in association with mad cow disease (bovine spongiform encephalopathy) in the United Kingdom; however, there have been scattered sporadic cases described with corneal transplantation as well as with implantation of cerebral electrodes.

CT may show no abnormality; however, atrophy (most commonly cortical) is the next most common presentation. On MRI, in addition to cortical atrophy, FLAIR hyperintensity in the deep gray matter nuclei, especially the caudate and putamen nuclei, as well as the thalami, is observed (Figures 90.1 and 90.5). Lesions are typically bilateral and are not associated with enhancement or significant mass effect. In addition, abnormalities involving the gray and white matter have been noted within the cerebral hemispheres. Several reported cases of sporadic Creutzfeldt–Jakob disease have shown increased signal intensity in the basal ganglia or cerebral cortex on diffusion-weighted images (reduced diffusion), as in this case (Figures 90.2 and 90.6). Ribbon-like areas of hyperintensity in the cerebral cortex on diffusion-weighted images also corresponded to the localization of periodic sharp-wave complexes on electroencephalogram.

REFERENCES

Hyare H, Thornton J, Stevens J, et al. High-b-value diffusion MR imaging and basal nuclei apparent diffusion coefficient measurements in variant and sporadic Creutzfeldt-Jakob disease. *AJNR Am J Neuroradiol.* 2010;31(3):521-526.

Lee H, Cohen OS, Rosenmann H, et al. Cerebral white matter disruption in Creutzfeldt-Jakob disease. *AJNR Am J Neuroradiol.* 2012;33(10):1945-1950.

Neuroradiology: THE REQUISITES. 4th ed. p 243.

CASE 91

Neurofibromatosis Type-2

1. **B.** This was a patient with known neurofibromatosis type-2 (NF2) with multiple meningiomas, bilateral vestibular schwannomas, and additional probable schwannomas.
2. **D.** NF2 is an autosomal dominant neurocutaneous syndrome, and patients with this disease have, *M*ultiple *I*nherited *S*chwannomas, *M*eningiomas and *E*pendymomas giving rise to the acronym *MISME*.
3. **B.** Merlin, or schwannomin, is a tumor suppressor protein encoded on the NF2 gene on chromosome 22q12.1. This provides molecular linkage between membrane proteins and cytoskeleton and modulates cell proliferation, differentiation, apoptosis, survival, motility, adhesion, and invasion. Inactivation or reduced expression has been demonstrated in a variety of systemic and central nervous system cancers including schwannomas, meningiomas, and ependymomas. Interactions between tumor cells and stroma may further alter molecular homeostasis and promote the evolution of malignant phenotypes.
4. **A.** Ependymoma. Note, 8 mm heterogeneous enhancing lesion along the posterior left lateral ventricle (Figures 91.1 and 91.2).

Comment

This case shows imaging findings characteristic of neurofibromatosis type-2, including bilateral vestibular schwannomas, as well as multiple dural-based, extra-axial, avidly enhancing masses, consistent with meningiomas. There are additional probable schwannomas, e.g., 6 mm right extraconal mass exerting a mass effect on the right lateral rectus muscle (Figures 91.3 and 91.4), an 8 mm enhancing mass in the region of the right foramen magnum (F), and 6 mm enhancing mass in the left Meckel's cave (Figure 91.3). Additional meningiomas and schwannomas were present along the optic nerve, cavernous sinus, and parasellar region, which are not shown. In the posterior fossa, there are two large enhancing extra-axial masses in bilateral cerebellopontine angles with the extension of enhancing tissue into the bilateral internal auditory canals most consistent with bilateral vestibular schwannomas (Figures 91.3 and 91.5). These exert mass effects over the brainstem and cerebellar hemisphere with distortion of the fourth ventricle with mild hydrocephalus. Notice that there is a superimposed meningioma abutting the left vestibular schwannoma. This left cerebellopontine angle mass that likely represents a combination of schwannoma and meningioma is seen extending posteriorly and inferiorly into the left hypoglossal canal, partially visualized on Figure 91.5. The 8 mm heterogeneous enhancing lesion in the region of the posterior left lateral ventricle presumably represents an ependymoma (noting that intracranial ependymoma would be unusual in NF2). There are lobulated soft tissue masses in the left scalp (arrows in Figures 91.4 and 91.6) likely representing scalp schwannomas.

Neurofibromatosis type-2 is an autosomal dominant disorder transmitted on chromosome 22. It typically presents in adolescence or young adulthood, and the most common clinical presentation is bilateral sensorineural hearing loss as a result of vestibular schwannomas. The radiologic hallmark of NF2 is the presence of bilateral vestibular schwannomas, as seen in this case. Otherwise, the diagnosis of NF2 can be made if a patient has a unilateral vestibular schwannoma and a first-degree relative with NF2, or if the patient has a first-degree relative with NF2 and at least two schwannomas, meningiomas, or ependymomas. Unlike NF1, cutaneous manifestations in NF2 are rare. CNS tumors are present in virtually 100% of patients with NF2. Schwannomas most commonly involve cranial nerve VIII. The trigeminal nerve is the next most common site for schwannomas, also seen in this case. Although most of these tumors are sporadic, those arising from more than one cranial nerve or from cranial nerves III through VI should prompt a search for NF2. Other imaging findings that may be present in NF2 include prominent calcifications along the choroid plexus, or occasionally along the cerebral or cerebellar cortex. Lesions within the spinal canal are common and include schwannomas and meningiomas. Intramedullary tumors are typically ependymomas.

REFERENCES

Borofsky S, Levy LM. Neurofibromatosis: types 1 and 2. *AJNR Am J Neuroradiol*. 2013;34(12):2250-2251.

Morrow KA, Shevde LA. Merlin: the wizard requires protein stability to function as a tumor suppressor. *Biochim Biophys Acta*. 2012;1826(2): 400-406.

Ruggieri M, Praticò AD, Serra A, et al. Childhood neurofibromatosis type 2 (NF2) and related disorders: from bench to bedside and biologically targeted therapies. *Acta Otorhinolaryngol Ital*. 2016;36(5):345-367.

Vargas WS, Heier LA, Rodriguez F, et al. Incidental parenchymal magnetic resonance imaging findings in the brains of patients with neurofibromatosis type 2. *Neuroimage Clin*. 2014;4:258-265.

Neuroradiology: THE REQUISITES. 4th ed. pp 293-295.

CASE 92

Progressive Multifocal Leukoencephalopathy (PML)

1. **A.** Asymmetric white matter involvement, subcortical and deep white matter involvement, and the absence of mass effect and enhancement, overall findings consistent with the diagnosis of progressive multifocal leukoencephalopathy (PML) in this immunocompromised patient.

2. **D.** PML lesions are due to reactivation of John Cunningham virus (JCV) which infects myelin-producing cells and oligodendrocytes.

3. **A.** PML lesions are asymmetric involving the periventricular and subcortical white matter, with little, or no mass effect and no enhancement. Note, the subcortical U-fibers are commonly involved. Typically, PML lesion presents a sharply demarcated border along the subcortical U-fibers and a hazy and ill-defined inner border (Figure 92.2). Corpus callosum may also be involved. Spectra of biopsy-proven PML lesions were characterized by significantly reduced NAA, presence of lipid and lactate, and by significantly increased Cho compared with controls.

4. **D.** Natalizumab therapy is associated with PML in multiple sclerosis patients with positive JC virus serology.

Comment

Before the AIDS epidemic, PML was largely seen in a spectrum of immunocompromised patients, including those with hematologic malignancies (leukemia and lymphoma), those who had undergone organ transplantation, patients taking immunosuppressive drugs, and those with autoimmune disorders. However, over the past few decades, the majority of cases of PML have been noted in patients with HIV infection. PML is caused by the infection of oligodendrocytes with a ubiquitous double-stranded DNA virus of the polyomaviridae family, John Cunningham virus

(JCV). Histologically, multifocal regions of demyelination involve the subcortical U-fibers, as seen in this case.

The clinical presentation of PML includes focal neurologic deficits (hemiparesis), visual symptoms, and especially progressive cognitive decline. The infection is rapidly progressive, with continued neurologic decline, CNS demyelination, and death usually occurring within 6 months to a year from the onset of symptoms.

MRI is far more sensitive than CT in defining the number and extent of lesions in PML. On CT, PML usually appears as focal regions of hypodensity within the white matter, usually without mass effect or enhancement. On MRI, increased T2W signal intensity with associated T1W hypointensity is noted in the involved white matter. PML has a predilection to involve the subcortical white matter, although the deep and periventricular white matter can also be involved. There is a slight preference for the involvement of the parietal and occipital white matter, but any area of the brain may be affected, including the cerebellum. Although single focal lesions may be seen, multifocal lesions typically occur and are usually asymmetric. Unilateral multifocal distribution may also occur. Mass effect or enhancement is less common in PML, occurring in 5% to 10% of cases.

REFERENCES

Cosottini M, Tavarelli C, Del Bono L, et al. Diffusion-weighted imaging in patients with progressive multifocal leukoencephalopathy. *Eur Radiol*. 2008;18(5):1024-1030.

Sahraian MA, Radue EW, Eshaghi A, et al. Progressive multifocal leukoencephalopathy: a review of the neuroimaging features and differential diagnosis. *Eur J Neurol*. 2012;19(8):1060-1069.

Usiskin SI, Bainbridge A, Miller RF, et al. Progressive multifocal leukoencephalopathy: serial high-b-value diffusion-weighted MR imaging and apparent diffusion coefficient measurements to assess response to highly active antiretroviral therapy. *AJNR Am J Neuroradiol*. 2007; 28(2):285-286.

Neuroradiology: THE REQUISITES. 4th ed. p 217.

CASE 93

Pituitary Hyperplasia

1. **C.** In this patient, there is a prominent pituitary gland with superior convexity and a maximum height of 11.1 mm abutting the undersurface of the optic chiasm. Note, the preservation of posterior pituitary bright spot (Figure 93.1) and a normal morphology of the infundibulum (Figure 93.2). There is homogenous contrast enhancement with no focal lesion suggestive of an adenoma (Figures 93.2–93.4). This is a case of pituitary hyperplasia that refers to diffuse enlargement of the gland that can be physiological (young menstruating females or pregnant/lactating women) or, secondary to end-organ failure, as in this patient with primary hypothyroidism. In inflammatory etiologies such as lymphocytic hypophysitis, normal posterior pituitary bright spots may be absent, and infundibulum may be thickened.

2. **C.** The arrow points to the oculomotor nerve (CNIII) in the CSF-filled oculomotor cistern (OMC) in the posterior portion of the roof of the cavernous sinus, which is an important neuroradiologic and surgical landmark and can be routinely identified on thin-section high-resolution MR images. The CNIII originates from midbrain nuclei and exits between the cerebral peduncles. After leaving the midbrain, the nerve passes between the posterior cerebral arteries and superior cerebellar arteries; it runs superior and medial to the tentorial edge, just inferolateral to the posterior communicating artery, and traverses the cavernous sinus into the superior orbital fissure and orbital apex.

3. **A.** The intrinsic high T1 signal of the posterior pituitary bright spot is believed to be from the storage of vasopressin. The hormone is synthesized in the hypothalamus and carried down the axons that form the stalk to the posterior pituitary bound to a vasopressin-neurophysin II-copeptin complex, a macroproteic structure that shortens T1 signal.

4. **D.** The dorsum sellae is the posterior process of the sphenoid bone and forms the posterior wall of the sella turcica. It contains fatty bone marrow that can mimic the posterior pituitary bright spot on T1-weighted imaging. All of the others can also appear as hyperintense signals on T1-weighted images and mimic a posterior pituitary bright spot.

Comment

Pituitary hyperplasia is an underrecognized manifestation that occurs fairly commonly in primary hypothyroidism. It occurs due to the lack of negative feedback on the pituitary gland and the hypothalamus. The clinical presentation and imaging findings can mimic a pituitary mass such as a macroadenoma. These patients can present with features of hypothyroidism, hyperprolactinemia, and even visual field defects if there is compression of the optic chiasm. It is important to be cognizant of this entity as the primary modality of treatment is thyroid hormone replacement and not surgery.

The differential diagnosis of a sellar mass includes pituitary adenomas, pituitary hyperplasia, either physiologic (young menstruating females or pregnant/lactating women) or pathologic (resulting from end-organ dysfunction), lymphocytic hypophysitis, other pituitary tumors such as craniopharyngiomas and germ cell tumors, etc.

The prognosis in these patients is usually good with improvement after thyroid hormone replacement therapy. Very few patients require surgery if there are compressive symptoms or inadequate response to thyroxine replacement therapy.

REFERENCES

Bonneville F, Cattin F, Marsot-Dupuch K, Dormont D, Bonneville JF, Chiras J. T1 signal hyperintensity in the sellar region: spectrum of findings. *Radiographics*. 2006;26(1):93-113. doi:10.1148/rg.261055045.
Han L, Wang J, Shu K, Lei T. Pituitary tumorous hyperplasia due to primary hypothyroidism. *Acta Neurochir (Wien)*. 2012;154(8):1489-1492.
Namburi RP, Karthik TS, Ponnala AR. Autoimmune hypothyroidism presenting as pituitary hyperplasia. *Indian J Pediatr*. 2014;81(9):937-939.
Papakonstantinou O, Bitsori M, Mamoulakis D, Bakantaki A, Papadaki E, Gourtsoyiannis N. MR imaging of pituitary hyperplasia in a child with growth arrest and primary hypothyroidism. *Eur Radiol*. 2000;10(3):516-518.
Neuroradiology: THE REQUISITES. 4th ed. pp 350, 352-353.

CASE 94

Cavernous Venous Malformations of the Orbit (Orbital Cavernous Hemangioma)

1. **E.** Cavernous venous malformations of the orbit, also known as orbital cavernous hemangiomas, are the most common vascular lesions of the orbit in adults.

2. **B.** The most common presenting symptom is proptosis, and according to one series, it was seen in all patients (100%), followed by visual impairment (60%), and orbital pain (60%). This lesion was however found incidentally in this patient who was being investigated for right submandibular sialadenitis.

3. **D.** Fluid-fluid levels on T2-weighted images are pathognomonic for a venous lymphatic malformation and are not seen in cavernous hemangioma. All other options are correct.

4. **C.** The arrow represents the superior oblique muscle. Its primary action is intorsion, with secondary and tertiary actions being depression and abduction. It is innervated by trochlear nerve (CN IV).

Comment

Cavernous venous malformations are the most common vascular lesions in adults. These occur most often in middle-aged women with slow and progressive enlargement over time causing painless proptosis, which is the most common presenting symptom. However, abrupt proptosis during puberty or pregnancy is reported, which is suggestive of hormone- or cytokine-mediated angiogenic factors leading to lesion growth. These are slow-growing lesions and are sometimes discovered incidentally at imaging evaluations for other indications as was the case in this patient.

A well-defined, round soft tissue density mass is seen in the intraconal left orbit (approximately at the 8 o'clock position), which is interposed but not connected to the inferior and medial rectus muscles. It is separate from the optic nerve with no proptosis. There is a tiny focus of relative hyperattenuation posteriorly (Figure 94.1), which could reflect microcalcification (phlebolith). The mass is isointense on T1 to adjacent extraocular muscles, hyperintense on T2, and demonstrates progressive enhancement on the postcontrast sequences. Note that coronal images (Figure 94.6) were obtained before axial postcontrast T1 (Figure 94.5)—findings characteristic of an orbital cavernous venous malformation (orbital cavernous hemangioma).

Pathologically, these are composed of dilated large vascular spaces (thus cavernous) lined by flattened and attenuated endothelial cells, bounded by a fibrous pseudocapsule, without prominent arterial supply (accounting for the relatively slow enhancement).

These lesions are usually managed conservatively, and surgical excision is reserved for those that cause severe proptosis or optic nerve compression.

REFERENCES

Golden N, Mahadewa TGB, Ryalino C. Surgical outcome of orbital cavernous hemangioma: a case series. *Open Access Surgery*. 2019;12:1-5.
Rootman DB, Heran MK, Rootman J, White VA, Leumsamran P, Yucel YH. Cavernous venous malformations of the orbit (so-called cavernous haemangioma): a comprehensive evaluation of their clinical, imaging, and histologic nature. *Br J Ophthalmol*. 2014;98(7):880-888.
Smoker WR, Gentry LR, Yee NK, Reede DL, Nerad JA. Vascular lesions of the orbit: more than meets the eye. *Radiographics*. 2008;28(1):185-204; quiz 325.
Tian YM, Xiao LH, Gao XW. Adhesion of cavernous hemangioma in the orbit revealed by CT and MRI: analysis of 97 cases. *Int J Ophthalmol*. 2011;4(2):195-198.
Neuroradiology: THE REQUISITES. 4th ed. pp 330-332.

CASE 95

Orbital Dermoid Cyst

1. **A.** Orbital dermoid cyst. There is a well-marginated mass in the lateral aspect of the left orbit with central low (fat) attenuation (HU-44 to -54). This is contiguous with the zygomaticofrontal suture. There is mild associated proptosis.

2. **B.** The most common presentation of an orbital dermoid cyst is usually as a painless subcutaneous mass that demonstrates slow growth over time.

3. **A.** Orbital dermoids are congenital lesions. These are squamous epithelium-lined sacs that result from abnormal migration of ectodermal cells and are the most common orbital mass in children.

4. **C.** Orbital dermoid cysts are most frequently associated with the zygomaticofrontal suture, as seen in this case. On coronal soft tissue image (Figure 95.3), a dumbbell-shaped dermoid is seen that straddles the left lateral orbital wall with an osseous channel (widened zygomaticofrontal suture) connecting the two lobes. Note that the deep lobe displaces the left lateral rectus muscle and causes mild proptosis.

Comment

Orbital dermoid cysts are benign congenital choristomas. They are the most common orbital mass in children and tend to occur in children younger than 6 years of age, with the vast majority of them noticed between birth and 3 months of age. Dermoid cysts originate secondary to abnormal ectodermal cell migration that becomes entrapped in aberrant locations, adjacent to suture lines, most commonly found along the zygomaticofrontal suture. Clinical presentation is with a slowly progressive painless subcutaneous mass.

CT is a commonly used modality for imaging orbital dermoid cysts. On CT, a dermoid typically presents as a low attenuation nonenhancing lesion. The central cavity may be heterogeneous as a result of keratin and other cystic debris. Most dermoid cysts, in contrast to an epidermoid and most other orbital masses, have the attenuation characteristics of lipids because of their sebaceous contents, as in this case. Dermoids may also straddle the orbital bones (most commonly the lateral orbital wall), as seen in this case, with a lateral component (marked by * in Figure 95.3). These so-called "dumbbell" dermoids must be imaged to assess the extent of the orbital component before excision. An estimated 85% of dermoids are associated with adjacent bony changes such as smooth pressure erosion near the affected suture, clefts, and full-thickness bony channels, likely representing widening of the suture, as marked by the arrow in Figure 95.4.

MRI is often used for evaluating dermoid cysts and has the added advantage of not exposing the patient to radiation, particularly in the pediatric age group. The lipid components of these lesions cause T1 shortening, often appearing as bright as the subcutaneous fat, with dark signal on fat-suppressed images and no contrast enhancement.

Complete surgical excision without the rupture of the cyst is the standard of care. Rupture of the cyst leads to a severe inflammatory reaction in surrounding tissues and potential recurrence. The overall prognosis remains good with isolated reports of malignancy masquerading as dermoid cysts.

REFERENCES

D'Amore A, Borderi A, Chiaramonte R, et al. CT and MR studies of giant dermoid cyst associated to fat dissemination at the cortical and cisternal cerebral spaces. *Case Rep Radiol.* 2013;2013:239258.

Howard BE, Masood MM, Clark JM, Thorp BD. Intraorbital dermoid cyst with zygomaticofrontal suture erosion in an adult. *J Craniofac Surg.* 2019;30(2):514-515.

Jung BY, Kim YD. Orbital dermoid cysts presenting as subconjunctival fat droplets. *Ophthalmic Plast Reconstr Surg.* 2008;24(4):327-329.

Neuroradiology: THE REQUISITES. 4th ed. pp 415-416.

CASE 96

Ruptured Dermoid Cyst

1. **F.** All of these will cause T1 shortening effect. Besides this list, proteinaceous material can also be hyperintense on T1.
2. **B.** Ruptured dermoid cyst. Axial T1-weighted images (Figures 96.1–96.3) demonstrating scattered small droplets of T1 hyperintense material (lipid) in the subarachnoid spaces of both hemispheres. The originating (ruptured) cyst

is difficult to identify but is most likely located in the suprasellar area (Figure 96.3). DWI can aid in distinguishing epidermoid cysts from dermoid cysts, as dermoid cysts do not restrict diffusion.

3. **A.** Chemical shift artifact is indicative of the presence of fat. Fat is hyperintense on fast spin echo T2W images. When there is a question, fat-suppressed T1W imaging may confirm the presence of fat. Chemical shift artifacts can be observed at the fat/water interface in the frequency encoding directions.
4. **A.** Chemical shift artifact on long TR images is identified by the presence of a hyperintense rim and a hypointense rim at opposite margins of the lesion in the frequency-encoding direction. These artifacts arise due to the difference in resonance of hydrogen protons in fat and water. The protons of fat resonate at a slightly lower frequency than those of water, and these are misregistered on the final image, creating the typical chemical shift artifact. High-field-strength magnets are particularly susceptible to this artifact.

Comment

Epidermoid and dermoid lesions are developmental anomalies that may be considered congenital inclusions within the neural tube related to incomplete disjunction of the neuroectoderm from the cutaneous ectoderm. Both lesions are of epidermal origin and may be associated with dermal sinuses or a bone defect. Dermoid cysts and teratomas are typically midline lesions, and both occur more commonly in men. In the intracranial compartment, they may be found in the parasellar or suprasellar region, as in this case. Within the posterior fossa, the superior cerebellar cistern and fourth ventricle are the most common locations.

On CT, dermoids are decreased in attenuation (< -120 Hounsfield units) because of their fat content. Calcification may be seen in the periphery of the lesion. On MRI, dermoids show the signal characteristics of fat, and chemical shift artifact is frequently present. When necessary, fat suppression can be applied to confirm the diagnosis. All scattered small droplets of T1 hyperintense material (lipid) in the subarachnoid spaces in this case were suppressed on the fat-saturated images (not shown). Other common MR imaging findings in these relatively uncommon lesions include the presence of fat-fluid levels within dermoid cysts, and peripheral enhancement. On the other hand, teratomas often have areas of solid enhancement.

Dermoid cysts may contain dermal appendages, including sebaceous and sweat glands, as well as hair follicles. They are often asymptomatic but may enlarge over time due to recurrent glandular secretions and/or recurrent desquamation of the epithelial lining of the cyst. When symptomatic, patients may have headaches, as the sebum results in an aseptic chemical meningitis. A serious complication of dermoid cysts is their propensity to rupture into the subarachnoid space, as in this patient, which may result in vasospasm with ischemia, and even death.

REFERENCES

Jacków J, Tse G, Martin A, Sąsiadek M, Romanowski C. Ruptured intracranial dermoid cysts: a pictorial review. *Pol J Radiol.* 2018;83:e465-e470.

Koh YC, Choi JW, Moon WJ, et al. Intracranial dermoid cyst ruptured into the membranous labyrinth causing sudden sensorineural hearing loss: CT and MR imaging findings. *AJNR Am J Neuroradiol.* 2012;33(5):69-71.

Liu JK, Gottfried ON, Salzman KL, et al. Ruptured intracranial dermoid cysts: clinical, radiographic, and surgical features. *Neurosurgery.* 2008;62(2):377-384.

Neuroradiology: THE REQUISITES. 4th ed. pp 53-55.

CASE 97

Fibromuscular Dysplasia—Complicated by Dissection and Pseudoaneurysm Formation

1. **D.** Beaded appearance of the internal carotid arteries greater on the left, typical of fibromuscular dysplasia (FMD). There is a dissection of the left cervical internal carotid artery (ICA) and an associated 9 mm pseudoaneurysm at the C1–C2 level. On the right, there is beading and mild ectasia at the same level.
2. **B.** Fibromuscular dysplasia is classified into five categories according to the vessel wall layer affected. Involvement of the media with hyperplasia or dysplasia is most frequent (60%–70%) and corresponds to a rarefaction of smooth media muscle cells replaced by fibrosis.
3. **D.** The renal arteries are most commonly affected in FMD.
4. **E.** Arterial tortuosity syndrome (ATS) is an extremely rare autosomal recessive connective tissue disorder characterized by lengthening (elongation) and twisting or distortion (tortuosity) of arteries throughout the body. According to a recent large study, no reports unequivocally document vascular dissections or ruptures. All other options are correct.

Comment

Fibromuscular dysplasia (FMD) is an idiopathic, noninflammatory, and nonatherosclerotic angiopathy of small and medium-sized arteries most commonly seen in young women with a female to male ratio of 3:1. It is a potentially serious disease, especially when it affects the craniocervical vasculature, where it can lead to severe stenosis, aneurysm/pseudoaneurysm formation, subarachnoid hemorrhage, dissection, or arterial occlusion. Imaging plays a critical role in diagnosis as the clinical symptoms are often nonspecific. It is most commonly seen in the renal arteries with a reported prevalence of 4%–6%. The cervical arteries (internal carotid and vertebral arteries) are the second most commonly affected with a prevalence of 0.3%–3%. FMD is classified into five categories, with a medial type being the most common.

Vascular imaging is necessary for diagnosis, and CTA has the best sensitivity/specificity ratio. Vascular loops, fusiform vascular ectasia, and a "string-of-beads" aspect are typical imaging findings, as seen in this case. According to one study, approximately 20% of patients with FMD had an arterial dissection. In 75% of cases, the dissection was located in the carotid artery, 22% in the renal artery, and 17% in the vertebral artery.

In the craniocervical vasculature, the cervical ICA is most commonly affected, and the proximal 2 cm of this vessel is usually spared due to architectural differences in this part of the vessel's wall. The extracranial vertebral artery and external carotid arteries may be involved; however, intracranial FMD is relatively uncommon. Intracranial FMD with a typical string-of-beads aspect (basilar artery, carotid, middle cerebral artery) is usually an intracranial extension of extracranial lesions. The incidence of intracranial aneurysms is increased in patients with a reported prevalence of ~17%.

In this case, there was a localized intimal dissection with pseudoaneurysm formation in the cervical left ICA with mild ectasia of the right ICA. Extracranial dissections commonly result from major or minor trauma, including chiropractic manipulation, or result from an underlying vascular abnormality or dysplasia. There was no reported history of trauma in this case.

Arterial tortuosity syndrome (ATS) is an extremely rare genetic connective tissue disorder characterized by lengthening (elongation) and twisting or distortion (tortuosity) of arteries throughout the body. Affected arteries are prone to developing aneurysms or areas of stenosis. Affected individuals may have distinctive facial features that are noticeable at birth or during early childhood. ATS can potentially cause severe life-threatening complications during infancy or early childhood, although individuals with milder symptoms have also been described. Arterial tortuosity syndrome is caused by mutations in the SLC2A10 gene and is inherited in an autosomal recessive manner.

REFERENCES

Beyens A, Albuisson J, Boel A, et al. Arterial tortuosity syndrome: 40 new families and literature review. *Genet Med*. 2018;20(10):1236-1245. [Erratum in: Genet Med. 2018 Sep 10.]
Varennes L, Tahon F, Kastler A, et al. Fibromuscular dysplasia: what the radiologist should know: a pictorial review. *Insights Imaging*. 2015;6(3): 295-307.
Neuroradiology: THE REQUISITES. 4th ed. pp 118, 120.

CASE 98

Left Thalamic Glioblastoma (GBM)

1. **D.** All of these primary brain tumors can have associated hemorrhage.
2. **A.** There is a large, necrotic, heterogeneously enhancing hemorrhagic mass centered in the left thalamus. Relative cerebral blood volume map (CBV) (Figure 98.7) derived from dynamic susceptibility contrast (DSC) MRI perfusion showing tumor with high perfusion, findings consistent with a high-grade glioma. Pathology demonstrated an IDH-negative glioblastoma.
3. **E.** Perfusion MRI (DSC and dynamic contrast-enhanced [DCE] techniques) plays an important role at almost all major clinical decision points in neuro-oncology, including initial diagnosis, prognosis, guidance for biopsy, as well as posttreatment monitoring.
4. **A.** DTI-FT helps in assessing the location of critical white matter tracts and aids in presurgical mapping of brain tumors. The convention for color coding is red: transverse fibers, green: anteroposterior fibers, and blue: craniocaudal fibers, corticospinal tracts in Figure 98.8.

Comment

This case illustrates a large, necrotic, heterogeneously enhancing hemorrhagic mass centered in the left thalamus, with mass effect over the third ventricle resulting in mild hydrocephalus, but no transependymal edema. Notice the significantly elevated relative cerebral blood volume (CBV) (Figure 98.7) on (DSC) MRI perfusion indicative of a high-grade glioma. Pathology revealed an IDH-negative glioblastoma, WHO grade 4. Most GBMs enhance and usually demonstrate heterogeneity because of the presence of necrosis or hemorrhage. Margins of the enhancing component are usually ill defined, and there is irregular thick peripheral enhancement due to central necrosis. Contrast is useful in identifying areas of blood–brain barrier breakdown, and for stereotactic biopsy planning, particularly for unresectable deep-seated tumors, as in this case. In addition, enhanced images may identify tumor spread to regions that otherwise would not be noticed on unenhanced images, such as the leptomeninges, subarachnoid space, or subependymal region along the ventricular margins.

In this less typical case, the GBM is centered in the deep gray matter (most GBMs are located in the frontal lobe, multiple lobes, followed by the temporal and parietal lobes). Metabolic and physiologic in vivo techniques such as MR spectroscopy and MR perfusion imaging allow correlation of metabolic activity with vascular properties and provide further insight into the underlying tumor biology and grade. In high-grade tumors, proton MR spectroscopy shows an elevated choline:NAA ratio (not performed in this case), and perfusion imaging shows markedly elevated rCBV (Figure 98.7), indicative of a high-grade neoplasm. For presurgical planning and identification of eloquent white matter tracts relative to the tumor DTI-FT is often requested by the neurosurgeon to reduce potential neurologic deficits, as in this case.

The left CST fibers (blue) are displaced anteriorly and laterally by the mass and are located within 5 mm from the anterior enhancing edge of the mass, and some of the visualized left-sided CST fibers were coursing through the FLAIR signal abnormality along the anterior margin of the mass (not shown).

The left arcuate fasciculus/superior longitudinal fasciculus (AF/SLF) fibers (green) are slightly displaced superolaterally by the mass.

The left inferior longitudinal fasciculus and inferior fronto-occipital fasciculus (ILF/IFOF) fibers (yellow) are slightly laterally displaced by the mass and are seen abutting the lateral enhancing edge of the mass. Similar to the CST, AF/SLF, some of the left-sided fibers course through the area of abnormal FLAIR signal.

REFERENCES

Essig M, Nguyen TB, Shiroishi MS, et al. Perfusion MRI: the five most frequently asked clinical questions. *AJR Am J Roentgenol.* 2013;201(3):W495-W510.

Mukherjee P, Berman JI, Chung SW, Hess CP, Henry RG. Diffusion tensor MR imaging and fiber tractography: theoretic underpinnings. *AJNR Am J Neuroradiol.* 2008;29(4):632-641.

Neuroradiology: THE REQUISITES. 4th ed. pp 21-22, 59-62.

CASE 99

Joubert's Syndrome

1. **B.** Joubert's syndrome. There is cerebellar vermian hypoplasia (Figure 99.1) with apposition of the cerebellar hemispheres in the midline, without fusion. Note the characteristic molar tooth configuration of the midbrain (Figure 99.2).
2. **B.** The posterior fossa typically shows a bat-wing-shaped morphology of the fourth ventricle (Figure 99.4) in patients with Joubert's syndrome and related anomalies.
3. **A.** The "molar tooth sign" is a diagnostic criterion for Joubert's syndrome and consists of elongated, thickened, and horizontally oriented superior cerebellar peduncles, deep interpeduncular cistern, and absence of decussation of the superior cerebellar peduncles. It was initially described in Joubert's syndrome but is now recognized to occur in a number of other conditions, e.g., nephronophthisis, hepatic fibrosis, Cogan's syndrome, and pontine tegmental cap dysplasia.
4. **A.** Rhombencephalosynapsis is characterized by the absence of the vermis and fusion of the cerebellar hemispheres, dentate nuclei, and superior cerebellar peduncles. The hallmark of Joubert's syndrome is separation or disconnection of the cerebellar hemispheres, which are apposed but not fused in the midline. In pontine tegmental cap dysplasia, there is a flattened ventral pons, vaulted pontine tegmentum (the "cap") that protrudes into the fourth ventricle, partial absence of the middle cerebellar peduncles, vermian hypoplasia, and absent inferior olivary prominence.

Comment

Congenital posterior fossa anomalies may result from inherited or acquired causes A malformed cerebellum may be hypoplastic (diminutive cerebellar volume), dysplastic (abnormal cerebellar foliation, fissuration, and architecture), or hypodysplastic (combination of hypoplasia and dysplasia). Each part of the cerebellum (vermis and hemispheres) may be hypoplastic and/or dysplastic,

resulting in global cerebellar involvement (uncommon) or predominantly vermian involvement.

The predominant abnormality in Joubert's syndrome is aplasia or hypoplasia of the vermis, particularly the superior portion. In addition, these patients have dysplastic cerebellar tissue, including heterotopic and dysplastic cerebellar nuclei; abnormal development of the inferior olivary nuclei; and absence of decussation of the superior cerebellar peduncles and pyramidal tracts. Joubert's syndrome is inherited with an autosomal recessive pattern and is characterized by hypotonia, ataxia, oculomotor apraxia, with variable intellectual disability, as in this case. At least 26 genes have been implicated, and all of these genes encode for proteins of the nonmotile primary cilia (ciliopathy), which play a key role in the development and functioning of various cells, including neurons, which in the CNS are implicated in neuronal cell proliferation and axonal migration in the cerebellum and brainstem. Compound heterozygous mutations in the centrosome and spindle pole associated protein 1 (CSPP1) gene were detected in this patient.

MR imaging in these patients show a characteristic molar tooth appearance of the midbrain which is the diagnostic criterion for Joubert's syndrome. Sagittal T1W images demonstrate a diminutive vermis (Figure 99.1). Axial images in particular show an enlarged fourth ventricle with a "bat-wing" shape (Figure 99.4). Because of dysgenesis of the vermis, the hallmark of Joubert's syndrome is separation or disconnection of the cerebellar hemispheres, which are apposed but not fused in the midline.

REFERENCES

Bosemani T, Orman G, Boltshauser E, Tekes A, Huisman TA, Poretti A. Congenital abnormalities of the posterior fossa. *Radiographics.* 2015;35(1):200-220.

Poretti A, Boltshauser E, Loenneker T, et al. Diffusion tensor imaging in Joubert syndrome. *AJNR Am J Neuroradiol.* 2007;28(10):1929-1933.

Poretti A, Huisman TA, Scheer I, Boltshauser E. Joubert syndrome and related disorders: spectrum of neuroimaging findings in 75 patients. *AJNR Am J Neuroradiol.* 2011;32(8):1459-1463.

Saleem SN, Zaki MS. Role of MR imaging in prenatal diagnosis of pregnancies at risk for Joubert syndrome and related cerebellar disorders. *AJNR Am J Neuroradiol.* 2010;31(3):424-429.

Neuroradiology: THE REQUISITES. 4th ed. pp 282-283.

CASE 100

Canavan Disease

1. **E.** Macrocephaly is a clinical-radiological term that refers to a generalized increase in head size, whereas megalencephaly is characterized by an abnormally large brain. All of the aforementioned conditions can present with macrocephaly.
2. **D.** This case demonstrates the typical clinical and imaging findings of Canavan disease with extensive white matter T2 hyperintensity involving the subarcuate U-fibers, and globus pallidi, with sparing of the putamina and corpus callosum (Figures 100.1 and 100.2). MRS reveals a markedly elevated NAA peak with elevated NAA:creatine ratio which is considered pathognomonic for Canavan disease.
3. **B.** Canavan disease is an autosomal recessive disorder due to a gene mutation on the short arm of chromosome 17 leading to deficiency of N-acetylaspartoacylase, a key enzyme in myelin synthesis, with resultant accumulation of N-acetylaspartate (NAA) in the brain, cerebrospinal fluid, plasma, and urine. However, metachromatic leukodystrophy (MLD) is the most common hereditary (autosomal recessive) leukodystrophy caused by deficiency of the enzyme arylsulfatase A.
4. **A.** Adrenoleukodystrophy (ALD) typically spares the subcortical U-fibers with a characteristic parieto-occipital periventricular

white matter involvement. More than 50% cases demonstrate peripheral contrast enhancement.

Comment

Leukodystrophies, or demyelinating disorders, represent a spectrum of inherited diseases that usually result in both abnormal formation and abnormal maintenance of myelin. Many of the more common of these rare disorders are inherited in an autosomal recessive pattern. In many of the leukodystrophies, specific enzyme deficiencies have been identified as the cause. These diseases cause abnormal growth or development of the myelin sheath, the fatty covering that acts as an insulator around nerve fibers in the brain. Myelin is made up of at least 10 different chemicals. Each of the leukodystrophies affects one (and only one) of these substances.

At the time of imaging, this 18-month-old boy had macrocephaly (head circumference in the 85th percentile). There were early difficulties with latching, but the parents did not notice any abnormalities until 6 months of age. The child was found to have elevated NAA on urine organic acid testing. Both parents were from Eastern Europe (Ashkenazi heritage), and maternal sister was a carrier of Canavan disease. The child was later found positive for the mutation in the ASPA gene (c.854>C; p. E285A) at which time he was formally diagnosed with Canavan disease.

Canavan disease is transmitted as an autosomal recessive disorder usually identified in infants of Ashkenazi Jewish descent and in Saudi Arabians. It is the result of a deficiency of *N*-acetylaspartoacyclase. Infants may have macrocephaly due to enlargement of the brain. On histologic evaluation, there is diffuse demyelination, and the white matter is replaced by microscopic cystic spaces, giving it a "spongy" appearance. In contrast to most of the other demyelinating syndromes, Canavan disease preferentially begins in the subcortical U-fibers and later spreads to diffusely involve the deep white matter. There may be sparing of the corpus callosum, internal capsules, and putamina, as in this case. There may be bilaterally symmetric T2W signal abnormalities in the globus pallidi, as in this case. The brainstem is involved in late disease. Usually, the ventricles remain normal or may be slightly small; however, in the late stages of the disease, when cerebral atrophy occurs, there may be proportionate enlargement of the ventricles and cerebral sulci. Diffusion-weighted imaging shows diffuse restriction, and MR spectroscopy shows a markedly elevated peak of NAA peak which is fairly specific and is only described in cases of Canavan disease.

Alexander disease is different from many of the leukodystrophies in that no familial pattern has been recognized. Like Canavan disease, it presents with macrocephaly in addition to developmental delay and spasticity. The deep white matter is usually involved early, and the internal capsules are typically involved (in contrast to Canavan disease, in which they are often relatively spared).

REFERENCES

Cakmakci H, Pekcevik Y, Yis U, et al. Diagnostic value of proton MR spectroscopy and diffusion-weighted MR imaging in childhood inherited neurometabolic brain diseases and review of the literature. *Eur J Radiol*. 2010;74(3):161-171.

Ibrahim M, Parmar HA, Hoefling N, Srinivasan A. Inborn errors of metabolism: combining clinical and radiologic clues to solve the mystery. *AJR Am J Roentgenol*. 2014;203(3):W315-W327.

Janson CG, McPhee SW, Francis J, et al. Natural history of Canavan disease revealed by proton magnetic resonance spectroscopy (1H-MRS) and diffusion-weighted MRI. *Neuropediatrics*. 2006;37(4):209-221.

Neuroradiology: THE REQUISITES. 4th ed. p 227.

Challenge

CASE 101

Bone Marrow Reconversion—Diffuse Replacement of Fat in the Marrow

1. **A.** There is T1 hypointensity of bone marrow in all of these cases from marrow reconversion.
2. **A.** All of these three patients have hematopoietic marrow reconversion. Hematopoietic (red) marrow has a high cell:fat ratio and is T1 hypointense; hence, option A is the correct choice. Prominence of sclerosis is a feature seen in myelofibrosis.
3. **F.** Hemoglobinopathies (such as sickle cell disease and thalassemia) and myeloproliferative disorders (leukemia, myelofibrosis, etc.) are all associated with extramedullary hematopoiesis.
4. **D.** The liver and spleen are the main sites of extramedullary hematopoiesis. Other organs such as the lungs, kidney, and the peritoneal cavity as well as lymph nodes can also become the sites of hematopoiesis when in diseased states.

Comments

The normal signal intensity of marrow is dependent on the ratio of cells, fat, and water. In children, hematopoietic (red) marrow has a high cell:fat ratio and is hypointense on T1W images. As we age, the amount of fat increases, and by early adulthood, the marrow has undergone fatty conversion (yellow marrow), and on T1W images, it becomes isointense to hyperintense to white matter. Unenhanced (nonfat saturated) T1W imaging is the best way to assess for marrow abnormalities, especially because it is part of all standard brain MR imaging protocols. Note, GRE images are not regarded as a standard for evaluating differences between the intensity of red and yellow bone marrow. Similarly, contrast administration is also not useful in routine evaluation of bone marrow. Yellow bone marrow does not show enhancement, and red bone marrow shows a minimal (<10%) enhancement, making the differences unimportant.

Hematopoietic (red) marrow is composed of approximately 40% fat, 40% water, and 20% protein; in contrast, inactive fatty (yellow) marrow contains approximately 80% fat, 10% to 15% water, and 5% protein. On the unenhanced T1W images, yellow marrow has high signal intensity relative to that of muscle; it approaches the intensity of subcutaneous fat. Cellular red marrow becomes hypointense to subcutaneous fat on T1 and is slightly hyperintense to the muscle (usually its signal intensity is slightly lower than that of yellow marrow) on T2.

Marrow conversion represents a normal process in which yellow marrow gradually replaces red marrow. At birth, marrow is predominantly red in both the appendicular and axial skeletons. In the appendicular skeleton, most of the marrow has undergone conversion by the time an individual is 21 years of age. Residual red marrow is found in the proximal metaphyses of the femurs and humeri. In the axial skeleton, in adults, a larger portion of the marrow remains hematopoietic compared with the appendicular skeleton.

Reconversion of bone marrow is a reverse process of natural replacement of red marrow with yellow marrow which can make imaging interpretation challenging and sometimes confusing. It can occur as a physiological response to increased hematopoietic needs of the body, including nonmedical (smoking) as well as medical conditions, as illustrated in these three cases: chronic idiopathic anemia in case 1, myelofibrosis in case 2, and beta thalassemia in case 3.

The differential diagnosis of diffuse replacement of the fatty marrow with hypointense tissue (cells or water) includes hematologic malignancies (lymphoma, leukemia, and myeloma); granulomatous disease (sarcoid and tuberculosis); chronic anemias, such as thalassemia, sickle cell disease, or chronic blood loss; and AIDS (hypointense marrow has been attributed to several factors, including chronic anemia and low CD4 counts). Metastases may diffusely replace the marrow (most common with breast carcinoma in women and prostate carcinoma in men). More often, metastatic disease presents with multiple focal lesions.

REFERENCES

Loevner LA, Tobey JD, Yousem DM, et al. MR imaging characteristics of cranial bone marrow in adult patients with underlying systemic disorders compared with healthy control subjects. *AJNR Am J Neuroradiol.* 2002;23(2):248-254.

Małkiewicz A, Dziedzic M. Bone marrow reconversion - imaging of physiological changes in bone marrow. *Pol J Radiol.* 2012;77(4):45-50.

Neuroradiology: THE REQUISITES. 4th ed. p 538.

CASE 102

Hemorrhagic Venous Infarction

1. **C.** Initial noncontrast head CT shows a large area of hypoattenuation in the left temporal lobe with focal areas of hemorrhage, findings very suspicious for a "hemorrhagic venous infarction." The next best imaging study to confirm this finding would be MRI and MR venography. Note, cerebral venous thrombosis (CVT) and venous ischemia should be considered in the assessment of confluent infarct or hemorrhage in atypical brain regions, crossing arterial territories, or infarcts with relative cortical sparing.
2. **B.** Parenchymal hemorrhages (Figure 102.3) and predominant vasogenic edema (minimal cytotoxic edema) in the left temporal lobe (Figures 102.4 and 102.5) extending to posterior perisylvian and deep white matter regions, with thrombosis involving the left transverse and sigmoid sinuses. The pattern is most consistent with hemorrhagic venous infarction.
3. **C.** Contrast-enhanced MRV is more sensitive in detecting CVT than TOF MRV. In addition, 3D contrast-enhanced gradient-recalled-echo T1W sequences are excellent for the diagnosis of CVT.

Comment

This case illustrates a hemorrhagic venous infarction in the left temporal lobe. Several findings on an initial head CT should raise the suspicion of a venous infarct: (1) the presence of hemorrhage, especially in the white matter with relative sparing of the overlying gray matter; (2) signal abnormality which is not in a typical arterial distribution; and (3) an infarct in a young patient. This patient had acute thrombosis of the left transverse and sigmoid sinus (Figures 102.6 and 102.7) in the setting of oral contraceptive use.

The most common predisposing factor is hypercoagulability in the context of a prothrombotic condition, e.g., pregnancy, postpartum status, cancer, or use of oral contraceptives as in this case. The time to the appearance of symptoms of CVT varies widely; subacute presentation (2–30 days) is the most common (50% of cases), as in this patient, followed by acute (<2 days) and chronic (>30 days) manifestation, occurring in 30% and 10% of cases, respectively.

Symptoms of venous occlusion are related to the rate at which collateral venous drainage is established, the location of the clot, and the rate of clot formation. Because of the network of venous collaterals in the brain, if the venous occlusive process is slow enough to allow time for collateral circulation to develop, the patient may remain asymptomatic. However, in the setting of acute occlusion of a large vein or dural venous sinus, venous congestion will result in back pressure that extends to the capillary bed, where the flow will be diminished such that there is ischemia and, if extensive enough, infarction. Associated parenchymal abnormalities are seen in 40%–60% of cases of CVT in subcortical territories that are not in the typical arterial vascular distribution. Unlike arterial infarctions, the anatomic territories for venous occlusive disease are also less consistent than arterial territories.

The diagnosis of CVT can be confirmed both on MRV and CTV. However, MRI is superior as it is able to visualize both the clot as well as the parenchymal sequelae. Treatment is usually with early initiation of anticoagulation. The presence of hemorrhage is generally not a contraindication but should be reviewed and decided on a case-by-case basis. This patient was also placed on anticoagulation (eliquis) with clinical improvement at 3 months. Follow-up MRV showed improvement but the only partial resolution of her thrombosis (not shown).

It is generally observed that complete recanalization is achieved more often in patients in whom CVT affects the superior sagittal sinus or the straight sinus than in those in whom it affects the transverse sinus or sigmoid sinus and that complete recanalization is not necessary for clinical recovery.

REFERENCES

Canedo-Antelo M, Baleato-González S, Mosqueira AJ, et al. Radiologic clues to cerebral venous thrombosis. *Radiographics*. 2019;39(6):1611-1628.

Kumral E, Polat F, Uzunkopry C, et al. The clinical spectrum of intracerebral hematoma, hemorrhagic infarct, non-hemorrhagic infarct, and non-lesional venous stroke in patients with cerebral sinus-venous thrombosis. *Eur J Neurol*. 2012;19(4):537-543.

Yamashita E, Kanasaki Y, Fujii S, et al. Comparison of increased venous contrast in ischemic stroke using phase sensitive MR imaging with perfusion changes on flow-sensitive alternating inversion recovery at 3 Tesla. *Acta Radiol*. 2011;52(8):905-910.

Neuroradiology: THE REQUISITES. 4th ed. pp 134-136.

CASE 103

Intracranial Vertebral Artery Dissection—Spontaneous

1. **D.** Noncontrast head CT shows acute subarachnoid hemorrhage (SAH) in the basilar cisterns and right Sylvian fissure (Figure 103.1) as well as hemorrhage in the fourth ventricle (Figure 103.2). Notice the irregularity of the V4 segment of the right vertebral artery just distal to the takeoff of the right PICA, with an associated 2 cm × 3 mm fusiform dissecting pseudoaneurysm.

2. **B.** Vertebral artery dissections are most commonly seen in the V2 (~35%) or in the V3 segments (~34%). Conventional angiography is considered the gold standard and may demonstrate focal caliber change, proximal or distal stenosis, or fusiform aneurysmal dilatation. Patients with intracranial extension are not treated with anticoagulation or antiplatelet agents because of the associated risk of subarachnoid hemorrhage. In patients who present with subarachnoid hemorrhage (as in this case), consideration should be given to operative or endovascular trapping or coiling of the dissected artery. Note a pipeline stent was placed in the right vertebral artery in this patient (not shown).

3. **A.** Cerebral vasospasm following SAH is seen in 40%–70% of patients and is a major cause of mortality and morbidity. It usually occurs after a few days from the onset of hemorrhage and peaks at days 4–7. Patients present with neurological deterioration attributable to vasospasm-induced ischemia often referred to as "delayed cerebral ischemia." In this patient, mild to moderate non-flow-limiting vasospasm is seen in the right PICA as well as the basilar artery (Figures 103.5 and 103.6).

4. **D.** All of these are recognized complications of intracranial vascular dissections. Intracranial extension of dissection has a high rate of SAH usually with a disastrous outcome. This patient passed away within 19 days of her initial presentation, despite aggressive management.

Comment

These images demonstrate intracranial dissection of the right vertebral artery with associated fusiform dissecting pseudoaneurysm. The most common presentation in these patients is with headache or neck pain, with a high frequency of associated subarachnoid hemorrhage seen in up to 50%. Although CT is not a sensitive study for detecting vascular injuries, it may identify patients at increased risk (those with skull base fractures or fractures of the vertebral bodies extending through the foramen transversarium, which houses the cervical vertebral artery). It is also important to recognize that vertebral artery dissections may also be spontaneous (i.e., no clear etiology or only minor trauma) and may occur in association with excessive vomiting, excessive straining, and coughing (as in this case).

CT and CT angiography (CTA) are often the first imaging studies that can rapidly demonstrate posterior fossa ischemia or associated SAH. CT may also identify an occluded vertebral artery that appears as hyperdense or mural thrombus (often with some surrounding stranding). Thin section images may sometimes show a characteristic "double lumen" appearance. CTA can demonstrate luminal irregularity, as well as associated pseudoaneurysms. MRI can detect small foci of ischemia on DWI, and fat-saturated T1W images are more sensitive to detecting intramural hematomas (crescent sign). Conventional angiography remains the gold standard and may demonstrate focal dilatation, proximal or distal stenosis, or associated aneurysms/pseudoaneurysms. Note that there might be segmental tapering related to intramural hematoma, but the hematoma itself is not visualized on angiography. Treatment and prognosis depend on multiple factors, but the presence of subarachnoid hemorrhage usually has an unfavorable prognosis with a high rate of rebleeding and poor outcomes.

REFERENCES

Lv X, Wu Z, Yang X, et al. Endovascular treatment of cerebral aneurysms associated with arteriovenous malformations. *Eur J Radiol*. 2012;81(6):1296-1298.

Park KW, Park JS, Hwang SC, Im SB, Shin WH, Kim BT. Vertebral artery dissection: natural history, clinical features and therapeutic considerations. *J Korean Neurosurg Soc*. 2008;44(3):109-115.

Rahal JP, Malek AM. Benefit of cone-beam computed tomography angiography in acute management of angiographically undetectable ruptured arteriovenous malformations. *J Neurosurg*. 2013;119(4):1015-1020.

Neuroradiology: THE REQUISITES. 4th ed. pp 33-34, 161-162.

CASE 104

Suprasellar Hypothalamic Germinoma

1. **A.** Approximately 2.0 × 1.1 × 1.1 cm cystic and solidly enhancing mass is seen involving the hypothalamus, in the floor of the third ventricle filling and expanding the infundibular

recess and charismatic recess (Figure 104.7). No calcification within the lesion on the CT (Figure 104.1), and no diffusion restriction (Figure 104.3). The pituitary gland appears separate; notice that the posterior pituitary bright spot is not visualized (Figure 104.7). Stalk appears essentially unremarkable. The demographics of this patient such as being a relatively young male point toward the preferred diagnosis of germinoma rather than a hypothalamic glioma. Optic tract gliomas are more frequently encountered in younger patients and are usually more diffuse with heterogeneous enhancement and hamartomas do not enhance.

2. **A.** Synchronous lesions in the hypothalamic and pineal regions account for 10% of all intracranial germ cell tumors.
3. **A.** Intracranial germinomas tend to occur in the midline, either in the pineal region (vast majority) or along the floor of the third ventricle/suprasellar region.
4. **C.** Germinomas in the pineal region have a marked male preponderance with a male-to-female ratio of 5–22:1, whereas hypothalamic germinomas affect males and females with equal frequency and commonly cause symptoms indicative of hypothalamic involvement, such as diabetes insipidus, or precocious puberty.

Comment

This case demonstrates a mixed solid and cystic avidly enhancing midline mass that was found to be a germinoma on pathology. Due to their marked cellularity and protein content, germinomas are typically hyperdense on an unenhanced CT and isointense to the brain on T2W MR imaging. Cystic change and calcification are uncommon, and these neoplasms typically show prominent enhancement. On diffusion-weighted imaging, these may restrict being hyperintense, with corresponding low signal on apparent diffusion coefficient maps, not seen in this case perhaps secondary to cystic change. These tumors can metastasize by subarachnoid seeding, and screening MRI of the spine should be performed.

Germinomas are most common in children and young adults, and they arise from primitive germ cells. The pineal gland is the most common site (80%–90%), followed by the suprasellar region (15%–30%). Clinical presentation from suprasellar masses is variable but may include diabetes insipidus, hypopituitarism, or visual symptoms related to compression of the optic chiasm. Germinoma is the most common pineal tumor, accounting for 65% of all pineal germ cell neoplasms and approximately 40% of all pineal region tumors. Other germ cell tumors include teratoma, embryonal carcinoma, and choriocarcinoma. Teratomas may be distinguished from other germ cell tumors due to the presence of fat, calcification, and cyst formation (the fat and calcification or bone may have characteristic appearances on imaging). Choriocarcinomas may be differentiated due to the high incidence of hemorrhage within these tumors. In addition, β-human chorionic gonadotropin is a good serum marker for choriocarcinoma. Less common germ cell tumors, including embryonal cell carcinoma, endodermal sinus (yolk sac) tumors, and teratomas, may have hormonal markers such as β-human chorionic-gonadotropin and α-fetoprotein. The mainstay of treatment is radiation therapy, with 80%–90% long-term cure rates. Leptomeningeal seeding or spillage during surgery are poor prognostic indicators.

REFERENCES

Dumrongpisutikul N, Intrapiromkul J, Yousem DM. Distinguishing between germinomas and pineal cell tumors on MR imaging. *AJNR Am J Neuroradiol*. 2012;33(3):550-555.
Saito R, Kumabe T, Kanamori M, et al. Early response to chemotherapy as an indicator for the management of germinoma-like tumors of the pineal and/or suprasellar regions. *J Clin Neurosci*. 2014;21(1):124-130.
Saleem SN, Said AH, Lee DH. Lesions of the hypothalamus: MR imaging diagnostic features. *Radiographics*. 2007;27(4):1087-1108.
Neuroradiology: THE REQUISITES. 4th ed. p 367.

CASE 105
Primary Orbital Lymphoma

1. **A.** Primary lymphoma of the orbit is one of the commonest orbital tumors and accounts for as much as half of all orbital malignancies.
2. **A.** Recent advances in molecular and cytogenetics have established that lymphoma can be associated with *Chlamydia psittaci* infection.
3. **A.** Orbital lymphoma involves mainly superior-lateral quadrant and the orbital structures inside. Eyelid and extraocular muscles are also commonly involved, as in this case.
4. **D.** Enophthalmos. Inward retraction of the globe (just like the skin of the involved breast) is a characteristic of metastatic scirrhous breast carcinoma due to infiltration and desmoplasia. This may occasionally be seen in metastases from gastrointestinal tract adenocarcinomas.

Comment

This patient demonstrates multiple solid enhancing lesions with diffusion restriction involving bilateral orbits (Figures 105.1–105.6), skull base/sphenoid sinus (Figures 105.3–105.5), calvarium and scalp (Figure 105.7–105.9), consistent with lymphomatous involvement. In addition, there is extensive meningeal enhancement, likely reflecting leptomeningeal as well as pachymeningeal involvement with lymphoma (Figure 105.9).

Primary lymphoma of the orbit is one of the most common orbital tumors and accounts for almost 50% of all orbital malignancies. Lymphoma of the orbit can be unilateral or bilateral, part of systemic disease, or can be isolated (primary) to the orbit. It is a B-cell non-Hodgkin lymphoma, and in most cases arises from mucosa-associated lymphoid tissue (MALT). Orbital lymphoma mainly involves superior-lateral quadrant and the orbital structures inside, such as the eyelid and extraocular muscles in the majority of cases (up to 40%), the conjunctiva in 33% of cases, and the lacrimal apparatus in 25% of cases. These lesions are usually managed with radiation therapy, and some higher-grade lesions also receive chemotherapy. Distant recurrences are reported in approximately 15% of cases. The recent identification of *Chlamydia psittaci* as a causative factor in the increasing incidence of orbital lymphomas has led to antibiotic therapy being used to reduce the size of the tumor and in some cases results in remission.

Clinical manifestations of ocular metastases and lymphoma are variable, depending on the site of involvement, ranging from asymptomatic to proptosis, diplopia, decreased vision, and less commonly, pain, red eye, and lid swelling. The symptoms of orbital metastasis may precede detection of the primary tumor in up to 25% of cases. In autopsy series, up to 7% of patients with known systemic carcinoma had metastases to the orbit. The presence of orbital metastases is an unfavorable prognostic sign, with an average mean survival time of less than 2 years. Management is palliative and may include radiation, chemotherapy, or surgery and is intended to preserve vision, provide symptomatic relief, and improve quality of life.

The most common location of orbital metastases is the globe. Ocular metastases characteristically involve the uveal region, resulting in thickening in this location on imaging. The intraconal retrobulbar disease is usually related to the direct extension of an ocular metastasis. In most cases, metastasis occurs through hematogenous spread. The most common tumors to metastasize to the globe are breast, followed by prostate carcinoma in adults.

Outside of the globe, orbital metastases most often are extraconal and are usually related to bone metastases (prostate carcinoma is most common). Extraosseous spread from a bone metastasis frequently invades the adjacent extraocular muscle.

REFERENCES

Haradome K, Haradome H, Usui Y, et al. Orbital lymphoproliferative disorders (OLPDs): value of MR imaging for differentiating orbital lymphoma from benign OPLDs. *AJNR Am J Neuroradiol*. 2014; 35(10):1976-1982.

Priego G, Majos C, Climent F, Muntane A. Orbital lymphoma: imaging features and differential diagnosis. *Insights Imaging*. 2012;3(4):337-344.

Rudoltz MS, Ayyangar K, Mohiuddin M. Application of magnetic resonance imaging and three-dimensional treatment planning in the treatment of orbital lymphoma. *Med Dosim*. 1993;18(3):129-133.

Neuroradiology: THE REQUISITES. 4th ed. p 337.

CASE 106

Aqueductal Stenosis

1. **C.** Aqueduct of Sylvius. There is a significant and disproportionate enlargement of the lateral ventricles and the third ventricle (Figures 106.1–106.3) with normal to small size of the fourth ventricle (Figure 106.4). High-resolution heavily T2-weighted images demonstrate a thin septum/web across the inferior aspect of the cerebral aqueduct (Figure 106.5) with an expanded funnel-shaped aqueduct above this level (Figure 106.3). Also notice that the floor of the expanded third ventricle is thinned and displaced inferiorly (Figure 106.5), with no flow across the aqueduct in phase-contrast CSF flow study (Figure 106.6).
2. **C.** Imaging findings in this case are consistent with aqueductal stenosis due to an obstructing web with chronic compensated hydrocephalus.
3. **C.** Aqueductal stenosis is the most common cause of congenital hydrocephalus. Acquired aqueductal stenosis may be intrinsic, related to clot or adhesions from prior hemorrhage or infection (meningitis/ventriculitis), or extrinsic from compression of the aqueduct related to tumors (tectal gliomas, pineal tumors, cerebellar neoplasms).
4. **C.** Congenital aqueductal stenosis may be seen as an inherited X-linked recessive disorder in boys. They can have adducted thumbs (bent toward the palm), with severe intellectual disability and spasticity. It is caused by mutations in the L1CAM gene and is inherited in an X-linked recessive manner.

Comment

This case demonstrates the characteristic findings of aqueductal stenosis from an obstructing web as seen in the high-resolution thin section images (Figure 106.5). There is prominent dilation of the lateral and third ventricles, with a relatively normal-sized fourth ventricle. There is upward convexity or bowing of the corpus callosum related to the lateral ventricular dilation, and there is inferior bowing of the floor of the third ventricle, with depression of the optic chiasm. Congenital aqueductal stenosis may be seen as an inherited X-linked recessive disorder in boys. Children may present with an enlarging head circumference. Blockage of the aqueduct may be caused by webs, septae, or gliosis.

Aqueductal stenosis is often acquired in relation to previous subarachnoid hemorrhage, meningitis or ventriculitis, or extrinsic compression from a mass or tumor. MRI is the modality of choice in evaluating affected patients. Three-dimensional (3D) constructive interference in the steady-state (CISS) sequence is extremely useful in distinguishing intrinsic aqueductal abnormalities from extrinsic mass or compression. The presence of aqueductal CSF

flow may also be evaluated by performing time-resolved 2D phase-contrast CSF flow imaging with velocity encoding (VENC) which relies upon location-specific sequential application of a pair of phase encoding pulses in opposite directions. Stationary protons will experience the same pulse at both times and therefore return no signal, whereas protons that have moved will experience different phase encoding pulses and will be visible.

Treatment is usually either with an endoscopic third ventriculostomy (ETV) or with ventriculoperitoneal shunting. However, in this patient, headaches subsequently resolved, there were no visual complaints, and no papilledema was found on fundoscopic exam. Overall, the clinic-radiological picture suggested that the patient had findings of raised ICP in the past, but his brain compensated for this problem over the years, and hence no surgical intervention was performed.

REFERENCES

Algin O, Turkbey B. Evaluation of aqueductal stenosis by 3D sampling perfection with application-optimized contrasts using different flip angle evolutions sequence: preliminary results with 3T MR imaging. *AJNR Am J Neuroradiol*. 2012;33(4):740-746.

Stadlbauer A, Salomonowitz E, Brenneis C, et al. Magnetic resonance velocity mapping of 3D cerebrospinal fluid flow dynamics in hydrocephalus: preliminary results. *Eur Radiol*. 2012;22(1):232-242.

Neuroradiology: THE REQUISITES. 4th ed. pp 286-287.

CASE 107

Cavernous Sinus Mass—Meningioma

1. **B.** The mass is centered in the left cavernous sinus.
2. **F.** The oculomotor nerve (CNIII), the trochlear nerve (CNIV), and the ophthalmic division of the trigeminal nerve (CNV1) lie in the lateral wall of the cavernous sinus in that order from superior to inferior. The maxillary division of the trigeminal nerve (CNV2) lies just inferior to the junction of the lateral and medial wall dura of the cavernous sinus. The abducens nerve (CNVI) and the sympathetic plexus around the carotid artery, on the contrary, lie within the cavity of the cavernous sinus in close relation to the ICA.
3. **A.** Meningiomas are one of the most common lesions to involve the cavernous sinus.
4. **A.** Meningioma of the cavernous sinus.

Comment

A variety of lesions can affect the cavernous sinus, including neoplasms primarily arising from bone (chondrosarcoma, chondroma, and chordoma) and bone metastases. Metastases and lymphoma primarily affecting the cavernous sinus and perineural spread of tumor are also common. Benign neoplasms include meningioma, schwannoma, and extension of a pituitary adenoma. A variety of vascular and inflammatory lesions may also involve the cavernous sinus.

Infectious processes include bacterial and fungal (actinomycosis, aspergillus, and mucormycosis) agents. In addition, the cavernous sinus may be affected indirectly by complications of infectious processes (e.g., cavernous sinus thrombosis). Tolosa–Hunt syndrome represents an idiopathic granulomatous inflammatory disorder that may affect the orbital apex and cavernous sinus. Histologically, Tolosa–Hunt syndrome is identical to orbital pseudotumor (differing only in location). It may present with painful ophthalmoplegia, deficits of the cranial nerves coursing through the cavernous sinus, and retro-orbital pain. Symptoms may last for days to weeks, and may be recurrent. Like orbital pseudotumor, it responds rapidly to steroid treatment. MRI may show abnormal signal intensity or an enhancing mass within the cavernous sinus.

There may be an extension into the orbital apex. Thrombosis of the cavernous sinus or superior ophthalmic vein may occur.

In this case, there is a mass within the left cavernous sinus that is relatively isointense to brain parenchyma on T2W imaging (Figure 107.1). Neoplastic processes that are hypointense on T2W imaging include lymphoma, meningioma, and less commonly, plasmacytoma and schwannoma. Sarcoid may also be hypointense on T2W imaging. Notice that the enhancement extends along the lateral dural margin, as well as posteriorly along the tentorial margin (Figure 107.3) (an appearance that may be seen with meningiomas, lymphoma, and sarcoid). The marked narrowing of the left cavernous internal carotid artery with preserved flow void (Figures 107.1 and 107.2) makes meningioma the best diagnosis. Biopsy through a left temporal craniotomy revealed a WHO grade 1 meningioma.

REFERENCES

Amemiya S, Aoki S, Ohtomo K. Cranial nerve assessment in cavernous sinus tumors with contrast-enhanced 3D fast-imaging employing steady-state acquisition MR imaging. *Neuroradiology.* 2009;51(7):467-470.
Mahalingam HV, Mani SE, Patel B, et al. Imaging spectrum of cavernous sinus lesions with histopathologic correlation. *Radiographics.* 2019;39(3):795-819.
Sughrue ME, Rutkowski MJ, Aranda D, et al. Factors affecting outcome following treatment of patients with cavernous sinus meningiomas. *J Neurosurg.* 2010;113(5):1087-1092.
Neuroradiology: THE REQUISITES. 4th ed. p 370.

CASE 108

Lhermitte–Duclos Disease (Dysplastic Gangliocytoma of the Cerebellum)

1. **D.** There are demarcated areas of T2W hyperintensity with preserved appearing cerebellar folia with mild mass effect and a classic "laminated" or "corduroy appearance" (Figures 108.1 and 108.2). Notice, no enhancement (Figure 108.7), mild diffusion hyperintensity from T2 shine-through effects (Figures 108.4 and 108.5), with no elevation of plasma volume (Figure 108.8) and no elevated choline on MRS (Figure 108.9). All findings are consistent with the diagnosis of dysplastic cerebellar gangliocytoma. SHH variant of medulloblastoma can sometimes appear similar but demonstrates restricted diffusion and avid contrast enhancement.
2. **D.** Lhermitte–Duclos disease (LDD) is a slowly progressive unilateral hamartomatous cerebellar tumor associated with mutations of the phosphatase and tensin homolog (PTEN) gene and is associated with Cowden syndrome which is an autosomal dominant multisystem disorder that increases the risk for benign and malignant neoplasms. In such cases, it is termed COLD syndrome (Cowden-Lhermitte–Duclos syndrome).
3. **A.** It is recognized as a WHO grade 1 tumor in the current WHO classification of CNS tumors.
4. **B.** LDD demonstrates high fluorodeoxy glucose (FDG) uptake on PET/CT. All others are incorrect.

Comment

Lhermitte–Duclos disease (LDD), also known as dysplastic cerebellar gangliocytoma, is a rare tumor of the cerebellum. The exact pathogenesis remains unknown, but LDD is considered to represent a complex hamartomatous malformation, not a true neoplasm, but it is still recognized as a WHO grade I tumor according to the current WHO classification of CNS tumors. When symptomatic, the patient typically presents with complaints related to mass effect in the second and third decades of life. It is associated with mutations of the phosphatase and tensin

homolog (PTEN) gene and is one of the PTEN hamartoma tumor syndromes which includes Cowden syndrome, an autosomal dominant multisystem disorder associated with an increased incidence of neoplasms in the endometrial, breast, colon, and thyroid. Intracranial meningiomas have also been noted with this syndrome.

Dysplastic gangliocytomas often occur in the cerebellar hemispheres. These lesions present as nonspecific hypoattenuating mass on CT. Calcification has been reported. On MRI, these lesions have a more characteristic appearance in which the gray and white matter of the cerebellar hemisphere are both involved and are thickened and hyperintense on T2W imaging, showing a somewhat characteristic "laminated" or "corduroy" appearance. They may exert a mass effect. Hydrocephalus may be present. Dysplastic gangliocytomas do not demonstrate significant enhancement, as in this case, but reported to show avid tracer uptake on FDG–PET. On pathologic evaluation, they usually appear as dysplasia with cellular disorganization of the normal laminar structure of the cerebellum, and hypertrophied granular cell neurons. Histologically, there is hypermyelination of axons, and pleomorphic ganglion cells replace the granular and Purkinje cell layers. Surgical resection is often curative in symptomatic cases. It is important to remember the association with COLD syndrome (Cowden–Lhermitte–Duclos syndrome), with increased risk of other neoplasms such as breast, endometrial, and thyroid cancers. Therefore, consider adding a recommendation for the evaluation of possible tumors in these locations in the radiology report.

REFERENCES

Calabria F, Grillea G, Zinzi M, et al. Lhermitte-Duclos disease presenting with positron emission tomography magnetic resonance fusion imaging: a case report. *J Med Case Rep.* 2012;6(1):76.
Cianfoni A, Wintermark M, Piludu F, et al. Morphological and functional MR imaging of Lhermitte-Duclos disease with pathology correlate. *J Neuroradiol.* 2008;35(5):297-300.
Nakagawa T, Maeda M, Kato M, et al. A case of Lhermitte-Duclos disease presenting high FDG uptake on FDG-PET/CT. *J Neurooncol.* 2007;84(2):185-188.
Thomas B, Krishnamoorthy T, Radhakrishnan VV, Kesavadas C. Advanced MR imaging in Lhermitte-Duclos disease: moving closer to pathology and pathophysiology. *Neuroradiology.* 2007;49(9):733-738.
Neuroradiology: THE REQUISITES. 4th ed. p 67.

CASE 109

Neurosarcoidosis

1. **E.** All of the following can present with basilar meningitis. Infections (e.g., tuberculosis, neurosyphilis, pyogenic infections, *Cryptococcus*), sarcoidosis, leptomeningeal seeding of primary malignancies (e.g., carcinomatosis from systemic malignancies or primary brain tumors), lymphoma, and chemical meningitis (e.g., ruptured dermoid).
2. **B.** This patient had known sarcoidosis with CNS and pulmonary involvement. These images demonstrate extensive nodular leptomeningeal enhancement throughout the subarachnoid spaces, in the basilar cisterns and around multiple cranial nerves and extending inferiorly along the spinal cord. Enhancement is also noted around the optic nerves, and infundibular stalk. The vast majority of patients with neurosarcoidosis generally have systemic disease. Leptomeningeal involvement is common. Pituitary and hypothalamic involvement is also common as is the involvement of perivascular spaces. In addition, patients can present with communicating hydrocephalus due to blockage of the cisterns from an inflammatory exudate. Occasionally, hydrocephalus may be secondary to mass effect from a parenchymal lesion or from entrapment of a ventricle related to ependymitis.

3. **B.** The following primary tumors can present with subarachnoid seeding, medulloblastoma, pineoblastoma, germinoma, glial neoplasms (glioblastoma, oligodendroglioma), as well as diffuse midline glioma.

Comment

Sarcoidosis is a systemic disorder characterized pathologically by noncaseating granulomas. A typical presentation is in the third and fourth decades of life, and it is slightly more common in females than in males. CNS involvement has been reported in up to 20% of cases, and isolated CNS involvement occurs in fewer than 2% to 4% of cases. Multiple patterns of CNS involvement are described. The most common is chronic meningitis with a predilection for the leptomeninges of the basal cisterns, as in this case. These patients may present with chronic meningeal symptoms, cranial neuropathies (especially involving the facial and optic nerves), or symptoms related to the involvement of the hypothalamus and pituitary stalk. Imaging findings are best demonstrated with MRI and include nodular leptomeningeal enhancement that can be seen throughout the subarachnoid spaces, as in this case. Another common pattern of CNS sarcoid is brain parenchymal involvement, with multiple regions of signal abnormality, that may occur as a result of direct extension from leptomeningeal disease; periventricular white matter lesions mimicking multiple sclerosis may be present because of disease extension along the perivascular spaces or related to sarcoid-induced small vessel vasculitis. There may be enhancing parenchymal granulomas which may be mistaken for a primary or metastatic tumor or tumefactive demyelination. Less commonly, the dural-based disease may be the predominant imaging finding and may be mistaken for a meningioma.

Gallium-67 scan is insensitive to detect CNS lesions but is sometimes used to detect systemic involvement in confusing cases. Corticosteroid therapy remains the mainstay of treatment with methotrexate being used sometimes as a second-line agent and imaging correlates poorly with treatment response.

Central nervous system tuberculosis may have a variety of clinical and radiologic presentations, including nodular tuberculous meningitis similar to neurosarcoidosis, cerebritis, tuberculoma, abscess formation, or a combination of these. CNS tuberculosis is normally related to hematogenous dissemination from a systemic source, such as the lung, genitourinary system, or gastrointestinal tract. Vasculitis may be seen in up to one-third of patients with basilar meningitis. This is because the vessels coursing through this inflammatory exudate may become directly involved. Consequences of arteritis include vasospasm and infarction.

REFERENCES

Dumas JL, Valeyre D, Chapelon-Abric C, et al. Central nervous system sarcoidosis: follow-up at MR imaging during steroid therapy. *Radiology.* 2000;214(2):411-420.
Prabhakar HB, Rabinowitz CB, Gibbons FK, et al. Imaging features of sarcoidosis on MDCT, FDG, PET and PET/CT. *AJR Am J Roentgenol.* 2008;190:1-6.
Smith JK, Matheus MG, Castillo M. Imaging manifestations of neurosarcoidosis. *AJR Am J Roentgenol.* 2004;182(2):289-295.
Neuroradiology: THE REQUISITES. 4th ed. pp 202-203, 562.

CASE 110

Epidermoid Cyst—Suprasellar Cistern

1. **C.** A lobulated near-CSF intensity mass in the suprasellar cistern with a high signal on DWI is consistent with an epidermoid cyst.
2. **A.** Cerebellopontine angle (CPA) cistern. Note that 40%–50% of epidermoid cysts are located in the CPA cistern and are the third most common lesions in this region, after vestibular schwannomas and meningiomas. Other locations include prepontine cistern, suprasellar cistern, cisterna magna, and the pineal region. Rarely, epidermoid cysts can be extradural which arise in the diploic space of the calvarium, in the temporal bone and petrous apex.
3. **B.** Epidermoid cysts are often indistinguishable from arachnoid cysts on many MR sequences, except for DWI/ADC which helps to differentiate them.
4. **A.** The unit is an "area" per "time" and is expressed in mm²/s.

Comment

Epidermoid cysts are congenital lesions that result from incomplete separation of the neural and cutaneous ectoderm at the time of closure of the neural tube. These cysts are lined by a single layer of stratified squamous epithelium, and they contain desquamated epithelium, keratin, and cholesterol crystals. Many of these cysts are incidental findings, but when symptomatic, epidermoid cysts typically present in the second to fourth decade of life. Men and women are equally affected. These are frequently asymptomatic, with headache being the most common presenting symptom. In the cerebellopontine cistern, they may present with dizziness, trigeminal neuralgia, and facial nerve weakness.

This case illustrates the typical appearance of an epidermoid cyst. There is a mass in the suprasellar cistern that exerts a mild mass effect on the adjacent brain stem. On T2W image (Figure 110.2), the lesion is isointense to CSF. On the unenhanced T1W images (not shown), these are mildly hyperintense to CSF, with a fine internal architecture. Unlike arachnoid cysts, which are typically isointense to CSF on T2 and FLAIR images, epidermoid cysts are hyperintense relative to CSF on these pulse sequences. Furthermore, this case illustrates hyperintensity on DWI with lower ADC values (compared to an arachnoid cyst), characteristic of these lesions (Figures 110.3 and 110.4). In contrast, there is no enhancement, as in this case (Figure 110.1). Other characteristic features of epidermoid cysts that distinguish them from arachnoid cysts (the major differential consideration here) are also presented in this case, including the lobulated and scalloped borders of this lesion and its insinuating nature, which fills and conforms to the shape of the space that it occupies.

Epidermoid cysts and dermoid cysts are of ectodermal origin. The epidermoid cyst has desquamated skin, whereas dermoid cysts also have skin appendages, such as hair follicles. Teratomas are true neoplasms that arise from ectopic pluripotent stem cells and by definition contain elements from all three embryological layers: endoderm, mesoderm, and ectoderm.

REFERENCES

Lakshmi M, Glastonbury CM. Imaging of the cerebellopontine angle. *Neuroimaging Clin N Am.* 2009;19(3):393-406.
Ren X, Lin S, Wang Z, et al. Clinical, radiological, and pathological features of 24 atypical intracranial epidermoid cysts. *J Neurosurg.* 2012; 116(3):611-621.
Neuroradiology: THE REQUISITES. 4th ed. pp 53, 444, 568.

CASE 111

Encephalocele

1. **D.** This case demonstrates a small encephalocele along the floor of the left middle cranial fossa, with a small portion of the inferior left temporal lobe protruding into the left mastoid air cells (Figures 111.1–111.4) with mild associated gliosis in the inferior left temporal lobe (Figure 111.3). There was fluid opacification of the left mastoid air cells, possibly due to CSF leak. Note, bilateral hippocampi are normal in volume and

signal intensity. On high-resolution temporal bone CT, an osseous defect was confirmed in the tegmen tympani and tegmen mastoideum, with left temporal encephalocele abutting the ossicles (Figures 111.5 and 111.6).

2. **E.** Small temporal encephaloceles are increasingly recognized as an etiology for seizures and can be caused by trauma, erosion of temporal bone by chronic suppurative otitis media/cholesteatoma formation, or iatrogenic from prior surgery or idiopathic (form spontaneously). These are also encountered as asymptomatic sequelae of idiopathic intracranial hypertension.

3. **C.** In individuals with temporal lobe epilepsy, and especially if seizure activity can be localized to the encephalocele, then surgical resection and repair have good clinical outcomes.

In this patient, EEG demonstrated left temporal slowing, possibly reflecting the source of the patient's seizures, and surgical repair was recommended.

4. **B.** CSF leak is the most common presentation in the postoperative setting.

Comment

This case illustrates a small left temporal encephalocele associated with fluid opacification of the left mastoid air cells. An osseous defect was confirmed on a high-resolution CT. EEG demonstrated left temporal slowing, confirming the source of the patient's seizures, and surgical repair was subsequently recommended.

Meningocele (encephalocele) refers to herniation of the meninges, CSF, or brain tissue through an osseous defect in the cranium and can be congenital or acquired. Congenital encephaloceles are due to an abnormality in the process of invagination of the neural plate and are more common in the frontoethmoidal region, particularly in the Vietnamese and southeastern Asian women. During embryogenesis, the dura around the brain contacts the dermis in the facial or nasion region as the neural plate regresses. When there is a failure of dermal regression, an encephalocele, dermoid cyst, sinus tract, or nasal glioma may develop. Note, a basal glioma is a misnomer in that the benign mass is composed of heterotopic glial tissue and is not a true tumor. Nasofrontal and sphenoethmoidal encephaloceles are frequently clinically occult, and the differential diagnosis is broad when this entity is seen through the nasoscope on office examination.

Most acquired meningoencephaloceles are seen in the setting of prior trauma or surgery and involve the nasal cavity, paranasal sinuses, or the temporal bone. Temporal bone encephaloceles may be asymptomatic for years but eventually produce conductive hearing loss, meningitis, cerebrospinal fluid (CSF) leaks, facial nerve weakness, or (rarely) seizures, as in this case. A combination of imaging modalities, including nuclear scintigraphy, CT, and MR imaging, can be used to assess CSF leaks and meningoencephaloceles. It is important to determine whether the CSF leak is due to a dural laceration or a meningocele (encephalocele). Dedicated thin section or volumetric T1 and T2W sequences are most useful in establishing this diagnosis by demonstrating a direct extension of brain tissue in the temporal bone. Surgical resection and repair have good clinical outcomes in patients with temporal lobe epilepsy, especially if seizure activity can be localized to the encephalocele.

REFERENCES

Campbell ZM, Hyer JM, Lauzon S, Bonilha L, Spampinato MV, Yazdani M. Detection and characteristics of temporal encephaloceles in patients with refractory epilepsy. *AJNR Am J Neuroradiol.* 2018;39(8):1468-1472.

Muñoz A, Hinojosa J, Esparza J. Cisternography and ventriculography gadopentate dimeglumine-enhanced MR imaging in pediatric patients: preliminary report. *AJNR Am J Neuroradiol.* 2007;28(5):889-894.

Pinzer T, Lauer G, Gollogly J, et al. A complex therapy for treatment of frontoethmoidal meningoencephaolcele in a developing third world country: neurosurgical aspects. *J Neurosurg.* 2006;104(5):326-331.

Neuroradiology: THE REQUISITES. 4th ed. pp 282, 415-416.

CASE 112

Facial Nerve—Inflammation (Bell's Palsy)

1. **C.** Bell's palsy. This case demonstrates linear enhancement of the distal canalicular segment of the right facial nerve, labyrinthine segment, geniculate ganglion, extending to the distal tympanic segment. Note, no appreciable enhancement is seen on the left side. Findings can be seen in inflammatory conditions, including viral infections, Lyme disease, as well as sarcoidosis. Neoplasm/metastatic disease is possible but presents with nodular enhancement and wouldn't improve in 6 days. Bell's palsy is the most common cause of facial paralysis and is the most likely diagnosis in this case.

2. **A.** Facial nerve (CNVII) is the only cranial nerve that can show postcontrast enhancement, attributed to the presence of perineural vascular plexus. The typical sites of enhancement include anterior genu (geniculate ganglion), posterior genu (between tympanic and mastoid segments), and some enhancement can also be seen in the tympanic and mastoid segments. Note, the labyrinthine segments, the cisternal, canalicular as well as extracranial segments do not enhance. The presence of enhancement in these regions implies pathology.

3. **C.** Crista falciformis, also known as the falciform crest, is a horizontal ridge that divides the lateral portion of the internal auditory canal (IAC) into superior and inferior portions.

4. **D.** The cochlear division of the vestibulocochlear nerve. The mnemonic "Seven up, Coke down" is useful to remember the relative position of nerves inside the IAC. In addition to crista falciformis, Bill bar is a vertical ridge of bone that divides the superior compartment of the IAC into an anterior and posterior compartment, thus dividing the IAC into four quadrants: anterosuperior (facial nerve), anteroinferior (cochlear), posterosuperior (superior vestibular nerve), and posteroinferior (inferior vestibular nerve).

Comment

This case shows linear enhancement of the right facial nerve (CNVII) on either side of the geniculate ganglion, from the distal canalicular segment to the distal tympanic segment, as well as enhancement of the facial nerve in the fundus of the IAC, known as the "fundal tuft sign." No appreciable enhancement is seen on the contralateral side. The patient presented with typical symptoms of Bell's palsy and was clinically improving at the time of imaging. Statistically, inflammatory processes (i.e., viral) are most likely. Other infectious etiologies associated with CNVII involvement, in addition to viral causes, include Lyme disease. In immunocompromised patients, especially those with HIV infection, cytomegalovirus can affect the nerves in the IAC. Other inflammatory processes that affect the cranial nerves here include neurosarcoidosis.

Neoplasms that may involve CNVII include schwannoma (unlikely in this case, given acute clinical presentation). Subarachnoid seeding of the tumor may involve the internal auditory canals and can be seen in lymphoma and carcinomatosis (lung, breast, or seeding of primary brain tumors). Perineural spread of malignancies along the facial nerve is often associated with destructive changes in the temporal bone, commonly arising from temporal bone squamous cell carcinoma, primary parotid malignancies, as well as skin cancers of the ear and cheek.

Frequently, imaging is not necessary for the workup of Bell's palsy. Imaging is reserved for atypical cases to assess for causes other than the viral disease in the following situations: (1) facial weakness that persists for a longer period than would be expected in an uncomplicated Bell's palsy, i.e., >6 weeks, (2) slowly progressive palsy, (3) facial palsy accompanied by spasm, (4) recurrent palsy, (5) bilateral symptoms, (6) unusual degrees of pain, and (7) and the presence of multiple cranial neuropathies or other neurologic symptoms.

Also, note that the pattern of enhancement does not correlate with prognosis and may persist for months after the resolution of symptoms. The diameter of the nerve is the key difference between Bell's palsy and tumors involving the nerve. In Bell's palsy, there is a smooth linear enhancement, with little or no enlargement and no focal nodularity, as in this case. Enlargement and nodularity of the intratemporal segments of the CNVII should raise suspicion for a neoplasm.

REFERENCES

Al-Noury K, Lofty A. Normal and pathological findings for the facial nerve on magnetic resonance imaging. *Clin Radiol.* 2011;66(8):701-707.
Jenke AC, Stoek LM, Zilbauer M, et al. Facial palsy: etiology, outcome and management in children. *Eur J Paediatr Neurol.* 2011;15(3):209-213.
Mohan S, Hoeffner E, Bigelow DC, Loevner LA. Applications of magnetic resonance imaging in adult temporal bone disorders. *Magn Reson Imaging Clin N Am.* 2012;20(3):545-572.
Neuroradiology: THE REQUISITES. 4th ed. pp 395-396.

CASE 113

Functional Magnetic Resonance Imaging (f-MRI)—Language Mapping

1. **C.** T2*. Oxygenated hemoglobin is diamagnetic, whereas deoxygenated hemoglobin is paramagnetic. Thus, the T2* time is different for the two of them, and the amount of oxygen used by active brain areas can be mapped in f-MRI experiments.
2. **B.** Language f-MRI was performed in this right-handed 24-year-old female with seizures for language lateralization. Multiple areas of activation are seen in the left inferior frontal gyrus (Broca area), and bilaterally in the temporal gyri (Wernicke area); overall greater activation is seen on the left side than on the right, suggesting left hemispheric dominance for language function.
   On the sentence completion task (Figure 113.1), left > right frontal operculum and posterior superior temporal/supramarginal activation was seen. On the word generation task (Figure 113.2), left > right frontal operculum and posterior superior temporal/supramarginal activation was seen. On the rhyming task (Figure 113.3), left frontal operculum and posterior superior temporal/supramarginal activation was seen. On the object naming task (Figure 113.4), there was robust bilateral occipital activation typical of this task. For f-MRI, it should be noted that lack of activation does not necessarily indicate a lack of function and not all activating areas are absolutely eloquent. According to the law of cerebral dominance, there is a left-sided hemispheric dominance for language processing in 95% of right-handed individuals and in 70% of left-handed individuals.
3. **D.** All of these statements are correct regarding f-MRI and language mapping.
4. **D.** In the dominant hemisphere, pars opercularis coupled with pars triangularis makes up the Broca's area which is well known for speech production.

Comments

Functional MRI (f-MRI) is one of the most commonly used functional neuroimaging techniques for studying the cerebral representation of language processing and is currently being used as a substitute for the more invasive Wada test. f-MRI utilizes "blood-oxygenation-level-dependent (BOLD) contrast taking advantage of the close relationship between local neuronal activity and blood flow, aka neurovascular coupling. When local neuronal activity increases, local blood flow also increases, leading to an increase in oxygenated hemoglobin (diamagnetic and is magnetically indistinguishable from brain tissue) that is disproportionate to the increased oxygen demand for neuronal activity. As a result, local susceptibility effects caused by the presence of paramagnetic deoxygenated hemoglobin decreases, leading to a signal intensity increase on T2*-weighted MR images in those brain areas that are active.

f-MRI is increasingly being used for presurgical language assessment in the treatment of patients with brain tumors, epilepsy, vascular malformations, etc. The American Society of Functional Neuroradiology (ASFNR) taskforce generated an adult language paradigm algorithm for presurgical language assessment including the following tasks: Sentence Completion, Word Generation, Rhyming, Object Naming, and/or Passive Story Listening. The use of tasks from different categories improves reliability for hemispheric dominance assessment, but at the cost of increased examination time. All of these tasks are easy to implement, analyze, and perform, which is essential for clinical care as well as patient-based clinical research.

Resting-state f-MRI (rs-fMRI) is similar to conventional f-MRI, but the main difference is that it does not require patients to perform a task or respond to a stimulus. Patients simply lie in the scanner for ~5–6 minutes with their eyes closed or staring at a fixed point while the whole-brain BOLD data are collected. T2*-weighted echo-planar images are obtained with 3–4 mm isotropic spatial resolution, TR values of 2–3 sec, and multiband acceleration (if available). A major benefit of its task-free nature is that rs-fMRI can be performed in all patient settings, including infants and children, patients with neurological deficits, and even those who are anesthetized. rs-fMRI has allowed the discovery of at least 20 distinct patterns of brain connections called resting state networks (RSNs). The most important RSN is the "default mode network" (most active at rest, involved with introspection and mind wandering), networks for visual and auditory processing, executive control, dorsal attention, and salience (identification of unusual/remarkable events). These networks have provided significant insights into the cognitive organization of the brain in health and disease.

REFERENCES

Glover GH. Overview of functional magnetic resonance imaging. *Neurosurg Clin N Am.* 2011;22(2):133-139, vii.
Lv H, Wang Z, Tong E, et al. Resting-state functional MRI: everything that nonexperts have always wanted to know. *AJNR Am J Neuroradiol.* 2018;39(8):1390-1399.
Smits M, Visch-Brink E, Schraa-Tam CK, Koudstaal PJ, van der Lugt A. Functional MR imaging of language processing: an overview of easy-to-implement paradigms for patient care and clinical research. *Radiographics.* 2006;26(suppl 1):S145-S158.
Neuroradiology: THE REQUISITES. 4th ed. pp 13-14, 61.

CASE 114

Reversible Cerebral Vasoconstriction Syndrome (RCVS)

1. **D.** Trauma is the most common cause of subarachnoid hemorrhage (SAH).
2. **C.** This patient presented with a thunderclap headache, with convexity nonaneurysmal subarachnoid hemorrhage (Figures 114.1 and 114.2) and multifocal narrowing and tapering of the left greater than right anterior and middle cerebral arteries (Figures 114.3–114.5) in keeping with postpartum angiopathy which is a subset of reversible cerebral vasoconstriction syndrome (RCVS).

3. **D.** RCVS typically manifests with multifocal vascular narrowings and convexity SAH. No aneurysms are found on cerebral angiography as in this case. RCVS can also present with lobar hemorrhage, watershed infarcts, and vasogenic edema.

4. **H.** Thunderclap headache is a severe headache that comes on suddenly and is often associated with nausea and vomiting. It can be life-threatening with many causes, as listed here. It is often referred to as the "worst headache of life" and comes "out of nowhere." The pain usually peaks within a minute, lasts about 5 minutes, and may go away, and is often the only warning symptom of a serious problem.

Comment

Reversible cerebral vasoconstriction syndrome (RCVS) is a clinicoradiologic syndrome presenting with sudden severe headache and segmental vasoconstriction of cerebral vasculature that usually resolves within 3 months. It is not a single entity but is considered a common presentation of multiple diverse disorders, all characterized by multifocal reversible cerebral vasoconstriction. RCVS now encompasses what was previously thought to be a group of distinct clinical entities, including Call-Fleming syndrome, coital thunderclap headache, drug-induced angiopathy, postpartum angiopathy, etc. The diagnosis of RCVS can be challenging, as segmental vasoconstriction can be absent early in the course of the disease and that the clinical symptoms overlap with other known CNS disorders such as aneurysmal SAH and primary angiitis of the CNS.

RCVS commonly affects patients aged 20–50 years, with a female predominance, and interestingly, the mean age of men tends to be a decade younger than that of females (fourth decade). The diagnostic criteria for RCVS were initially proposed by Calabrese et al. but are now slightly modified by the International Headache Society and include the following: (1) severe, acute headaches, (2) uniphasic disease course, with no new symptoms after 1 month of onset, (3) no evidence for aneurysmal SAH, (4) normal or near-normal findings on CSF analysis, (5) multifocal segmental cerebral vasoconstriction, and (6) reversibility of angiographic abnormalities within 12 weeks of onset. Though these criteria have not been prospectively verified, they could still prove to be useful to clinically diagnose RCVS and to increase awareness of this entity.

The exact pathophysiology of RCVS remains unknown; however, alterations in cerebral vascular tone leading to vasoconstriction likely underlie the development of the syndrome. Most patients with RCVS have a good outcome with no permanent sequelae, while a small minority will experience a more fulminant course culminating in permanent disability or death. Current treatment recommendations include withdrawal of any suspected exogenous triggers, and intensive care unit–level care, with analgesics, blood pressure control, and seizure prophylaxis. Treatment with calcium channel blockers has been found to be efficacious and is preferred as a reasonable first-line therapy. Short course glucocorticoid therapy has also been advocated.

REFERENCES

Calabrese LH, Dodick DW, Schwedt TJ, et al. Narrative review: reversible cerebral vasoconstriction syndromes. *Ann Intern Med.* 2007;146:34-44.

Miller TR, Shivashankar R, Mossa-Basha M, Gandhi D. Reversible cerebral vasoconstriction syndrome, part 1: epidemiology, pathogenesis, and clinical course. *AJNR Am J Neuroradiol.* 2015;36(8):1392-1399.

Neuroradiology: THE REQUISITES. 4th ed. pp 122, 221.

CASE 115

Ganglioglioma

1. **A.** Gangliogliomas are WHO grade 1 CNS tumors that typically occur in the temporal lobes and present with seizures.

2. **B.** Gangliogliomas are composed of ganglion cells (neuronal element) and glial cells (neoplastic element) and can occasionally dedifferentiate into a higher-grade tumor such as an anaplastic gangliogliomas (WHO grade 3) and a glioblastoma (WHO grade 4). On imaging, a cystic mass with an enhancing mural nodule is seen in <50% of cases. BRAF V600E mutations are encountered in up to 60% of cases.

3. **D.** All of these listed tumors are known to have BRAF V600E mutations. BRAF is a proto-oncogene, encoding for a serine/threonine protein kinase, and mutations of BRAF are the most common alteration of the RAS/MAPK pathway. These mutations have been identified in a variety of CNS tumors as listed here.

Comment

Gangliogliomas are slow-growing, low-grade benign tumors that most commonly affect children and young adults. Gangliogliomas have a predominance of glial tissue and typically occur in the cerebrum, most commonly arising in the temporal lobe (as in this case), followed by the frontal lobe, parietal lobe, occipital lobe, and region of the hypothalamus and the third ventricle. They may also be infratentorial, arising within the cerebellum, brain stem, or in the spinal cord. Gangliogliomas are typically circumscribed tumors that occur superficially in the brain parenchyma, with little or no surrounding edema. They are usually cystic (purely cystic or cystic with solid components), although solid tumors without cyst formation are also reported. Calcification is frequently present in up to 30%, and these neoplasms may demonstrate variable contrast enhancement, ranging from mild to marked. However, contrast enhancement need not be present.

Because gangliogliomas are composed of both glial (usually astrocytes) and neural elements, they may undergo malignant transformation. When neuronal elements make up the majority of the mass, the neoplasm is referred to as a ganglioneuroma. Gangliocytomas are composed of mature ganglion cells. They rarely have glial elements and therefore have no potential for malignant change. These are also related to ganglioneurocytoma which also have small mature neoplastic neurons.

In locations where a complete resection is possible, the prognosis is generally good, but if complete resection is not possible, e.g., tumors located in the brain stem or spinal cord, then local recurrence is commonly seen.

In children and young adults, the main differential considerations for ganglioglioma on imaging studies include low-grade astrocytoma, juvenile pilocytic astrocytoma, dysembryoplastic neuroepithelial tumor (DNET), and pleomorphic xanthoastrocytoma (PXA).

REFERENCES

Caseiras GB, Chheang S, Babb J, et al. Relative cerebral blood volume measurements of low-grade gliomas predict patient outcome in a multi-institution setting. *Eur J Radiol.* 2010;73(2):215-220.

Compton JJ, Laack NN, Eckel LJ, et al. Long-term outcomes for low-grade intracranial ganglioglioma: 30-year experience from the Mayo Clinic. *J Neurosurg.* 2012;117(5):825-830.

Neuroradiology: THE REQUISITES. 4th ed. pp 66-69.

CASE 116

Fourth Ventricular Neoplasm—Choroid Plexus Papilloma (CPP)

1. **B.** Choroid plexus papillomas (CPPs) occur mainly in children, with a predilection for the lateral ventricles, while in adults, these are more frequently found in the fourth ventricle.

Ependymomas are overall most frequent in the posterior fossa in children, and in adults, they are frequently supratentorial.

2. **B.** In children, CPPs most often occur in the trigone of the lateral ventricles.
3. **D.** Hemangioblastoma is the most common primary intra-axial infratentorial tumor in adults. These are otherwise uncommon tumors and comprise only about 1%–2.5% of all intracranial tumors and approximately 10% of all posterior fossa tumors.
4. **C.** CPPs are WHO grade 1 tumors, atypical CPPs are WHO grade 2 tumors, and choroid plexus carcinomas are WHO grade 3 tumors.

Comment

Choroid plexus papillomas (CPPs) are epithelial tumors arising from the surface of the choroid plexus. Unlike most other brain tumors, which are more common in the posterior fossa in children and supratentorial compartment in adults, the relationship is reversed for CPPs. In adults, CPPs most often (70%) occur in the fourth ventricle, whereas in children, these most commonly (80%) occur in the atria/trigone of the lateral ventricles. Overall, CPPs are uncommon tumors and account for ~1% of all brain tumors, 2%–6% of pediatric brain tumors, and 0.5% of adult brain tumors.

CPPs commonly present with hydrocephalus (in up to 80% of all cases), as a result of overproduction of CSF or obstructive hydrocephalus related to adhesions from proteinaceous or hemorrhagic material blocking the subarachnoid cisterns or ventricular outlets. In addition, large tumors cause focal expansion of the ventricle they arise in and may also cause trapping. These tumors are composed of vascularized connective tissue and frond-like papillae lined by a single layer of epithelial cells.

This case demonstrates a heterogeneous, but avidly enhancing circumscribed mass in the fourth ventricle measuring 2.1 × 3.2 × 3.6 cm. Notice the CSF clefts along the anterior, lateral as well as posterior aspects of the mass (Figures 116.1–116.4). There is no restricted diffusion (Figure 116.5) and no susceptibility (Figure 116.6). Associated obstructive hydrocephalus with transependymal edema is seen along the left temporal horn (Figure 116.4). Pathology showed an atypical CPP (WHO grade 2). Most commonly, CPPs are indolent, WHO grade 1 tumors, and the more aggressive choroid plexus carcinomas are WHO grade 3 tumors.

Hemangioblastomas are usually not within the fourth ventricle and usually have prominent flow voids, not seen in this case. An ependymoma could have been a reasonable alternative diagnosis in this case, but usually they are encountered in younger adults. Intracranial ependymomas are overall most frequently seen in the posterior fossa (~60%). Supratentorial ependymomas are a type of location-specific ependymomas and account for 30% of all ependymomas. They share a similar pathological spectrum to posterior fossa ependymomas, with the exception that the RELA fusion-positive ependymoma subtype is usually supratentorial and is not found in the posterior fossa. Approximately 50% of infratentorial ependymomas extend into the cerebellopontine angle cisterns and foramen magnum via the fourth ventricle outflow tracts (foramina of Magendie and Luschka).

Calcification, hemorrhage, and cysts are frequently present in both CPPs and ependymomas. On MRI, hypointensity may correspond to calcium, vessels, or blood products. Tumors that are very cystic will be hyperintense on T2W images, whereas those with large areas of old blood products may be hypointense. Both neoplasms may enhance avidly or heterogeneously, depending on the degree of cyst formation, calcification, and hemorrhage. When contained in the fourth ventricle, CPPs and ependymomas may be difficult to distinguish, as in this case. The age of the patient usually helps in limiting the playing field. In the pediatric

population, ependymoma is the best choice. Other intraventricular neoplasms are more common in adults.

REFERENCES

de Castro FD, Reis F, Guerra JG. Intraventricular mass lesions at magnetic resonance imaging: iconographic essay - part 1. *Radiol Bras*. 2014;47(3):176-181.
Dangouloff-Ros V, Grevent D, Blauwblomme T, et al. Choroid plexus neoplasms: toward a distinction between carcinoma and papilloma using arterial spin-labeling. *AJNR Am J Neuroradiol*. 2015;36(9):1786-1790.
Neuroradiology: THE REQUISITES. 4th ed. pp 49-51.

CASE 117

Glioma of the Tectum (Quadrigeminal Plate)

1. **D.** These images demonstrate a 10-mm lesion within the anterior aspect of the superior colliculus of the tectum causing compensated obstructive hydrocephalus, most consistent with a low-grade neoplasm (tectal glioma), which are usually low-grade astrocytomas.
2. **D.** The quadrigeminal plate, also known as the tectal plate or tectum, is constituted by the paired superior and inferior colliculi.
3. **D.** Surgical interventions and biopsy can have significant morbidity in this region and is usually not performed unless the lesion is significantly larger and or contrast enhancing. Usually, CSF diversion, either an endoscopic third ventriculostomy (ETV) or a VP shunt, is sufficient. ETV was performed in this case with relief of presenting symptoms with stable tectal findings on follow-up imaging.
4. **D.** Tectal beaking refers to the fusion of the midbrain colliculi into a single beak pointing posteriorly and invaginating into the cerebellum and is seen with Chiari type II malformations.

Comment

These images show diffuse dilatation of the lateral and third ventricles with no surrounding T2 signal abnormality to suggest the presence of transependymal egress of CSF, consistent with a compensated obstructive hydrocephalus. There is a 10-mm T2/FLAIR hyperintense (Figures 117.3 and 117.4), T1 hypointense, nonenhancing lesion (Figure 117.6) along the anterior aspect of the superior colliculus of the tectum (Figure 117.2), which likely represents a low-grade neoplasm (tectal glioma). There is resultant compression of the aqueduct of Sylvius, which is typically seen in patients with tectal gliomas. In the vast majority of patients, the clinical presentation is that of obstructive hydrocephalus, as was seen in this case. Gliomas arising from the tectum are usually low-grade astrocytomas. They may be solid or cystic masses and have a wide spectrum of enhancement characteristics, ranging from none to prominent. According to a large study, contrast enhancement was seen in 40% and cystic changes in 14%, the presence of both was significantly correlated with lesions ≥3 cm². They found that larger lesions (≥3 cm²), the presence of contrast enhancement, and cystic changes at presentation were risk factors for progression. In patients where the tissue was available, 83% showed features similar to pilocytic astrocytoma and 17% aligned best with diffuse astrocytoma. BRAF duplication (a marker of KIAA1549-BRAF fusion) and BRAF V600E mutation were detected in 25% and 7.7%, respectively. No case had histone H3 K27M mutation. Given the usual indolent course and risks associated with resection or biopsy in such an eloquent area, the general recommendation is close observation after CSF diversion for hydrocephalus.

The midbrain is separated into the tegmentum and the tectum, which are portions of the midbrain anterior and posterior to the aqueduct of Sylvius, respectively. The tectum (roof) consists of the quadrigeminal plate that contains the paired superior and inferior colliculi. The tectum is affected more frequently by extrinsic rather than intrinsic lesions. It is often compressed (particularly the superior colliculi), along with the aqueduct of Sylvius, by pineal region masses, such as meningiomas in adults, germ cell tumors (germinoma, embryonal carcinoma, choriocarcinoma, and teratoma), tumors of pineal origin (pineoblastoma and pineocytoma), and aneurysms of the vein of Galen, which may result in Parinaud's syndrome. In this case, * denotes the normal pineal gland in Figure 117.2. Occasionally, the tectum may be affected by demyelinating disease, vascular abnormalities, or trauma. In addition, the tectum may be abnormal in congenital malformations, most notably, Chiari II malformation, in which there may be a spectrum of abnormalities, ranging from collicular fusion to tectal beaking.

REFERENCES

Griessenauer CJ, Rizk E, Miller JH, et al. Pediatric tectal plate gliomas: clinical and radiological progression, MR imaging characteristics, and management of hydrocephalus. *J Neurosurg Pediatr.* 2014;13(1):13-20.

Liu APY, Harreld JH, Jacola LM, et al. Tectal glioma as a distinct diagnostic entity: a comprehensive clinical, imaging, histologic and molecular analysis. *Acta Neuropathol Commun.* 2018;6(1):101.

Neuroradiology: THE REQUISITES. 4th ed. pp 3, 282-286.

CASE 118

Intradiploic Epidermoid Cyst (Recurrent)

1. **C.** Findings consistent with prior right parietal calvarial resection and placement of methacrylate cranioplasty. Large intermediate-attenuation soft tissue surrounding the methacrylate cranioplasty which appears encapsulated extending into the overlying scalp, and with inward bowing of the adjacent dura with associated mild mass effect upon the adjacent lateral right frontoparietal gyri. The calvarial cortex surrounding the lesion appears smoothly remodeled. No appreciable enhancement is seen in association with the lesion.

   Since 2012, there has been modest growth of an encapsulated proteinaceous cystic lesion at the surgical site surrounding and now displacing the cranioplasty material, extending into the scalp and with mild inward bowing of the dura as described. Given the history, this is favored to reflect residual/recurrent epidermoid cyst.

   Along the right parietal cranioplasty, there is an expansile T2/FLAIR hyperintense lobulated lesion with restricted diffusion and a lack of internal enhancement. This lobulated medial lesion measures 5.8 × 3.6 × 5.2 cm and displaces the cranioplasty laterally from the normal calvarial contour. Recurrent right parietal calvarial epidermoid surrounding the right cranioplasty slowly enlarging over time and laterally displacing the cranioplasty as above.

2. **A.** Epidermoid cysts are benign intracranial tumors that are predominantly located in the cerebellopontine angle, accounting for ~1% of intracranial tumors. Intradural epidermoid cysts are far more common than intradiploic epidermoid cysts. All other statements are correct.

3. **D.** Epidermoid cysts can be congenital (most common pathogenesis), and the tumor can be traced back to two possible origins: congenital or acquired [7]. Congenital epidermoid cysts that account for the vast majority of the tumor are attributed to anomalous implantation of ectodermal cells during the closure of the neural tube between the third and fifth week of embryonic life [3,8]. Acquired epidermoid cysts are thought to be the result of displacement of epithelial tissue secondary to previous lumbar puncture or trauma [9–14]. As for the patient, she did not have any trauma.

4. **D.** Inclusion of ectodermal cells rests during embryonic development; less commonly, it has been suggested that they may be acquired by traumatic implantation of ectodermal tissue into the bone. Langerhans cell histiocytosis (LCH) is a rare multisystem disease seen in young children characterized by clonal proliferation of Langerhans cells. The most commonly affected "system" is the skeletal system, which is involved in nearly 80% of cases, and the most commonly affected bone or group of bones in children is the skull. In particular, the frontal bone is most involved in this demographic. All of the other alternatives in the question are also common sites of involvement in LCH. Notably, the mandible is the most commonly affected bone in adults with LCH.

Comment

Epidermoid and dermoid cysts of the skull are rare. Both are proposed to occur as a result of the inclusion of epithelial cells during the closure of the neural tube between the third and the fifth week of gestation. However, the development of epidermoid cysts secondary to the implantation of epithelial cells after trauma has been suggested as the cause in approximately 25% of cases. Epidermoid cysts account for fewer than 2% of intracranial and cranial tumors. Approximately 25% occur in the skull, whereas the remaining 75% are intradural. Dermoid cysts are even less common. Epidermoid cysts tend to present in young adults, whereas dermoid cysts are present in children and young adolescents.

Approximately 10% of calvarial epidermoid cysts are incidental lesions; the remaining 90% are symptomatic. The most common presentation is an enlarging scalp mass; however, pain or headache is present in approximately 20% of cases. The most common location of these cysts is the parietal bone, followed by the frontal and temporal bones. Approximately 70% of these lesions involve both the inner and outer tables of the skull. Involvement of only the outer cortical table or, less commonly, the inner table may occur. On plain films, epidermoid cysts typically appear as lytic lesions with sclerotic borders. The differential diagnosis includes hemangioma, eosinophilic granuloma, and leptomeningeal cysts, especially in childhood. Other lytic lesions, particularly in adults, cannot be definitively differentiated on plain films alone. These lesions are typically hyperintense on T2W imaging; however, on unenhanced T1W imaging, their signal characteristics are variable. High T1W signal intensity may be due to the presence of blood products, protein, debris, crystals, or fat.

REFERENCES

Demir MK, Yapicier O, Onat E, et al. Rare and challenging extra-axial brain lesions: CT and MRI findings with clinico-radiological differential diagnosis and pathological correlation. *Diagn Interv Radiol.* 2014; 20(5):448-452.

Ding S, Jin Y, Jiang J. Malignant transformation of an epidermoid cyst in the temporal and prepontine region: report of a case and differential diagnosis. *Oncol Lett.* 2016;11(5):3097-3100.

Li J, Qian M, Huang X, Zhao L, Yang X, Xiao J. Repeated recurrent epidermoid cyst with atypical hyperplasia: a case report and literature review. *Medicine (Baltimore).* 2017;96(49):e8950.

Neuroradiology: THE REQUISITES. 4th ed. pp 2, 53-55.

CASE 119

Posterior Circulation Ischemia due to Subclavian Steal

1. **C.** The brachiocephalic artery.
2. **C.** Retrograde flow down the right vertebral artery. Figure 119.4, an arch aortogram, shows that the origin of the right subclavian artery is occluded.

3. **B.** "Subclavian steal" and is more commonly found on the left.
4. **D.** On standard two-dimensional time-of-flight MR angiography, there is usually a stationary superior saturation pulse that is used to suppress the signal from the neck veins. Because in subclavian steal there is retrograde flow in the involved vertebral artery, this saturation pulse has to be removed or an inferior saturation pulse should be applied.

Comment

Subclavian steal results from occlusion or a hemodynamically significant stenosis of the subclavian artery proximal to the origin of the vertebral artery, or stenosis of the brachiocephalic artery. Subclavian steal occurs much more commonly on the left than on the right. There is a retrograde flow of blood down the ipsilateral vertebral artery (stealing blood from the circle of Willis) to provide collateral blood supply to the arm (bypassing the occlusion or stenosis of the proximal subclavian artery).

In patients with a subclavian steal, symptoms and signs may be related to decreased blood flow to the arm (decreased pulse, reduced blood pressure, decreased temperature, or claudication) or to neurologic symptoms due to periodic ischemia in the posterior circulation. Note that no acute ischemia was evident in the posterior circulation in this case, negative DWI; see Figure 119.1.

Neurologic symptoms include transient attacks, dizziness, and visual symptoms. Similar neurologic symptoms may occur with high-grade stenoses or occlusions of the proximal vertebral artery; however, the arm is not symptomatic. Subclavian stenosis can often be diagnosed on physical examination. Imaging studies that may help to confirm the diagnosis include Doppler ultrasound and MR angiography studies, which may correctly demonstrate retrograde flow down the involved vertebral artery. On arch aortography, early arterial films show occlusion or stenosis of the proximal left subclavian artery, whereas delayed films demonstrate retrograde flow, as was seen in this case; see Figures 119.6 and 119.7. Neurointerventional techniques may be used to treat symptomatic patients and include percutaneous transluminal angioplasty or positioning of stents.

REFERENCES

Jung KH, Kim JM, Lee ST, et al. Brain response characteristics associated with subclavian steal phenomenon. *J Stroke Cerebrovasc Dis.* 2014; 23(3):157-161.
Sheehy N, MacNally S, Smith CS, et al. Contrast-enhanced MR angiography of subclavian steal syndrome: value of the 2D time-of-flight "localizer" sign. *AJR Am J Roentgenol.* 2005;185(4):1069-1073.
Neuroradiology: THE REQUISITES. 4th ed. pp 3, 94.

CASE 120

CNS Vasculitis—Primary Angiitis of the CNS (PACNS)

1. **D.** All of the above. The corpus callosum has a rich arterial supply and is rarely affected by infarcts. The majority of the corpus callosum is supplied by the pericallosal arteries (branches of the anterior cerebral artery) and the posterior pericallosal arteries (branches of the posterior cerebral artery), with additional supply from the anterior communicating artery, via either the subcallosal artery or median callosal artery.
2. **B.** MRI shows multifocal infarcts of varying ages in bilateral cerebral white matter, deep gray nuclei, corpus callosum as well as in the left cerebellum (Figures 120.1–120.4). Note, the enhancement of a subacute infarct in the genu of corpus callosum (Figure 120.6) with vessel wall enhancement of the right A2 ACA and left P2/P3 PCA (arrows in Figures 120.5

and 120.6) with multifocal segmental narrowing confirmed on conventional angiography (Figures 120.8 and 120.9). Constellation of findings is most suggestive of an inflammatory vasculopathy such as a small vessel vasculitis.
3. **D.** Imaging findings of PACNS are nonspecific, with infarctions seen in more than 50% of patients. MRI is very sensitive, but not "specific" for the diagnosis of PACNS. It is also said that a normal MRI essentially excludes this diagnosis.
4. **A.** Rarely, intravascular lymphoma may mimic PACNS.

Comment

This case demonstrates multifocal infarcts of varying chronicity spanning multiple vascular territories also involving the corpus callosum, where infarcts are rare, because of its rich arterial supply. Dedicated high-resolution vessel wall imaging sequences demonstrated focal narrowing and vessel wall enhancement of the right A2 ACA and left P2/P3 PCA. Mild circumferential enhancement was also seen in the left distal vertebral artery (not shown). Subsequent conventional angiography confirmed segmental narrowing suggestive of an inflammatory vasculopathy.

The clinical presentation of CNS vasculitis remains variable, ranging from headache, changes in mental status, and meningitis to hemorrhagic or ischemic stroke, as in this case. The vasculitides that can affect the CNS include infectious and noninfectious causes. Infectious etiologies include tuberculosis, which frequently involves the vessels around the basal cisterns. There are several classifications of noninfectious vasculitis that result from inflammatory infiltrates, both within and surrounding the vessel walls, that lead to regions of segmental narrowing and dilation on conventional catheter angiography. Among the noninfectious causes of vasculitis are necrotizing vasculopathies, such as primary angiitis of the CNS (PACNS), polyarteritis nodosa (PAN), Kawasaki disease, sarcoidosis, and granulomatosis with polyangiitis (GPA). Vasculitis is occasionally associated with collagen vascular diseases, such as systemic lupus erythematosus and rheumatoid arthritis; however, this is less frequent than is reported. More often, the cause of ischemic events in these patients is related to a hypercoagulable state, such as antiphospholipid antibodies (lupus anticoagulant and anticardiolipin antibodies). Certain recreational drugs have also been associated with vasculitis and infarcts, including amphetamines, ecstasy, and cocaine.

Even with the technical advances in MR angiography and CT angiography, conventional catheter angiography is still best for showing the changes in vasculitis in the cerebral arteries. A normal (negative) finding on the angiogram does not exclude CNS vasculitis. If vasculitis is highly suspected clinically, a biopsy is indicated to make the diagnosis. Even in cases in which angiography findings are positive, a biopsy may still be necessary to confirm the diagnosis.

This patient continued to have progressive neurological decline. CSF serology showed lymphocytic pleocytosis, elevated protein, and low glucose. AQP4-IgG was negative. The ANA and ANCA panels were negative. Transthoracic echocardiography was unrevealing for an embolic source. Fluorescein angiography did not find evidence of vasculitis; punch dermal biopsies did not identify intravascular lymphoma. The patient ultimately underwent a right frontal biopsy, which revealed brain parenchyma with perivascular and intraparenchymal T-cell and macrophage infiltration and reactive gliosis and was offered empiric treatment for CNS vasculitis versus neuroinflammatory process with Cytoxan, but subsequently passed away one month later.

REFERENCES

Abdel Razek AA, Alvarez H, Bagg S, et al. Imaging spectrum of CNS vasculitis. *Radiographics.* 2014;34(4):873-894.
Obusez EC, Hui F, Hajj-Ali RA, et al. High-resolution MRI vessel wall imaging: spatial and temporal patterns on reversible cerebral

vasoconstriction syndrome and central nervous system vasculitis. *AJNR Am J Neuroradiol*. 2014;35(8):1527-1532.

Türe U, Yaşargil MG, Krisht AF. The arteries of the corpus callosum: a microsurgical anatomic study. *Neurosurgery*. 1996;39(6):1075-1084; discussion 1084-1085.

Neuroradiology: THE REQUISITES. 4th ed. pp 3, 116-123.

CASE 121

Air Embolism with Acute Right Cerebral Infarct

1. **A.** Intracranial air. Note, the use of lung windows may help in improving the detection of intracranial air as shown in Figure 121.4.
2. **D.** Cerebral air embolism. This patient was completing his dialysis, and while disconnecting from his tunneled HD catheter, he developed neurological symptoms of rightward eye deviation and unresponsiveness. Head CT revealed multiple air emboli within the right cerebral hemisphere (Figures 121.1–121.3).
3. **C.** The treatment of established neurological damage due to cerebral air embolism is hyperbaric oxygenation therapy.

Comment

Cerebral air embolism is a known complication of hemodialysis, laparoscopy, open heart surgery, lung biopsy, image-guided procedures, childbirth (cesarean section), endoscopic retrograde cholangiopancreatography (ERCP), trauma and central line catheterization, etc.

Our patient was completing his dialysis, and while disconnecting from his tunneled HD catheter, he had rightward eye deviation and unresponsiveness. CT head and CTA head and neck revealed multiple R>L supratentorial cerebral air emboli. The patient underwent a 4-hour session of hyperbaric oxygenation therapy with subsequent improvement in cerebral air. TTE demonstrated an interatrial communication at rest, which would explain his pneumocephalus. The tunneled dialysis catheter was subsequently exchanged with no clear abnormalities.

In addition to the aforementioned causes, cerebral air embolism may also result from a paradoxical intracardiac shunt, as seen in this patient. Cerebral air emboli usually occur on the right side because air preferentially flows into the first branch of the aortic arch, the brachiocephalic artery, and it is said that an injection of 2–3 ml of air into the cerebral circulation can be fatal. When a cerebral air embolism is suspected, the patient's head should be quickly lowered (Trendelenburg position), and the patient should be turned to the left lateral decubitus position to trap air in the apex of the ventricle and prevent further ejection into the pulmonary arterial system.

The treatment of cerebral air embolism is supportive. Endotracheal intubation, ventilation, and administration of oxygen to maintain and improve oxygenation and decrease the size of gas bubbles are recommended. Antiseizure medications are given to suppress seizures. Hyperbaric oxygenation therapy helps by raising ambient pressure around the gas bubble and increasing the gradient for nitrogen out of the bubble and for oxygen into the bubble. Normovolemia should be attained with infusion of colloids. Use of anticoagulation and corticosteroids is not recommended.

REFERENCES

Jeon SB, Kang DW. Neurological picture. Cerebral air emboli on T2-weighted gradient-echo magnetic resonance imaging. *J Neurol Neurosurg Psychiatry*. 2007;78(8):871.

Schlimp CJ, Bothma PA, Brodbeck AE. Cerebral venous air embolism: what is it and do we know how to deal with it properly? *JAMA Neurol*. 2014;71(2):243.

Wieczorek M, Lukat M, Hoeltgen R, et al. Investigation into causes of abnormal cerebral MRI findings following PVAC duty-cycled, phased RF ablation of atrial fibrillation. *J Cardiovasc Electrophysiol*. 2013;24(2):121-128.

Neuroradiology: THE REQUISITES. 4th ed. pp 3, 87-89.

CASE 122

Sinonasal Undifferentiated Carcinoma (SNUC) with Intracranial Extension

1. **A.** A large extra-axial heterogeneous mass centered in the anterior skull base, with osseous erosions, extension inferiorly into the nasal cavity, with cystic and solid components, marked intracranial mass effect, and a 9 mm leftward midline shift. Pathology was consistent with a sinonasal undifferentiated carcinoma (SNUC).
2. **B.** Eighty percent of all maxillary antral carcinomas are squamous cell carcinomas.
3. **A.** Malignant transformation occurs in approximately 5% to 10% of cases.
4. **C.** The term nasal glioma is a misnomer in that it is a benign slowly growing mass composed of heterotopic glial tissue. Unlike meningoceles (encephaloceles), nasal gliomas do not have CSF spaces that communicate with the intracranial subarachnoid spaces, and hence do not demonstrate pulsation or enlargement on Valsalva. Nasal gliomas are isodense relative to the normal brain on CT, bright on T2 secondary to gliosis, with a bifid crista galli and a prominent foramen cecum. Surgical resection is often curative.

Comment

This case shows a large, aggressive sinonasal undifferentiated carcinoma (SNUC) with erosion of the anterior skull base and intracranial extension with extensive edema in bilateral frontal lobes, ventricular effacement, mass effect, and leftward midline shift.

Malignant tumors of the sinonasal tract are rare, accounting for 3% of head and neck cancers. The majority arise in the maxillary sinus, approximately 20% arise in the ethmoid sinuses, and the remainder (<1%) originate in the frontal and sphenoid sinuses. Squamous cell carcinoma is the most common histologic type, seen in ~80% of cases. Nickel and chrome refining processes have been implicated in the development of all types of malignancy of the paranasal sinuses, and exposure to wood dust has been associated specifically with adenocarcinoma of the ethmoid. Up to a fivefold increased risk of sinonasal carcinoma has been observed with heavy smoking. Clinical presentation of sinus malignancies is nonspecific and often mimics benign disease. Approximately 10% of patients are asymptomatic. Delay in diagnosis is common. Up to 75% of all paranasal sinus tumors are stage T3 or T4 at the time of diagnosis. Resectability and treatment are determined by the presence of orbital invasion, intracranial spread, dural invasion, and perineural spread.

SNUC is a rare cancer of the nasal cavity or paranasal sinuses. Initial symptoms range from a bloody nose, runny nose, double vision, and bulging eye to chronic infections and nasal obstruction. It has been associated with papillomas in the nasal cavity, which are benign, but can undergo malignant degeneration. A history of radiation therapy for other cancers has been associated with the development of SNUC, although most patients have not had previous radiation therapy.

REFERENCES

Christopherson K, Werning JW, Malyapa RS, et al. Radiotherapy for sinonasal undifferentiated carcinoma. *Am J Otolaryngol*. 2014;35(2):141-146.

Donald PJ. Sinonasal undifferentiated carcinoma with intracranial extension. *Skull Base*. 2006;16(2):67-74.

Yoshida E, Aouad R, Fragoso R, et al. Improved clinical outcomes with multi-modality therapy for sinonasal undifferentiated carcinoma of the head and neck. *Am J Otolaryngol*. 2013;34(6):658-663.

Neuroradiology: THE REQUISITES. 4th ed. pp 12, 432-435.

CASE 123

Ectopic Posterior Pituitary and Nonvisualization of the Infundibulum—Hypopituitarism

1. **C.** An ectopic posterior pituitary gland. Nodular T1 hyperintense focus is seen along the median eminence (floor of the third ventricle) without a clear distal portion of the infundibulum inserting onto the top of the pituitary gland in the sella turcica.
2. **D.** The infundibulum (pituitary stalk) is not visualized.
3. **C.** Patients with ectopic posterior pituitary gland most commonly present with features of growth hormone deficiency (pituitary dwarfism).
4. **D.** The focal spot of hyperintense T1 signal in the posterior aspect of the sella turcica results from the storage of vasopressin, a hormone synthesized by the hypothalamus. To enable its descent from the hypothalamus to the posterior pituitary lobe, it is bound to a macroproteic structure, "vasopressin–neurophysin II–copeptin complex," which shortens the T1 signal. This focus of high signal intensity may be observed outside the sella when the hypothalamohypophysial axis is interrupted, as seen in this case.

Comment

The posterior pituitary develops from the neuroectoderm of the diencephalon. Pituitary gland function is controlled by the hypothalamus via the infundibular stalk. Nerve fibers from nuclei in the hypothalamus course into the infundibulum to reach the posterior pituitary gland. Normally, the anterior pituitary gland and the pituitary stalk are well defined. The posterior pituitary is usually identified as a hyperintense "bright" spot on T1W MR images. This hyperintensity has been attributed to the storage of vasopressin that is transported from the hypothalamus to the posterior pituitary bound to a macroproteic structure, "vasopressin–neurophysin II–copeptin complex," which shortens the T1 signal.

An ectopic posterior pituitary gland may result from aberrant neuronal migration during embryogenesis, transection of the pituitary, or an insult to the pituitary stalk due to ischemia, anoxia, or compression leading to reorganization of the proximal neurons of the neurohypophysis. Breech delivery and perinatal anoxia have been associated with the transection of the pituitary stalk and hypopituitarism. However, many patients with hypopituitarism and ectopic posterior pituitary have uncomplicated perinatal courses. This patient was diagnosed with panhypopituitarism at the age of two months after an apneic episode. He was on hydrocortisone as well as long-term growth hormone treatment. On imaging, besides ectopic posterior pituitary and nonvisualization of the infundibulum (Figures 123.1–123.4), there were features suggestive of aberrant neuronal migration with fenestrated flax, cortical dysplasia involving the cingulate gyri (Figures 123.5 and 123.6), and gray matter heterotopias (not shown). There was thinning of the posterior body of the corpus callosum with a small splenium (Figures 123.1 and 123.2), a paucity of occipital white matter with periventricular T2 hyperintensity and prominence of the occipital horns, reflecting a sequela of prior insult such as PVL (not shown).

The exact etiology of an ectopic posterior pituitary is not fully understood, with possible implications of the HESX1 gene. Regardless of the underlying cause, an ectopic posterior pituitary

results from the incomplete downward extension of the infundibulum resulting in frequent growth hormone deficiency, and even panhypopituitarism, as seen in the current case.

An ectopic posterior pituitary and nonvisualization of the stalk on MR imaging are associated with decreased function of the anterior pituitary (hypopituitarism). Posterior pituitary hormone deficiency in the presence of an ectopic posterior pituitary is uncommon, suggesting that this ectopic tissue functions normally to produce antidiuretic hormone.

REFERENCES

Bonneville F, Cattin F, Marsot-Dupuch K, Dormont D, Bonneville JF, Chiras J. T1 signal hyperintensity in the sellar region: spectrum of findings. *Radiographics*. 2006;26(1):93-113.

Maghnie M, Lindberg A, Koltowska-Haggstrom M, et al. Magnetic resonance imaging of CNS in 15,043 children with GH deficiency in KIGS (Pfizer International Growth Database). *Eur J Endocrinol*. 2013; 168(2):211-217.

Secco A, Allegri AE, Di Lorgi N, et al. Posterior pituitary (PP) evaluation in patients with anterior pituitary defect associated with ectopic PP and septo-optic dysplasia. *Eur J Endocrinol*. 2011;165(3):411-420.

Takahashi T, Miki Y, Takahashi JA, et al. Ectopic posterior pituitary high signal in preoperative and postoperative macroadenomas: dynamic MR imaging. *Eur J Radiol*. 2005;55(1):84-91.

Neuroradiology: THE REQUISITES. 4th ed. pp 10, 349-351.

CASE 124

Radiation Necrosis After Treatment of High-Grade Glioma (Glioblastoma)

1. **B.** This case shows an enlarged heterogeneous mass in the resection bed with a very low relative cerebral blood volume (rCBV) (Figure 124.5) and plasma volume (Vp) (Figure 124.6), consistent with radiation necrosis. Progressive neoplasm typically shows elevated rCBV corresponding to the regions of enhancement.
2. **A.** The first contrast-enhanced MRI should ideally be performed within two days after surgery in order to assess the extent of resection, but no later than 72 hours after surgery, before vascularized enhancing granulation tissue develops.
3. **C.** The standard of care treatment for glioblastoma (GBM) includes maximal safe surgical resection, followed by radiation therapy plus concomitant and maintenance temozolomide (TMZ). The addition of bevacizumab to standard treatment with TMZ revealed no improvement in overall survival (OS). Tumor-treating fields (TTFields) plus TMZ represent a major advance for the treatment of GBM, with recent clinical trials demonstrating improvement in OS as well as progression-free survival (PFS) with no deleterious effects on the quality of life (QOL), and should be considered as a standard for patients with newly diagnosed GBM with no contraindications.
4. **A.** IDH-mutated gliomas occur in younger patients and have a better prognosis than IDH wild-type gliomas irrespective of WHO grade. IDH-mutated gliomas occur preferentially in the frontal lobe. IDH wild-type gliomas occur in older patients and have a poor prognosis. Among lower-grade gliomas, the T2-FLAIR mismatch sign represents a highly specific imaging biomarker for the IDH-mutant, 1p/19q noncodeleted molecular subtype.

Comment

Glioblastoma (GBM) is the most common primary malignant brain tumor in adults. Standard of care treatment includes maximal safe surgical resection, followed by radiation therapy plus concomitant and maintenance temozolomide (TMZ). The addition of bevacizumab to standard treatment with TMZ revealed no improvement in overall survival (OS). In newly diagnosed GBM, methylation of the O6-methylguanine-DNA methyltransferase (MGMT) promoter has been shown to predict the response to TMZ. Tumor-treating fields (TTFields) plus TMZ represent a major advance for the treatment of GBM, with recent clinical trials demonstrating improvement in OS as well as progression-free survival (PFS) with no deleterious effects on the quality of life (QOL). GBM has an extremely poor prognosis, and hence treatment paradigms should go beyond improving survival with the aim of preserving and improving the QOL of patients.

Neuroimaging plays an integral role in the initial diagnosis, prognosis, as well as in the assessment of treatment response in neuro-oncology. Typically, granulation tissue develops within the first three days after surgery and may enhance. Therefore, in patients with enhancing tumors before surgical resection, it is especially important to perform the first postoperative MRI within 48 hours after surgery. The finding of enhancing tissue on these initial postoperative scans should raise a concern about residual neoplasm. Because T1W-hyperintense hemorrhage is usually present in the resection bed, it is important to compare enhanced images with unenhanced T1W images obtained in the same plane as the postcontrast images. Postoperative changes and granulation tissue typically decrease in size over time. In contrast, the residual tumor grows.

This patient typically highlights the phenomenon of treatment-related necrosis, aka "pseudoprogression," which is generally seen within six months after completion of chemoradiotherapy and is more commonly seen in patients who have MGMT-methylated tumors. Conventional MRI is limited in the differentiation of residual or recurrent tumors from treatment-related changes. True tumor progression generally demonstrates increased rCBV, increased Vp, and elevated choline on MR spectroscopy. Pseudoresponse is seen in the setting of bevacizumab administration (antiangiogenic therapy) with a marked decrease in enhancement secondary to vascular normalization and decreased vessel diameter and permeability and is not a true antitumoral effect.

In this case with predominant radiation necrosis with low rCBV and Vp, despite increasing enhancement over serial examinations, pathologic examination showed less than 5% viable neoplasm.

REFERENCES

Fatterpekar GM, Galeigo D, Narayana A, et al. Treatment-related change versus tumor recurrence in high-grade gliomas: a diagnostic conundrum—use of dynamic susceptibility contrast-enhanced (DSC) perfusion MRI. *AJR Am J Roentgenol.* 2012;198(1):19-26.

Gonçalves FG, Chawla S, Mohan S. Emerging MRI techniques to redefine treatment response in patients with glioblastoma. *J Magn Reson Imaging.* 2020;52(4):978-997. doi:10.1002/jmri.27105.

Reddy K, Westerly D, Chen C. MRI patterns of T1 enhancing radiation necrosis versus tumour recurrence in high-grade gliomas. *J Med Imaging Radiat Oncol.* 2013;57(3):349-355.

Stupp R, Taillibert S, Kanner A, et al. Effect of tumor-treating fields plus maintenance temozolomide vs maintenance temozolomide alone on survival in patients with glioblastoma: a randomized clinical trial [published correction appears in JAMA. 2018;319(17):1824]. *JAMA.* 2017;318(23):2306-2316. doi:10.1001/jama.2017.18718.

Neuroradiology: THE REQUISITES. 4th ed. pp 2, 82-86.

CASE 125

Diffuse Midline Glioma, H3 K27M–Mutant

1. **C.** MRI brain demonstrates a 3×2×3 cm hemorrhagic expansile pontine lesion with associated edema and mass effect on the prepontine cistern. Stereotactic biopsy of this tumor was consistent with diffuse midline glioma, H3 K27M–mutant.
2. **A.** The majority of these tumors are found in young children and are located in the pons.
3. **F.** Besides pons, they can also be seen in other midline locations, such as the thalamus, hypothalamus, third ventricle, pineal region, cerebellum, other parts of the brain stem, and spinal cord.
4. **C.** Diffuse midline glioma H3 K27M–mutant is a new entity recently added to the 2016 update of the WHO classification of CNS tumors, which represents the majority of diffuse intrinsic pontine gliomas (DIPGs). These are aggressive tumors with poor prognosis and are considered WHO grade IV tumors regardless of their histological features.

Comment

This case shows the characteristic appearance of a diffuse midline glioma H3 K27M–mutant, with a large expansile hemorrhagic mass in the pons bulging into the prepontine cistern and around the basilar artery (note effacement of the prepontine cistern and invagination [encasement] of the basilar artery). The enhancement pattern of diffuse midline gliomas is quite variable, ranging from no enhancement to avid heterogeneous enhancement, as in this case.

Diffuse midline glioma H3 K27M–mutant is a specific entity added to the 2016 update of the WHO classification of CNS tumors, which represents the majority of diffuse intrinsic pontine gliomas (DIPGs). The K27M mutation occurs in either of two genes, H3F3A or HIST1H3B, which encode the histone H3 variants, H3.3 and H3.1, respectively. While the K27M mutation appears quite specific for diffuse gliomas arising in midline structures, a separate missense variant (G34R or G34V) in H3F3A can sometimes be found within peripheral cerebral hemispheric gliomas predominantly in teenage and young adult patients. These mutations result in decreased methylation of the histone tails, resulting in altered gene expression patterns thought to block glial differentiation and promote gliomagenesis.

The majority of these tumors are found in young children and are located in the pons but can also be seen elsewhere in other midline structures. They are aggressive tumors with poor prognosis and are considered WHO grade IV tumors regardless of histological features.

Presenting symptoms include cranial nerve deficits, motor or sensory deficits, ataxia, abnormal eye movements, somnolence, and hyperactivity. Hydrocephalus is a late finding, with the exception of tumors arising in immediate proximity to the aqueduct.

MRI is the imaging modality of choice for the evaluation of brainstem abnormalities. Its multiplanar capabilities, improved resolution, and a relative absence of scanning artifacts frequently present on CT scans have resulted in improved detection of abnormalities in the posterior fossa. In addition, MRI is useful for planning stereotactic biopsy and radiation therapy. Because of the infiltrative nature and characteristic location of brainstem gliomas, radiation therapy remains the main therapeutic option. In cases in which the tumor is exophytic, the exophytic portion can be resected.

REFERENCES

Aboian MS, Solomon DA, Felton E, et al. Imaging characteristics of pediatric diffuse midline gliomas with histone H3 K27M mutation. *AJNR Am J Neuroradiol.* 2017;38(4):795-800.

Louis DN, Perry A, Reifenberger G, et al. The 2016 World Health Organization classification of tumors of the central nervous system: a summary. *Acta Neuropathol.* 2016;131(6):803-820.

Neuroradiology: THE REQUISITES. 4th ed. pp 2, 58-59.

CASE 126

Textiloma or Gossypiboma—Retained Surgical Sponge

1. **D.** Textiloma. Follow-up MRI (Figure 126.5) demonstrates rim-enhancing lesions adjacent to the surgical cavity with no elevation of relative cerebral blood volume (CBV), on fused CBV and postcontrast T1 maps (Figure 126.6). Functional MRI and diffusion fiber tractography were also performed for surgical planning which demonstrated left hemispheric dominance of language function and proximity of the posterior aspect of the left SLF to the posterior aspect resection cavity and new enhancing lesions (Figure 126.7). These were surgically resected, and pathology demonstrated dense fibrous tissue, consistent with dura, and gelfoam with reactive changes. Patient never received radiation therapy, so radiation necrosis is not a good choice. Lack of elevated CBV argues against malignant transformation and evolving subacute ischemia is usually seen earlier usually within 4–6 weeks of initial resection.

2. **E.** Postoperative textiloma due to hemostatic material and subsequent granuloma formation can mimic recurrent tumor, radiation necrosis, and even postoperative abscess.

3. **D.** Floseal consists of a bovine-derived gelatin matrix component and a human-derived thrombin component and is increasingly used for hemostasis in neurosurgical procedures. Floseal has a distinctive pseudoair hypoattenuation on CT and T2-hypointense speckles in a T2-hyperintense background with trapped microbubbles giving rise to GRE susceptibility. Its unique space-occupying appearance should not be mistaken for the retained surgical sponge (retained foreign body or a gossypiboma), which is a hyperdense serpiginous structure on CT. On MRI, it appears as a T2 hypointense serpentine foreign body with susceptibility effects on GRE.

Comment

A variety of hemostatic agents are routinely used to control intraoperative bleeding in many surgical subspecialties, including neurosurgery. These include cellulose, gelatin, and collagen-based agents; thrombin; and fibrin glue. These agents effectively achieve hemostasis with various limitations. Fibrin glue requires a dry surface, obviating its use in an excessively oozing field. Gelatin (Gelfoam) expands up to 320% with the absorption of fluid and may compress the neural tissue, therefore, necessitating removal after achieving hemostasis which risks rebleeding. Meticulous lining of the surgical bed with cellulose (Surgicel) is time-consuming and sometimes impossible through a narrow surgical corridor. Hemostatic agents can be mistakenly left behind during operations. Such foreign materials cause foreign body reactions in the surrounding tissue (called textilomas or gossypibomas).

Complications caused by these foreign bodies are well known, but cases are rarely published because of medicolegal implications. Some textilomas cause infection or abscess formation in the early stage, whereas others remain clinically silent for many years. Such foreign bodies can often mimic tumors or abscesses clinically or radiologically. There are reports of other hemostatic materials (Gelfoam [Pfizer, New York, NY], Surgicel [Johnson & Johnson, New Brunswick, NJ] causing foreign body reactions that cannot be distinguished from recurrent tumors on MRI. The MRI appearance of foreign materials left behind during surgery can differ, depending on the type of material left behind, the time elapsed since surgery, and the type of foreign body reaction that occurs. There are two types of foreign body reactions: (1) aseptic fibrous reaction, which involves adhesion formation, or encapsulation; and (2) granuloma formation, or an exudative reaction, which leads to abscess formation.

This patient developed irregular rim-enhancing lesions at the surgical site almost one year after the initial surgery. Imaging findings were confusing, and the diagnosis of a textiloma was confirmed on pathology.

REFERENCES

Ho LM, Merkle EM, Kuo PC, et al. Imaging appearance of surgical sponges at 1.5T MRI: an in vitro study. *Eur J Radiol*. 2011;80(2):514-518.

Learned KO, Mohan S, Hyder IZ, Bagley LJ, Wang S, Lee JY. Imaging features of a gelatin-thrombin matrix hemostatic agent in the intracranial surgical bed: a unique space-occupying pseudomass. *AJNR Am J Neuroradiol*. 2014;35(4):686-690.

Manzella A, Filho PB, Albuquerque E, et al. Imaging of gossypibomas: pictorial review. *AJR Am J Roentgenol*. 2009;193(6):94-101.

Montemurro N, Murrone D, Romanelli B, Ierardi A. Postoperative textiloma mimicking intracranial rebleeding in a patient with spontaneous hemorrhage: case report and review of the literature. *Case Rep Neurol*. 2020;12(1):7-12.

Neuroradiology: THE REQUISITES. 4th ed. pp 2, 82-85.

CASE 127

Hamartoma of the Hypothalamus (Tuber Cinereum Hamartoma)

1. **B.** At the tuber cinereum (floor of the third ventricle), between the optic chiasm and mammillary bodies. It is splaying the optic chiasm and the pituitary gland and infundibulum are normally seen. Note, the lesion is abutting the basilar artery and the brainstem posteriorly.

2. **D.** Gelastic seizures and precocious puberty.

3. **C.** These lesions usually follow the signal characteristics of gray matter on T1W imaging, but may be hyperintense on T2 and FLAIR imaging, as in the present case (Figures 127.1 and 127.2). They typically do not enhance (Figures 127.4 and 127.6). It is proposed that T2 hyperintensity correlated with the proportion of glial cells within the lesion.

4. **D.** The differential diagnosis of hypothalamic hamartomas includes all of these; however, the anatomic location of a tuber cinereum hamartoma, its imaging appearance, and the clinical history are highly specific.

Comment

The hypothalamus may be affected by a spectrum of pathologies, including developmental lesions, primary tumors, systemic tumors that involve the CNS (such as lymphoma), vascular malformations, and inflammatory processes, including granulomatous disease. MRI findings, combined with the patient's clinical presentation and age, are usually able to distinguish among the differential possibilities.

This case illustrates the characteristic appearance of a hypothalamic hamartoma (tuber cinereum hamartoma). The mass is isointense relative to gray matter on T1W imaging, is hyperintense to adjacent gray matter on T2W and FLAIR imaging, and sits just anterior to the mammary bodies at the level of the floor of the third ventricle. Mild T2W hyperintensity relative to gray matter, absence of contrast enhancement, and stability in lesion size are the classic MRI imaging findings of these hamartomas. MRI and MR spectroscopy (reduced *N*-acetylaspartate and increased myoinositol) suggest decreased neuronal density and gliosis in these lesions compared with normal gray matter. Hamartomas are benign nonneoplastic lesions that are likely congenital. Many are asymptomatic, but symptoms may be more common in children and with larger lesions, and typically include gelastic seizures ("fits of laughter") and central precocious puberty. Knowledge of this lesion and its radiologic and clinical presentations allows the specific diagnosis to be established in most cases. Occasionally, atypical imaging findings (marked hyperintensity on T2W imaging or lesions larger than 2.5 cm) raise the possibility of a hypothalamic glioma, which usually demonstrates postcontrast enhancement. In such cases, follow-up imaging at several-month intervals can be obtained (hamartomas should not grow). Giant lesions with a cerebriform appearance, resembling a "brain-within-a-brain" architecture have also been described.

REFERENCES

Amstutz DR, Coons SW, Kerrigan JF, et al. Hypothalamic hamartomas: correlation of MR imaging and spectroscopic findings with tumor glial content. *AJNR Am J Neuroradiol.* 2006;27(4):794-798.

Cox M, Ahn J, Kandula V, Piatt J. Giant hypothalamic hamartoma. *Appl Radiol.* 2017;46(5):31A-31B.

Kameyama S, Murakami H, Masuda H, et al. Minimally invasive magnetic resonance imaging-guided stereotactic radiofrequency thermocoagulation for epileptogenic hypothalamic hamartomas. *Neurosurgery.* 2009;65(3):438-449.

Neuroradiology: THE REQUISITES. 4th ed. pp 10, 358-366.

CASE 128

Clival Chordoma

1. **B.** Palsy of cranial nerve VI. The most common presenting complaint is diplopia from abducens nerve involvement in the Dorello's canal.
2. **D.** Chordomas are found along the axial skeleton and are relatively more common in the sacrum (50%).
3. **D.** Chordomas arise in the midline as they arise from notochordal remnants. On the other hand, chondrosarcoma arises from petro-occipital synchondrosis and is therefore paramidline in location. Both chordoma and chondrosarcoma cause bone destruction, are hyperintense on T2 and show postcontrast enhancement.
4. **C.** Giant cell tumor.

Comment

Chordomas arise in locations where notochordal remnants are found. They occur most commonly in the sacrum (50%), followed by the clivus (35%) and the spine, especially the upper cervical spine, C1–2 (15%). Although chordomas are considered benign neoplasms, based on their histologic appearance, they grow quite invasively, particularly at the skull base, where they can invade multiple skull base foramina, cavernous sinuses, or extend into the posterior and middle cranial fossa. CT and MRI play complimentary roles in assessing skull base tumors. On CT, calcification is seen in 50% of cases, and the regions of bone erosion or destruction are clearly delineated. Multiplanar MRI allows complete evaluation of the soft tissue extent of the lesion and its relationship with adjacent vital brain structures. On MRI, the signal characteristics of chordomas are variable. These tumors are typically hypointense to isointense to the brain on T1W imaging and are normally hyperintense on T2W imaging. There may be marked heterogeneity due to cellularity, vascularity, or calcification. Most chordomas enhance, although some predominantly cystic tumors have minimal enhancement. In our experience, tumors arising at the C1–2 regions have been associated with less enhancement and more cystic-type changes.

The differential diagnosis includes chondroid lesions (chondrosarcoma), metastatic disease, multiple myeloma, and lymphoma.

The presence of a calcified matrix usually limits the differential diagnosis to chordoma versus chondrosarcoma. Chordomas generally tend to be midline lesions, whereas chondrosarcomas tend to be more paramidline. Clinical symptoms of chordomas and chondrosarcomas may be quite similar at the skull base, including headache and cranial neuropathies (frequently affecting cranial nerve VI). Clinical presentation is usually in the second through fourth decades of life.

Surgical resection is usually the first line of treatment, with radiation therapy offered for recurrent cases. Recurrence, including seeding along the operative tract, is common. Similar to giant cell tumors, chordomas may metastasize in 7%–14% of patients with nodal, pulmonary, bone, cerebral, or abdominal visceral involvement. Prognosis is typically poor due to the locally aggressive nature of these tumors. Histological subtype has an impact on prognosis with chondroid chordoma having the best prognosis and dedifferentiated chordoma having the worst prognosis, and the more common conventional chordoma having an intermediate prognosis.

REFERENCES

Golden LD, Small JE. Benign notochordal lesions of the posterior clivus: retrospective review of prevalence and imaging characteristics. *J Neuroimaging.* 2014;24(3):245-249.

Erdem E, Angtuaco EC, Van Hemert R, Park JS, Al-Mefty O. Comprehensive review of intracranial chordoma. *Radiographics.* 2003;23(4):995-1009.

Yeom KW, Lober RM, Mobley BC, et al. Diffusion-weighted MRI: distinction of skull base chordoma from chondrosarcoma. *AJNR Am J Neuroradiol.* 2013;35(5):1056-1061.

Neuroradiology: THE REQUISITES. 4th ed. pp 10, 374-376.

CASE 129

Perineural Spread of Skin Cancer—Squamous Cell Carcinoma

1. **C.** Perineural spread of the tumor, along the greater auricular nerve to the facial nerve in the parotid gland extending to the auriculotemporal branch, foramen ovale, Meckel's cave, to the cisternal segment of the right trigeminal nerve. Also, note that enhancement of the facial nerve overlying the accessory lobe of the right parotid gland.
2. **A.** Imaging of perineural tumor spread is best accomplished with contrast-enhanced MRI, due to its higher soft tissue resolution and less artifacts when compared with CT.
3. **B.** Adenoid cystic carcinoma has perineural spread in 50% of cases.
4. **A.** The auriculotemporal branch. The auriculotemporal nerve is a sensory branch of the posterior division of the mandibular nerve. Perineural spread of head and neck malignancies e.g., squamous cell carcinoma as in this case, can occur along the auriculotemporal branch, which can spread to the facial nerve from the mandibular division (V3) of the trigeminal nerve, or vice versa.

Comment

This case illustrates the classic imaging appearance of the perineural spread of skin carcinoma (squamous cell carcinoma in this patient). The patient, who was previously treated for recurrent laryngeal cancer, subsequently developed skin cancer (squamous cell carcinoma) and presented with right facial weakness and pain. Contrast-enhanced axial T1W images (Figures 129.1 and 129.5) demonstrate perineural tracking of carcinoma along the right greater auricular nerve to the parotid gland allowing extension to the seventh cranial nerve with perineural tracking along the seventh nerve within the gland, and to the auriculotemporal branch, foramen ovale, Meckel's cave, to the cisternal segment of the fifth cranial nerve. Additionally, this case illustrates that the tumor may spread along branches of the auriculotemporal nerve, through the foramen ovale into Meckel's cave.

Perineural spread of the tumor represents tracking of the tumor along nerve sheaths, frequently discontinuous and remote from the site of the primary neoplasm and should be distinguished from perineural tumor invasion, which is a histopathological finding, describing neoplastic infiltration of a nerve at the site of the original tumor.

Perineural tumor spread occurs with a spectrum of tumors, including skin cancers (basal cell and desmoplastic melanoma are notorious for this tendency, but squamous cell carcinoma is common and may also have perineural spread, as was seen in this case); squamous cell carcinoma of the head and neck (in particular, nasopharyngeal cancer); primary salivary neoplasms (most notably, adenoid cystic carcinoma); lymphoma in the periorbital region; and other skull base neoplasms. Because the perineural spread of the tumor may not be symptomatic, the radiologist must always be on the hunt for this in appropriate clinical scenarios.

Perineural spread is a significant adverse prognostic indicator in the staging of head and neck cancers and influences treatment decision-making. Lesions believed to be resectable for cure may be deemed unresectable and radiation fields may need to be expanded. Therefore, a comprehensive knowledge of the pertinent anatomy of the cranial nerves, and the typical imaging features of perineural tumor spread is essential in the imaging surveillance of head and neck cancers.

REFERENCES

Budak MJ, Weir-McCall JR, Yeap PM, et al. High-resolution microscopy-coil MR imaging of skin tumors: techniques and novel clinical applications. *Radiographics.* 2015;35(4):1077-1090.
Ong CK, Chong VF. Imaging of perineural spread in head and neck tumours. *Cancer Imaging.* 2010;10 Spec no A(1A):S92-S98.
Panizza B, Warren T. Perineural invasion of head and neck skin cancer: diagnostic and therapeutic implications. *Curr Oncol Rep.* 2013;15(2):128-133.
Neuroradiology: THE REQUISITES. 4th ed. pp 14, 501.

CASE 130

Multiple System Atrophy Cerebellar Type (MSA-C) (Olivopontocerebellar Degeneration)

1. **B.** Ataxia.
2. **B.** In MSA-C, there is a predominance of cerebellar symptoms, whereas in MSA-P, there is a predominance of parkinsonian signs and symptoms. All other options are correct.
3. **D.** All of these conditions are known to cause cerebellar degeneration. Substance abuse (alcohol), medications (anticonvulsants, such as phenytoin), paraneoplastic syndromes, and some chemotherapeutic agents, to name a few.
4. **A.** Autosomal recessive and chromosome 9, respectively.

Comment

Multiple system atrophy cerebellar type (MSA-C) also known as olivopontocerebellar degeneration is an adult-onset, sporadic, progressive neurodegenerative disorder and is one of the clinical manifestations of multiple systemic atrophy (MSA). Initially, in 1969, the term MSA was proposed to encompass three unrelated diseases: (1) olivopontocerebellar atrophy (OPCA), (2) Shy-Drager syndrome (SDS), and (3) striatonigral degenerative disease (SND). Subsequently, MSA was classified as an α-synucleinopathy

together with Parkinson's disease (PD) and dementia with Lewy bodies (DLB). Patients with predominant parkinsonism are designated MSA-P, and those with predominant cerebellar ataxia are designated MSA-C.

MSA-C typically presents with cerebellar ataxia and bulbar dysfunction. Unlike SDS and SND (the other two manifestations of MSA), autonomic dysfunction and parkinsonism are less prominent.

There is greater involvement of the pons, cerebellum, and middle cerebellar peduncles in MSA-C, while putaminal volume loss outweighs pontocerebellar atrophy in MSA-P. In MSA-C, there is disproportionate atrophy of the cerebellum and brainstem (as seen in the current case). In MSA-C, there is often cruciform T2/FLAIR hyperintensity within the pons, termed the "hot-cross bun" sign. Middle cerebellar peduncle atrophy is typical and may be associated with abnormal T2/FLAIR signals within the peduncles. In MSA-P T2/SWI, hypointensity can be seen in the posterior putamen. A thin stripe of hyperintensity has also been described on the lateral aspect of the putamen on T2W images. Unfortunately, no effective treatment is currently available, with relentless progression of the disease culminating in death usually within 10 years of diagnosis.

REFERENCES

Schöls L, Amoiridis G, Przuntek H, Frank G, Epplen JT, Epplen C. Friedreich's ataxia. Revision of the phenotype according to molecular genetics. *Brain.* 1997;120(Pt 12):2131-2140.
Watanabe H, Riku Y, Hara K, et al. Clinical and imaging features of multiple system atrophy: challenges for an early and clinically definitive diagnosis. *J Mov Disord.* 2018;11(3):107-120.
Neuroradiology: THE REQUISITES. 4th ed. pp 7, 239-245.

CASE 131

Huntington's Disease (HD)

1. **B.** There is volume loss in bilateral caudate nuclei, consistent with the diagnosis of Huntington's disease. This patient underwent genetic testing that revealed 43 repeats.
2. **D.** The most consistent feature in HD is volume loss of the striatum, caudate nucleus, and putamina.
3. **D.** In NBIA, there is progressive iron accumulation in the globus pallidi and pars reticulata of the substantia nigra, which is seen as hypointensity on T2W MRI images and susceptibility on SWI/T2* images.
4. **A.** Ceruloplasmin. Wilson's disease is a disorder that results from abnormal ceruloplasmin metabolism, as a result of a variety of mutations in the ATP7B gene. This leads to increased levels of copper, which has toxic effects on hepatocytes with copper deposition in many organs, such as the liver and the brain.

Comment

A variety of disease processes affect the extrapyramidal nuclei (basal ganglia, thalami) as well as the nuclei in the brainstem. These conditions are most commonly degenerative or metabolic, and many are inherited. Among the neurodegenerative processes that can affect the deep gray matter are Huntington's disease, Wilson's disease, and neurodegeneration with brain iron accumulation (NBIA), previously known as Hallervorden–Spatz syndrome. Toxic exposure may also result in abnormalities of the deep gray matter. Lesions in these structures typically result in movement disorders that can occur in isolation or in combination and include the following subtypes: abnormalities in muscle tone, involuntary movements, abnormal postural reflexes, and the inability to carry out voluntary movements. Toxic exposures that affect the basal ganglia include carbon monoxide, ethylene glycol, toluene, etc. Although there is wide variation in the deep gray matter structures involved, many diseases have a characteristic involvement of specific structures.

Huntington's disease (HD) is an autosomal dominant progressive and fatal neurodegenerative disease caused by an expanded trinucleotide CAG sequence in the huntingtin gene (HTT) on chromosome 4. Clinical manifestations typically include involuntary movement (choreoathetosis), rigidity, dementia, and emotional instability. Cognitive deficits are believed to be due to abnormal connectivity between the deep gray matter and the cortex. The disease typically presents in the fourth or fifth decade of life. The disease is progressive, with death occurring 15 to 20 years after its onset. On imaging, as in this case, Huntington's disease is characterized by atrophy of the caudate nuclei, which results in ballooning of the frontal horns of the lateral ventricles ("box-like" configuration). There is also prominent putaminal volume loss which is generally not easily recognized on visual inspection but seen well on morphometry. MRI shows signal changes in these nuclei. These changes may be hyperintense on T2W images, which is believed to be related to gliosis; other cases show T2W hypointensity, which is likely related to iron deposition. Other major imaging findings include cortical atrophy. There is no treatment that is currently available for this disease.

REFERENCES

Apple AC, Possin KL, Satris G, et al. Quantitative 7T phase imaging in premanifest Huntington disease. *AJNR Am J Neuroradiol.* 2014; 35(9):1707-1713.

Doan NT, van der Bogaard SJ, Dumas EM, et al. Texture analysis of ultrahigh field T2*-weighted MR images of the brain: application to Huntington's disease. *J Magn Reson Imaging.* 2014;39(3):633-640.

Negi RS, Manchanda KL, Sanga S. Imaging of Huntington's disease. *Med J Armed Forces India.* 2014;70(4):386-388.

Neuroradiology: THE REQUISITES. 4th ed. pp 7, 248.

CASE 132

Multiple Sclerosis and Glioblastoma

1. **C.** In this patient with multiple sclerosis (MS), a follow-up MRI shows a new large heterogeneously enhancing bilobed mass centered at the anterior corpus callosum extending into the adjacent frontal lobes (left more than right), measuring up to 4.5 cm. There are extensive surrounding FLAIR signal abnormalities and mass effects. Notice the elevated relative cerebral blood volume (rCBV) on dynamic susceptibility contrast MR perfusion imaging (Figure 132.6). These findings are in keeping with high-grade glioma.

2. **B.** TDLs usually present with relatively little mass effect or surrounding edema. These lesions typically have an open or incomplete ring enhancement and low rCBV. Elevation of choline is consistently found in acute MS lesions. Note, Cho is a marker for cell membrane turnover and is not specific for neoplasms. Elevations in choline and lactate are consistently seen in TDLs.

3. **E.** The incidence of progressive multifocal leukoencephalopathy (PML) in the non-HIV setting is increasing and has been reported in all of the aforementioned conditions.

Comment

"Tumefactive" multiple sclerosis (MS), high-grade glioma (GBM), and occasionally an abscess can appear similar on imaging, particularly in the absence of clinical history. MS typically occurs in younger patients, and there are often additional clinical or imaging findings to suggest this diagnosis. On close questioning, patients often have neurologic symptoms that are spaced both in time and in location. Furthermore, MR imaging may demonstrate white matter lesions separate from the mass that are suggestive of MS, as seen on baseline MRI (Figures 132.1 and 132.2) in this patient. On follow-up imaging, there was development of a large heterogeneously enhancing mass centered in the corpus callosum and extending into bilateral frontal lobes with extensive edema, mass effect, and corresponding elevated rCBV. Pathology was consistent with an IDH wild-type glioblastoma.

Advanced MR imaging sequences may be of value in differentiating between a TDL and neoplastic processes such as high-grade glioma and lymphoma. Perfusion imaging, as in this case, shows markedly elevated rCBV corresponding to the areas of enhancement in this large necrotic mass, suggesting a high-grade glioma or GBM rather than TDL. Nonspecific spectroscopic findings in TDL include elevation of choline, lactate, and lipid peaks and a decrease in *N*-acetylaspartate. These spectroscopic characteristics reflect the histologic correlation of marked demyelination in the absence of significant inflammation. Gliomas also consistently show reductions in *N*-acetylaspartate and increases in phospholipids, reflecting the replacement of normal neuronal tissue with a proliferating cellular process. Increases in lactate are not uncommon as a result of tissue ischemia and necrosis.

Progressive multifocal leukoencephalopathy (PML) is also a demyelinating condition that results from the reactivation of John Cunningham virus (JC virus) infecting oligodendrocytes in patients with compromised immune systems. Its incidence is increasing, and besides HIV/AIDS, it is also reported in MS patients taking immunosuppressive monoclonal antibody therapy, such as natalizumab (Tysabri).

REFERENCES

Coban G, Mohan S, Kural F, et al. Prognostic value of dynamic susceptibility contrast-enhanced and diffusion-weighted MR imaging in patients with glioblastomas. *AJNR Am J Neuroradiol.* 2015;36(7):1247-1252.

Crombe A, Saranthan M, Ruet A, et al. MS lesions are better detected with 3D T1 gradient-echo than with 2D T1 spin-echo gadolinium-enhanced imaging at 3T. *AJNR Am J Neuroradiol.* 2015;36(3):501-507.

Saindane AM, Cha S, Law M, Xue X, Knopp EA, Zagzag D. Proton MR spectroscopy of tumefactive demyelinating lesions. *AJNR Am J Neuroradiol.* 2002;23(8):1378-1386.

Neuroradiology: THE REQUISITES. 4th ed. pp 6, 206-217.

CASE 133

Adrenoleukodystrophy (ALD)

1. **D.** Adrenoleukodystrophy (ALD). There is a confluent, symmetric posterior predominant white matter abnormality with the involvement of the splenium of the corpus callosum with relative cortical and subcortical U-fiber sparing. Notice different zones, with T1 hypointensity in the central zone (Figure 133.6) and thin peripheral enhancement (Figures 133.6 and 133.7).

2. **A.** Active demyelination and perivascular inflammation. In patients with ALD, the affected white matter typically has three zones. The *central zone* appears hypointense on T1W images, and markedly hyperintense on T2W images. This zone corresponds to irreversible gliosis and scarring. The *intermediate zone* appears isointense to slightly hypointense on T2W images and shows thin peripheral contrast enhancement which represents active inflammation and breakdown

of the blood–brain barrier. The *peripheral zone* represents the leading edge of demyelination and appears moderately hyperintense on T2W images and demonstrates no contrast enhancement.

3. **C.** X-linked inheritance classically affects young males.
4. **D.** Canavan disease is an autosomal recessive disorder caused by a mutation on the short arm of chromosome 17 leading to deficiency of *N*-acetylaspartoacylase, which is a key enzyme in myelin synthesis, with resultant accumulation of N-acetylaspartate (NAA) in the brain.

Comment

X-linked adrenoleukodystrophy is one of the most common adult-onset leukodystrophies related to a single enzyme deficiency (acyl-coenzyme A synthetase) within intracellular peroxisomes. This enzyme is necessary for β oxidation in the breakdown of very-long-chain fatty acids that accumulate in erythrocytes, plasma, and fibroblasts, as well as the CNS white matter and adrenal cortex. Boys typically present between the ages of 4 and 10 years. The clinical presentation may include behavioral disturbance, visual symptoms, hearing loss, seizures, and eventually spastic quadriparesis. Patients often present with adrenal insufficiency (Addison's disease), which may occur before or after the development of neurologic symptoms. This patient presented with seizures and a long history of slowly progressive cognitive difficulties since childhood. The diagnosis of X-linked adrenoleukodystrophy was confirmed by typical MRI findings and elevated very-long-chain fatty acids. Notably, several maternal uncles had a similar phenotype prior to early death.

As in other demyelinating and dysmyelinating disorders, MRI is the imaging modality of choice for the detection of white matter abnormalities. In adrenoleukodystrophy, the most common pattern of white matter disease is bilaterally symmetric abnormalities within the parietal and occipital white matter, extending across the splenium of the corpus callosum. The disease may continue to progress anteriorly to involve the frontal and temporal lobes. The regions of active demyelination, usually along the margins, may show contrast enhancement. Less typical presentations include predominantly frontal lobe involvement or holohemispheric involvement. Adrenoleukodystrophy also involves the cerebellum, spinal cord, and peripheral nervous system. As a rule, most children will have prominent supratentorial involvement, whereas adults will have more pronounced spinal cord involvement (adrenomyeloneuropathy). MR spectroscopy shows evidence of neuronal loss as manifested by decreased NAA and the presence of lactate.

Bone marrow transplantation is thought to be favorable in the early stages of the disease. The pattern of involvement also determines prognosis, with combined frontal and parieto-occipital usually heralding rapid disease progression, whereas isolated cerebellar or corticospinal tract involvement generally has a slower progression.

REFERENCES

Loes DJ, Fatemi A, Melhem ER, et al. Analysis of MRI patterns aids prediction of progression in X-linked adrenoleukodystrophy. *Neurology*. 2003;61(3):369-374.
McKinney AM, Nascene D, Miller WP, et al. Childhood cerebral X-linked adrenoleukodystrophy: diffusion tensor imaging measurements for prediction of clinical outcome after hematopoietic stem cell transplantation. *AJNR Am J Neuroradiol*. 2013;34(3):641-649.
van der Voorn JP, Pouwels PJ, Powers JM, et al. Correlating quantitative MR imaging with histopathology in X-linked adrenoleukodystrophy. *AJNR Am J Neuroradiol*. 2011;32(3):481-489.
Neuroradiology: THE REQUISITES. 4th ed. pp 6, 225-226.

CASE 134

Cytomegalovirus Meningitis and Ventriculitis (Ependymitis) in a Patient with HIV/AIDS

1. **B.** In this patient, there is more enhancement in the left internal auditory canals than in the right internal auditory canals (Figures 134.3 and 134.4), with thin ependymal enhancement along the bilateral lateral ventricles, posterior third ventricle, and fourth ventricle (Figures 134.1, 134.2, and 134.5). Notice the tiny amount of restricted diffusion in the dependent right occipital horn (Figure 134.6). These findings are most consistent with meningitis and ventriculitis in this immunocompromised patient.
2. **D.** Meningitis is the most common underlying condition responsible for ventriculitis.
3. **C.** Cytomegalovirus (CMV) meningitis and ventriculitis usually present with no mass effect, however hydrocephalus may be present. All others are correct.
4. **D.** Congenital CMV infection presents with bilateral ventricular subependymal calcification, ventricular enlargement, periventricular hypodensity on CT or hyperintensity on T2W MRI, atrophy, and migrational anomalies such as pachygyria or polymicrogyria.

Comment

Cytomegalovirus (CMV) is present in latent form in almost 80% of the American population, as indicated by the presence of antibodies. Reactivation usually results in a subclinical or mild flu-like syndrome. In immunocompromised patients, reactivation can result in disseminated infection, usually involving the respiratory and gastrointestinal tracts; however, it rarely can also infect the entire nervous system. In the CNS, CMV may cause meningoencephalitis and ventriculitis (ependymitis). Symptoms may be acute or chronic, developing over months. Patients may have fever, altered mental status, and progressive cognitive decline. Patients may also present with cranial neuropathies (as in this case). It is almost always seen in the context of profound immunosuppression, as in the current case, where the CD4 count at the time of diagnosis was 10. A lumbar puncture showed 1120 white blood cells with 90% segmented neutrophils, glucose 11, and protein > 600. Serum and CSF were positive for CMV by polymerase chain reaction (PCR).

MRI is the diagnostic study of choice in assessing immunocompromised patients suspected of having CNS infections. Imaging may show atrophy; high signal intensity in the periventricular white matter, typically not associated with significant mass effect; and retinitis (frequently seen in the AIDS population) in patients with CMV infection. When present, subependymal high-signal intensities with diffusion restriction and ependymal enhancement are important in establishing the diagnosis of CMV and help in differentiating CMV ventriculitis from other causes of meningoencephalitis in HIV-infected patients. CSF PCR has high sensitivity and specificity in diagnosing CMV infection. Treatment depends on disease severity. Severe disease is treated with a combination of intravenous ganciclovir and foscarnet.

REFERENCES

John KJ, Gunasekaran K, Sultan N, Iyyadurai R. Cytomegalovirus ventriculoencephalitis presenting with hydrocephalus in a patient with advanced HIV infection. *Oxf Med Case Reports*. 2019;2019(10):omz104.
Smith AB, Smirniotopoulos JG, Rushing EJ. From the archives of the AFIP: central nervous system infections associated with human immunodeficiency virus infection: radiologic-pathologic correlation. *Radiographics*. 2008;28(7):2033-2058. doi:10.1148/rg.287085135. Erratum in: Radiographics. 2009;29(2):638.
Neuroradiology: THE REQUISITES. 4th ed. pp 5, 184-192.

CASE 135

Central Neurocytoma

1. **A.** Heterogeneous cystic-solid partially enhancing mass in the left lateral ventricle touching the left lateral ventricular wall and the septum pellucidum, with internal foci of calcification (Figure 135.1) and ventricular entrapment. These imaging findings are most consistent with a central neurocytoma.
2. **A.** Oligodendroglioma. Electron microscopy and immunohistochemistry show neurosecretory granules and the neuronal marker synaptophysin, respectively, which are characteristic of central neurocytoma. Note that IDH mutations and 1p19q co-deletion are absent, which are a defining feature of oligodendrogliomas.
3. **A.** In children, the atria of the lateral ventricles. In adults, the fourth ventricle.
4. **A.** The atria of the lateral ventricles.

Comment

Central neurocytomas typically have a homogeneous cell population with neuronal differentiation. These benign neuroepithelial neoplasms occur in young and middle-aged adults. Patients may be asymptomatic or may present with headache and signs of increased intracranial pressure, frequently due to hydrocephalus, as in this case. Central neurocytomas arise most commonly within the body of the lateral ventricle (less frequently, the third ventricle), adjacent to the septum pellucidum and foramen of Monroe. They have a characteristic attachment to the superolateral ventricular wall. Most are confined to the ventricles, although a parenchymal extension may rarely occur. These features may help to distinguish neurocytomas from other intraventricular tumors, such as astrocytoma, giant cell astrocytoma, ependymoma, intraventricular oligodendroglioma, and meningioma. Preoperative diagnosis of central neurocytoma may help in planning therapy, because this tumor has a better prognosis than other intraventricular tumors arising in this area.

On CT and MR imaging, neurocytomas typically are heterogeneous masses that contain multiple cysts. They are well demarcated, with smooth, lobulated margins and moderate vascularity. Most neurocytomas have calcifications, as seen in this case. On MRI, the more solid component of these tumors tends to follow the signal characteristics of gray matter. Signal voids may be related to calcification or tumor vascularity. Contrast enhancement is variable, ranging from none to moderate. On imaging and conventional pathologic evaluation (microscopy), these tumors are frequently reminiscent of oligodendrogliomas. The distinction between these two neoplasms is important because central neurocytomas have a more benign course and the treatment may differ. Although neurocytomas have a favorable prognosis, malignant variants and recurrences may rarely occur.

REFERENCES

Donoho D, Zada G. Imaging of central neurocytomas. *Neurosurg Clin N Am*. 2015;26(1):11-19.
Tlili-Graiess K, Mama N, Arifa N, et al. Diffusion-weighted MR imaging and proton MR spectroscopy findings of central neurocytoma with pathological correlation. *J Neuroradiol*. 2014;41(4):243-250.
Neuroradiology: THE REQUISITES. 4th ed. pp 2, 49-52.

CASE 136

Cytokine Storm-Related Corpus Callosal Injury

1. **E.** Cytokine storm-related corpus callosal injury. This patient had extremely elevated markers for acute-phase reactants, suggesting an autoimmune injury from a cytokine storm. Ischemic stroke of the corpus callosum is extremely rare given the redundant blood supply including the anterior communicating artery, the pericallosal artery, and the posterior pericallosal artery.
2. **B.** Corpus callosum is susceptible to cytokine-induced injury due to the high density of cytokines, glutamate, and other receptors present within this region. An increased amount of glutamate leads to excitotoxic action on multiple glutamate receptors, sodium–potassium pumps, and aquaporins, resulting in an influx of water, manifesting as diffusion restriction, as seen in this patient.
3. **D.** Marchiafava–Bignami disease (MBD) is a rare complication of chronic alcoholism characterized by acute demyelination and necrosis of the central fibers of the corpus callosum (with relative sparing of upper and lower edges). Many patients do not recover and die, but prompt administration of parenteral thiamine (vitamin B complex) has been shown to result in improvement.
4. **E.** All of these conditions can present with "cytotoxic lesions of the corpus callosum (CLOCC)" typically involving the splenium.

Comment

Neurologic involvement is well-recognized in coronavirus disease 2019 (COVID-19) and appears to affect more severely infected patients. The most common CNS manifestations are acute infarcts with large clot burden and intracranial hemorrhage. However, additional patterns are also encountered, including disseminated leukoencephalopathy, hypoxic injury, meningitis and encephalitis, cytotoxic lesions of the corpus callosum (CLOCC), olfactory bulb involvement, cranial nerve enhancement, spinal manifestations, and long-term diffusion-tensor imaging changes of the brain. CLOCC has been described with COVID-19 particularly in children with multisystem inflammatory syndrome associated with COVID-19. CSF RT-PCR is usually negative for SARS-CoV-2 infection as was the case in this patient. These lesions likely relate to inflammatory damage from the coincident cytokine storm and high level of cytokine and glutamate receptors in the corpus callosum, most commonly in the splenium and rarely in the entire corpus callosum as in this case.

Marchiafava–Bignami disease (MBD) is a toxic demyelinating disorder initially described by two Italian pathologists. They identified it at autopsy in three patients with chronic alcoholism who presented with status epilepticus that subsequently progressed to a coma. All three patients consumed large quantities of red wine. This has also been described in patients with significant nutritional deficiencies, and it has been described in other populations and with other alcoholic beverages. This diagnosis should be considered in patients with acute encephalopathy or progressive dementia and alcoholism. It is most commonly seen in men and usually occurs in the third to fifth decade. On pathologic evaluation, MBD is typified by demyelination and necrosis, and it occurs most commonly in the central fibers of the corpus callosum. The acute form of this disease presents with seizures, motor or cognitive disturbances or a hemispheric disconnection syndrome (apraxia, hemialexia, dementia), and coma, and it is often fatal. Prompt treatment with parenteral thiamine is recommended.

REFERENCES

Hillbom M, Saloheimo P, Fujioka S, et al. Diagnosis and management of Marchiafava-Bignami disease: a review of CT/MRI confirmed cases. *J Neurol Neurosurg Psychiatry*. 2014;85(2):168-173.
Moonis G, Filippi CG, Kirsch CFE, et al. The spectrum of neuroimaging findings on CT and MRI in adults with COVID-19. *AJR Am J Roentgenol*. 2021;217(4):959-974.
Starkey J, Kobayashi N, Numaguchi Y, Moritani T. Cytotoxic lesions of the corpus callosum that show restricted diffusion: mechanisms, causes, and manifestations. *Radiographics*. 2017;37(2):562-576.
Neuroradiology: THE REQUISITES. 4th ed. pp 6, 222.

CASE 137

Metastatic Neuroendocrine Tumor (Carcinoid) to the Orbital Extraocular Muscles

1. **C.** Metastatic disease to the extraocular muscles (EOMs). There is mild right > left proptosis. Multiple enhancing masses are seen involving bilateral EOMs, e.g., on the right, the medial rectus is markedly enlarged, measuring 2.6 × 1.5 cm with mass effect over the right optic nerve (Figures 137.1 and 137.2). Smaller masses are seen on the left with a 1.2 × 0.8 cm mass in the lateral rectus muscle. These findings favor metastatic disease in this patient with a neuroendocrine tumor (carcinoid) of the terminal ileum. In thyroid orbitopathy, the tendinous insertions on the globe are typically spared (involvement is seen in this case, e.g., right medial rectus); moreover, there are discrete masses along the muscle bellies, rather than fusiform enlargement that is typical of thyroid orbitopathy.
2. **B.** Pain! Patients may also have exophthalmos, lid swelling, chemosis, and restricted ocular motility. Note, idiopathic orbital inflammation is usually unilateral (bilateral in ~10%).
3. **F.** Metastases to the EOMs are well-described in a variety of primary tumors, including breast, prostate, kidney, lung, and melanoma.
4. **B.** Enophthalmos. Inward retraction of the globe (similar to the skin of the affected breast) is the characteristic of metastatic scirrhous breast carcinoma.

Comment

Neuroendocrine tumors (NETs) arise from neuroendocrine cells throughout the body and are classified according to their site of origin, commonly in the lungs or gastrointestinal tract. The terms carcinoid tumor and carcinoid cancer are old ways of describing slow-growing NETs. This case represents metastatic NET to the orbit, specifically, to the EOMs. There is a tendency for both intraorbital, extramuscular, and EOM metastatic disease in patients with NETs. Uveal tract metastases are more commonly noted in bronchial lesions, whereas EOM metastases are more common in gastrointestinal primary tumors, as was the case in this patient. The metastatic potential of NETs is related to tumor size, usually seen in tumors larger than 1 cm. In symptomatic patients with intestinal NETs, more than 90% have metastatic disease, most commonly in the lymph nodes and liver.

Although a relatively rare neoplasm, it has an unusual propensity to metastasize to the orbits. It is suggested that in patients with known NET, well-defined, round, or fusiform masses of the EOM should strongly suggest metastatic involvement. The most common location for orbital metastases is the globe, usually involving the uveoscleral region.

Other common tumors that metastasize to the globe are breast and lung carcinoma in adults. Outside of the globe, orbital metastases are most often extraconal in the adjacent bony orbit. Intraconal metastatic disease is usually related to the direct extension of an ocular metastasis. Clinical manifestations are variable; some patients may be asymptomatic, whereas others may have proptosis, blurred vision, pain, or ophthalmoplegia, depending on the site of involvement.

REFERENCES

Gupta A, Chazen JL, Phillips CD. Carcinoid tumor metastases to the extraocular muscles: MR imaging and CT findings and review of the literature. *AJNR Am J Neuroradiol.* 2011;32(7):1208-1211.

Matsuo T, Ichimura K, Tanaka T, Takenaka T, Nakayama T. Neuroendocrine tumor (carcinoid) metastatic to orbital extraocular muscle: case report and literature review. *Strabismus.* 2010;18(4):123-128.

Neuroradiology: THE REQUISITES. 4th ed. pp 9, 324-342.

CASE 138

Human Herpesvirus-6 (HHV-6) Infection After Organ Transplantation

1. **D.** Human herpesvirus-6 (HHV-6) encephalitis. There is symmetric T2 (Figure 138.1) and FLAIR (Figure 138.2) hyperintensity in the bilateral mesial temporal lobes (bilateral hippocampi and amygdalae) with high signal intensity on DWI (Figure 138.3), and low apparent diffusion coefficient (ADC) (not shown).
2. **A.** Both HHV-6 and herpes simplex virus are members of the herpes family and have several similarities. However, in patients with HHV-6 encephalopathy, lesions are usually limited to the mesial temporal lobe, whereas in patients with HSE, extratemporal involvement is frequently seen. In the early stages, patients with HHV-6 encephalopathy usually have normal findings on head CT, but patients with HSE had abnormal swelling and decreased attenuation of the affected regions.
3. **D.** HHV-6 encephalitis is a rare CNS infection secondary to the reactivation of human herpesvirus 6 in immunosuppressed patients.
4. **C.** Arterial supply of the hippocampus is dependent on the collateral branches of the posterior cerebral artery and the anterior choroidal artery, forming the superficial hippocampal arteries that in turn lead to deep intrahippocampal arteries.

Comment

Human herpesvirus-6 (HHV-6) is a double-stranded DNA virus. More than 90% of the general population is seropositive for HHV-6 by 2–3 years of age. It is excreted by the salivary glands and may be passed to infants from their mothers. HHV-6 has a strong affinity for the CNS and has been detected by a polymerase chain reaction in up to one-third of the normal brain specimens, suggesting that the brain might be a latent viral site. Recently, HHV-6 encephalopathy has been reported in immunocompromised patients, especially patients who have undergone hematopoietic stem cell or solid-organ transplantation (lung and liver), receiving high-dose chemotherapy or immunosuppressants. Infection has typically been identified within 4 weeks of the transplantation. The pathogenesis is considered to be reactivation of the recipient's latent HHV-6 infection, and not infection from the donor. Immunocompromised patients are at risk for a spectrum of disease processes that may affect the CNS, and their symptoms are frequently nonspecific. Common neurologic symptoms in HHV-6 infection include disorientation, confusion, and short-term memory loss. Coma, hypopnea, and seizures have also been reported.

Early MRI findings, as in this case, include high signal intensity on T2 and FLAIR, and DWI in the mesial temporal lobe structures (hippocampus and amygdala). The DWI abnormality is accompanied by hypointensity on apparent diffusion coefficient (ADC) maps. Enhancement is usually not present. HHV-6 encephalopathy tends to exclusively involve the mesial temporal lobe and thus resembles HSE which usually has extratemporal sites of involvement. Note, acyclovir is not effective against HHV-6 because it lacks virus-specific thymidine kinase. Ganciclovir and foscarnet are found to be effective against HHV-6, but serious side effects, including myelosuppression and nephrotoxicity, may occur. Therefore, these drugs are not usually given prophylactically. Early diagnosis is critical to prevent serious neurologic sequelae. Mesial temporal involvement seen on MRI in a transplant recipient receiving preventive treatment with acyclovir is highly suggestive of HHV-6–associated encephalopathy.

REFERENCES

Noguchi T, Yoshiura T, Hiwatashi A, et al. CT and MRI findings of human herpesvirus 6-associated encephalopathy: comparison with findings of herpes simplex virus encephalitis. *AJR Am J Roentgenol.* 2010;194(3):754-760.

Tatu L, Vuillier F. Structure and vascularization of the human hippocampus. *Front Neurol Neurosci.* 2014;34:18-25.

Vu T, Carrum G, Hutton G, et al. Human herpesvirus-6 encephalitis following allogeneic hematopoietic stem cell transplantation. *Bone Marrow Transplant.* 2007;39(11):705-709.

Neuroradiology: THE REQUISITES. 4th ed. pp 5, 184-187.

CASE 139

Barrow Type A Direct Carotid-Cavernous Fistula of Left ICA Into Cavernous Sinus

1. **B.** Dilated engorged facial veins.
2. **A.** Carotid-cavernous fistula (CCF). There are multicompartmental intracranial hemorrhages (Figure 139.1), skull base, and otic capsule sparing left temporal fracture (Figure 139.2), enlarged cavernous sinuses and superior ophthalmic veins (Figure 139.3), engorged extraocular muscles, and increased vascularity of periorbital soft tissues and a barrow type A direct carotid-cavernous fistula (CCF).
3. **A.** Barrow classification divides CCF into, direct (type A) and indirect (types B–D). A direct connection between the cavernous internal carotid artery, and the cavernous sinus, type A, remains the most common type of CCF.
4. **C.** Cavernous sinus schwannomas most commonly arise from the trigeminal nerve (CN5).

Comment

There are two basic types of carotid–cavernous fistulas, direct (type A) and indirect (types B–D), each of which has a different etiology. Type A is most common where there is a direct connection between the cavernous internal carotid artery and the cavernous sinus. Indirect fistulae (types B–D), otherwise known as a dural arteriovenous fistula, is a shunt between meningeal branches of the cavernous internal carotid artery (type B), meningeal branches of the external carotid artery (type C), or meningeal branches of both the intracavernous carotid artery and the external carotid artery (type D) with the cavernous sinus.

The typical clinical presentation of a CCF is ophthalmologic symptoms, including pulsatile proptosis, pain, chemosis, and a palpable orbital bruit. This is because the cavernous sinus directly communicates with the ophthalmic veins, and an abnormal shunt between the sinus and the internal carotid artery can transmit arterial pressure to these veins. In addition, arterial perfusion to the globe is decreased, leading to visual loss. Direct CCFs are most commonly the result of head trauma, as in this patient; however, spontaneous CCFs may be seen in a spectrum of disorders, including atherosclerosis in elderly individuals, rupture of a carotid–cavernous aneurysm, or in association with underlying vascular dysplasias.

The clinical presentation and imaging findings are diagnostic of a direct CCF. CT and MRI often show enlargement of the superior ophthalmic vein, cavernous sinus, or petrosal venous plexus. Proptosis, periorbital soft tissue swelling, and diffuse enlargement of the extraocular muscles are commonly present, as in this case. MR angiography and catheter angiography show direct communication between the cavernous internal carotid artery and the cavernous sinus as well as early filling of the ipsilateral cavernous sinus, superior or inferior ophthalmic veins, and petrosal venous complex. In high-flow lesions, the contralateral venous system may opacify, as in this case, through intercavernous communications and the petrosal venous complex.

In this case, the left carotid injection shows a barrow type A direct CCF involving the posterior genu of the left cavernous internal carotid artery with significant venous shunting into the cavernous sinus, subsequently draining into the inferior petrosal sinuses and internal jugular veins. Additionally, there is retrograde flow into the left superior petrosal sinus, as well as dilated bilateral superior ophthalmic veins. There is minimal flow beyond the CCF, supplying the left hemisphere (Figures 139.6 and 139.7). Right common carotid artery injection in this patient shows a patent anterior communicating artery with robust cross-filling of the left anterior and middle cerebral artery territories (Figure 139.8). Contralateral injection of the right carotid artery and injection of the vertebrobasilar system are important in evaluating collateral flow, particularly if the involved internal carotid artery must be sacrificed to close the fistula, as was necessary in this case (Figures 139.9 and 139.10).

Management of these lesions in the majority of cases usually involves interventional neuroradiologic procedures. The goal of treatment is to eliminate flow through the fistula as well as to maintain internal carotid patency when possible. Treatment of direct and indirect fistulas may differ. Direct CCFs are usually treated transarterially with detachable coils or balloon embolization, with flow directed through the fistula into the cavernous sinus, tamponading the hole in the internal carotid artery. In the event that a transarterial route is not possible or is ineffective, a transvenous approach using platinum coils may be warranted. This can be achieved either via the femoral route or surgically via the superior ophthalmic vein. Gamma knife radiosurgery has also been shown to be effective in treating indirect dural arteriovenous fistulas.

REFERENCES

Chen CC, Chang PC, Shy CG, Chen WS, Hung HC. CT angiography and MR angiography in the evaluation of carotid cavernous sinus fistula prior to embolization: a comparison of techniques. *AJNR Am J Neuroradiol.* 2005;26(9):2349-2356.

Goyal A, Sharma S. Traumatic carotid-cavernous fistula: excellent demonstration on 3D CT angiography. *BMJ Case Rep.* 2013;2013:bcr2013 201707.

Mahalingam HV, Mani SE, Patel B, et al. Imaging spectrum of cavernous sinus lesions with histopathologic correlation. *Radiographics.* 2019;39(3): 795-819.

Miller NR. Dural carotid-cavernous fistulas: epidemiology, clinical presentation, and management. *Neurosurg Clin N Am.* 2012;23(1):179-192.

Neuroradiology: THE REQUISITES. 4th ed. pp 9, 332-333.

CASE 140

Astrocytoma IDH-Mutant—CNS WHO Grade 2 (Gliomatosis Pattern of Tumor Growth).

1. **D.** Astrocytoma CNS WHO grade 2. Axial T2 (Figure 140.1) FLAIR (Figure 140.2) and post-contrast T1 (Figure 140.3) images demonstrate a poorly defined, infiltrating, T2 and FLAIR hyperintense, nonenhancing mass in the left frontal lobe extending across the genu of the corpus callosum into the contralateral white matter with a mass effect over the frontal horns of the lateral ventricles.
2. **D.** In the 5th edition (2021) update to the WHO classification of CNS tumors, the term hemangiopericytoma has been retired and folded into a solitary fibrous tumor. Similarly, gliomatosis cerebri is no longer considered a distinct entity and is thought of as a growth pattern. The term primitive neuroectodermal tumor (PNET) was previously used to denote a highly malignant tumor belonging to the group of small round-cell tumors of neuroectodermal origin. Since 2016, this term has no longer been included in the diagnostic lexicon.
3. **C.** Gliomatosis cerebri is no longer recognized as a distinct entity. In 2016, it was redefined as merely a pattern of exceptionally widespread tumor growth that can be displayed by

any of the infiltrating gliomas. In the supratentorial compartment, the term is reserved for tumors that involve at least three cerebral lobes.

4. **D.** For the first time, molecular features have been explicitly added to the grading schema, and supersede histological features. Hence, an IDH-wild-type astrocytoma with low-grade histologic features will be classified as grade 4 (glioblastoma) if there is the presence of EGFR amplification, TERT promoter mutation, or the combined gain of chromosome 7 and loss of chromosome 10.

Comment

This case illustrates the typical radiologic appearance of an infiltrating glioma with a gliomatosis pattern of tumor growth. There is an extensive abnormality within the bilateral left more than the right frontal and left temporal lobes with cortical infiltration, gyral swelling, and extension across the genu of the corpus callosum that is also expanded. There is sulcal effacement and mass effect over the bilateral frontal horns. There are no regions of necrosis, and no post-contrast enhancement (Figure 140.3). The patient underwent craniotomy and partial resection of the mass with an integrated diagnosis of astrocytoma IDH-mutant—CNS WHO grade 2.

The WHO classification of CNS tumors, now into its 5th edition, published in 2021, builds on the prior version by placing greater emphasis on molecular markers both in terms of classification and grading which is reflected in a "layered report structure" wherein histological features, grading and molecular information are combined to form an "integrated diagnosis." New tumor types and subtypes are introduced, some based on novel diagnostic technologies such as DNA methylome profiling. Roman numerals have been replaced by Arabic numerals. The term anaplastic has been dropped in favor of grading only, e.g., what was previously known as an "anaplastic astrocytoma" is now referred to as an "astrocytoma, IDH-mutant, CNS WHO grade 3."

In addition, previously known diffuse astrocytoma, anaplastic astrocytoma, or secondary glioblastoma now all come under the one diagnosis, based on the presence of IDH mutation and the absence of 1p19q co-deletion and are graded 2, 3, or 4 based on histological and molecular features. Importantly, a grade 4 tumor is no longer a glioblastoma, but rather just an astrocytoma, IDH mutant WHO CNS grade 4. Molecular features supersede histological features, e.g., an IDH-wild-type astrocytoma with low-grade histologic features will be classified as a grade 4 glioblastoma if there is the presence of EGFR amplification, TERT promoter mutation, or the combined gain of chromosome 7 and loss of chromosome 10.

The most common presenting symptom of astrocytoma is seizures, but patients can also present only with altered mental status or a change in personality, as in this case. Although this tumor may affect patients of any age, it most commonly presents in young adults with a median age of 36 years. Treatment depends on clinical presentation, tumor grade, as well as the size and location with an overall better prognosis compared to grade 3 and grade 4 tumors.

REFERENCES

Johnson DR, Guerin JB, Giannini C, Morris JM, Eckel LJ, Kaufmann TJ. 2016 Updates to the WHO brain tumor classification system: what the radiologist needs to know. *Radiographics*. 2017;37(7):2164-2180.

Louis DN, Perry A, Reifenberger G, et al. The 2016 World Health Organization classification of tumors of the central nervous system: a summary. *Acta Neuropathol*. 2016;131(6):803-820.

Louis DN, Perry A, Wesseling P, et al. The 2021 WHO classification of tumors of the central nervous system: a summary. *Neuro Oncol*. 2021; 23(8):1231-1251.

Neuroradiology: THE REQUISITES. 4th ed. pp 2, 61.

CASE 141

Atypical Teratoid/Rhabdoid Tumor (AT/RT)

1. **D.** Atypical teratoid/rhabdoid tumors classically have low ADC values. Other common posterior fossa tumor in children that is cellular and shows low ADC values is medulloblastoma. Some anaplastic ependymomas may have elements that demonstrate low ADC values.

2. **D.** All of the above. Primary AT/RTs are rare and aggressive childhood embryonal neoplasms that can occur at any site within the CNS. These are most often reported as being infratentorial and intra-axial, but extra-axial lesions are usually situated in the cerebellopontine angle, as seen in this case. The tumor can also be multifocal with both infra- and supratentorial involvement.

3. **A.** The hallmark genetic alterations are mutations of SMARCB1 (INI1, SNF5, BAF47) or (rarely) SMARCA4 (BRG1), both members of the SWItch/sucrose nonfermentable chromatin remodeling complex.

Comment

Atypical teratoid/rhabdoid tumors (AT/RTs) are rare, aggressive embryonal tumors that comprise approximately 1%–2% of all pediatric brain tumors. Approximately 90% of all cases arise in children before 3 years of age, but rarely, AT/RTs can occur in older children and in adults older than 20 years of age in <2% of cases. AT/RT is a pathologic diagnosis, with a specific genetic/molecular alteration, as defined in 98% of cases, by loss of SMARCB1/INI1 expression. On the epigenetic level, AT/RTs are heterogeneous, and fall under three molecular subgroups: AT/RT–myelocytomatosis oncogene (MYC), AT/RT-tyrosine (TYR), and AT/RT–sonic hedgehog (SHH). These can occur at any location within the neuraxis, although most often reported as being infratentorial and intra-axial. Extra-axial lesions are usually situated in the cerebellopontine angle, as in this case.

On imaging, these are hypercellular and heterogeneous tumors with hemorrhage, peripherally localized cysts, high cellularity, seen as low T2 and apparent diffusion coefficient (ADC) signal, as well as a distinct band like "wavy" enhancement (present in 38% of cases). MRI screening of the entire neuraxis is useful for staging, as the leptomeningeal spread is present in 15%–30% of patients at diagnosis. This case shows a markedly heterogeneous and avidly enhancing ill-defined mass in the left cerebellopontine angle, with extension into the internal auditory canal (IAC) and mass effect over the left middle cerebellar peduncle and brainstem. Notice the areas of reduced diffusion within the mass on the axial DWI image (Figure 141.3) suggesting high cellularity. The differential diagnosis includes a malignant schwannoma and atypical meningioma. The imaging appearance would be very unusual for a meningioma, given the extension into the IAC and poorly demarcated margins.

The current standard of care is maximal safe resection, followed by intensive adjuvant chemotherapy. Postoperative craniospinal radiation improves overall survival but is often deferred because the majority of patients are less than 3 years of age, in a critical period of neurodevelopment, and therefore at risk for long-term neurocognitive sequelae. Even with multimodality treatment regimens, the median time to relapse is less than 6 months, and the median overall survival is less than 18 months.

REFERENCES

Ho B, Johann PD, Grabovska Y, et al. Molecular subgrouping of atypical teratoid/rhabdoid tumors-a reinvestigation and current consensus. *Neuro Oncol*. 2020;22(5):613-624.

Louis DN, Perry A, Wesseling P, et al. The 2021 WHO classification of tumors of the central nervous system: a summary. *Neuro Oncol*. 2021; 23(8):1231-1251.

Nowak J, Nemes K, Hohm A, et al. Magnetic resonance imaging surrogates of molecular subgroups in atypical teratoid/rhabdoid tumor. *Neuro Oncol.* 2018;20(12):1672-1679.
Neuroradiology: THE REQUISITES. 4th ed. pp 2, 64.

CASE 142

Amyotrophic Lateral Sclerosis (ALS) — Lou Gehrig's Disease

1. **C.** There is bilaterally symmetric high signal intensity within bilateral corticospinal tracts (Figures 142.1–142.4), consistent with the diagnosis of ALS.
2. **C.** ALS is a relentlessly progressive disorder characterized by the death of motor neurons (Betz cells in the cortex) with secondary Wallerian degeneration.
3. **C.** Decussation of the fibers of the pyramidal tract occurs at the level of the lower medulla.
4. **B.** Death usually results from pulmonary causes (respiratory failure, infections).

Comment

Amyotrophic lateral sclerosis (ALS) (Lou Gehrig's disease or Charcot disease) is the most common neurodegenerative disorder involving motor neurons. It occurs in approximately 1 in every 100,000 people annually. Most cases are sporadic, although autosomal dominant transmission may occur. ALS is typically present in the age group of 40 and 70, with a median age of 55 years at the time of diagnosis. Clinical manifestations include hyperreflexia, weakness of the hands and forearms, spasticity, and cranial neuropathies. There is a progressive loss of motor strength, with the preservation of intellectual and sensory function. The hypoglossal nerve is most commonly affected, and its involvement may be detected on imaging as denervation atrophy with fatty replacement of the tongue.

ALS typically involves the corticospinal tracts and motor neurons. Progression is usually relentless, with death frequently occurring within 3 to 6 years of disease onset. The cause is unknown. It is very difficult to diagnose this in its early stages, but based on the EI Escorial criteria, the principle goal is to rule out other neurological diseases that have a similar presentation. In extreme cases, abnormal T2W signal intensity may extend from the cortex, along the precentral gyrus of the motor strip (pyramidal Betz's cells or upper motor neurons); through the corona radiata, the posterior part of the posterior limb of the internal capsule, the cerebral peduncles, and brainstem; and down to the ventral and lateral portions of the spinal cord. Abnormal T2W and GRE/SWI hypointensity in the precentral gyrus, believed to be related to the deposition of iron or other minerals, may be present along the cerebral cortex in the motor strip, as in this case, Figure 142.5 (orange arrows; note, normal signal in cerebral cortex more anteriorly as shown by white arrows). Note that both of these features can be present in varying degrees in normal controls; hence, an appreciation of what is excessive is critical and needs an experienced neuroradiologist.

MR spectroscopy of the precentral gyrus region has shown a strong correlation between reduced *N*-acetylaspartate and glutamate levels and elevated choline and myoinositol levels and disease severity. MRI of the spinal cord may show signal abnormality and atrophy along the corticospinal tracts.

The most commonly used antiglutamate agent riluzole, which appears to slow the disease progression, has been shown to extend median survival in patients with bulbar onset of disease.

REFERENCES

Bensimon G, Lacomblez L, Meininger V. A controlled trial of riluzole in amyotrophic lateral sclerosis. ALS/Riluzole Study Group. *N Engl J Med.* 1994;330(9):585-591.
Cervo A, Cocozza S, Sacca F, et al. The combined use of conventional MRI and MR spectroscopic imaging increases the diagnostic accuracy in amyotrophic lateral sclerosis. *Eur J Radiol.* 2015;84(1):151-157.
Nelles M, Block W, Träber F, Wüllner U, Schild HH, Urbach H. Combined 3T diffusion tensor tractography and 1H-MR spectroscopy in motor neuron disease. *AJNR Am J Neuroradiol.* 2008;29(9):1708-1714.
Neuroradiology: THE REQUISITES. 4th ed. pp 7, 239-247.

CASE 143

Pleomorphic Xanthoastrocytoma (PXA)

1. **D.** PXA. The appearance of a solid, relatively well-circumscribed, avidly enhancing nodule with a peripheral eccentric cystic component and surrounding vasogenic edema located in the superficial left insula (Figures 143.1–143.4), in a young patient is most consistent with PXA. Notice the markedly elevated rCBV (Figure 143.5) despite the low-grade nature of this tumor. Contrast enhancement is uncommon with DNETs, rare in dysplastic gangliocytoma, and not seen in MVNTs.
2. **A.** More than half of all PXAs are located in the temporal lobe (as in this patient) with the remainder seen in the frontal and parietal lobes.
3. **D.** Seizures.
4. **B.** The most frequently found mutated gene in PXAs is BRAF, which encodes an intracellular component of the MAPK pathway. All of these other mutations are also seen in PXAs but with less frequency.

Comment

Pleomorphic xanthoastrocytoma (PXA) is a rare primary brain tumor thought to originate from subpial astrocytes or their precursors. It typically presents in children and young adults with equal frequency in boys and girls and is most commonly diagnosed in the second decade (mean age at diagnosis is 29 ± 16 years), as in this case. It occurs most commonly in the temporal lobe and frequently presents with seizures. These tumors may be well demarcated, with a solid avidly enhancing nodular component with peripheral cystic changes, seen in more than 50% of cases. These tend to be superficial, cortically based and may have leptomeningeal enhancement as a result of direct invasion of the meninges and surrounding vasogenic edema. In this case, no clear leptomeningeal enhancement was visible on imaging, but on histopathology, most of the tumor growth was seen in the subarachnoid space, with a final diagnosis of pleomorphic xanthoastrocytoma, WHO grade 2. Due to their superficial location and slow growth, PXAs may exhibit a "reactive" dural tail and/or superficial remodeling of the adjacent calvarium.

The differential diagnosis of a cortically based enhancing mass with meningeal involvement includes an inflammatory mass, granulomatous disease (sarcoid), lymphoma, metastases, meningioma, and other primary brain tumors such as oligodendroglioma and PXA.

The most frequently found mutated gene in PXAs is BRAF, and PXAs are commonly divided into *BRAF mutated* and *BRAF wild-type* which has both diagnostic and potential therapeutic implications.

WHO grade 2 PXAs generally have a favorable prognosis following complete surgical resection, with a 5-year survival of over 90%. Local recurrence and malignant transformation (to WHO grade 3) are encountered in up to 20% of cases with a substantially worse prognosis and a 5-year survival rate of only 40%–50%.

REFERENCES

Moore W, Mathis D, Gargan L, et al. Pleomorphic xanthoastrocytoma of childhood: MR imaging and diffusion MR imaging features. *AJNR Am J Neuroradiol.* 2014;35(11):2192-2196.

Shaikh N, Brahmbhatt N, Kruser TJ, et al. Pleomorphic xanthoastrocytoma: a brief review. *CNS Oncol.* 2019;8(3):CNS39.

Yu S, He L, Zhuang X, Luo B. Pleomorphic xanthoastrocytoma: MR imaging findings in 19 patients. *Acta Radiol.* 2011;52(2):223-2237.

Neuroradiology: THE REQUISITES. 4th ed. pp 2, 55-57.

CASE 144

Primary Leptomeningeal Melanomatosis

1. **A.** Blooming or susceptibility artifact is encountered on GRE/SWI sequences in the presence of paramagnetic substances that affect the local magnetic milieux. Melanin is weakly diamagnetic, and hence SWI provides a little additional diagnostic benefit over the standard T1W sequence and does not demonstrate signal loss or blooming. Signal transition of SWI may indicate secondary phenomena such as microbleeds and/or metal scavenging.

2. **A.** On precontrast T1W images, the superficial hyperintense signal is secondary to T1 shortening due to the indirect paramagnetic properties of melanin as a metal scavenger. Notice the T2 hypointensity in the spine in Figure 144.5.

3. **B.** Sagittal and axial T1 pre-contrast (Figures 144.1 and 144.3) and (Figure 144.2) axial post-contrast FLAIR images of the brain demonstrate communicating hydrocephalus and multiple areas of leptomeningeal signal abnormality, with corresponding T1 hyperintensity (yellow arrows). Imaging of the thoracic spine shows a T2 hypointense nodule along the surface of the spinal cord (Figure 144.5) with post-contrast enhancement on axial (Figure 144.6) and sagittal (Figure 144.7) T1W images (yellow arrows). A brain biopsy confirmed the diagnosis of leptomeningeal melanomatosis in this case. There was an absence of cutaneous or ocular melanoma, with a negative systemic oncologic workup.

Comment

Primary CNS melanocytic tumors are neoplasms originating from melanocytes, which are derived from the neural crest and migrate to the leptomeninges during embryogenesis. These can be diffuse or circumscribed. The diffuse meningeal melanocytic neoplasms can be either meningeal melanocytosis or meningeal melanomatosis, whereas circumscribed meningeal melanocytic neoplasms are meningeal melanocytoma and meningeal melanoma. Meningeal melanocytosis is the benign form of primary melanocytic tumor that represents the proliferation of melanocytic cells within the subarachnoid space. On pathological examination, if there is atypia, necrosis, or significant mitotic activity, then a diagnosis of meningeal melanomatosis is made.

Primary leptomeningeal melanomatosis is an extremely rare and aggressive cancer with no standardized treatment and a median overall survival of 4 months from diagnosis. The diagnosis of primary leptomeningeal melanomatosisis is highly challenging as presenting symptoms, and imaging findings are often nonspecific, as in this case.

Because melanocytosis in the CSF may be associated with high protein content, an unenhanced CT may show a hyperdense exudate in the subarachnoid spaces that may be mistaken for acute hemorrhage. On MRI, unenhanced T1W and FLAIR images may show hyperintense lesions along the leptomeninges, with regions of T2W hypointensity and prominent enhancement, as was seen in this case. In this patient, CSF examination showed several large, highly atypical epithelioid cells. Systemic oncologic workup was negative, but the final diagnosis was confirmed on brain biopsy. Biopsy results were BRAF negative, and given the extent of the disease and poor prognosis, the patient was transitioned to hospice care.

REFERENCES

Baumgartner A, Stepien N, Mayr L, et al. Novel insights into diagnosis, biology and treatment of primary diffuse leptomeningeal melanomatosis. *J Pers Med.* 2021;11(4):292.

Louis DN, Perry A, Wesseling P, et al. The 2021 WHO classification of tumors of the central nervous system: a summary. *Neuro Oncol.* 2021;23(8):1231-1251.

Pirini MG, Mascalchi M, Salvi F, et al. Primary diffuse meningeal melanomatosis: radiologic-pathologic correlation. *AJNR Am J Neuroradiol.* 2003;24(1):115-118.

Straub S, Laun FB, Freitag MT, et al. Assessment of melanin content and its influence on susceptibility contrast in melanoma metastases. *Clin Neuroradiol.* 2020;30:607-614.

Neuroradiology: THE REQUISITES. 4th ed. pp 17, 608-610.

CASE 145

Dural Arteriovenous Fistula (dAVF)

1. **A.** There is extensive T2/FLAIR hyperintense signal abnormality involving the left greater than right thalami (Figure 145.1), with central areas of diffusion hyperintensity (Figure 145.2), few foci of susceptibility suggesting microhemorrhages (Figure 145.3) and associated patchy enhancement (Figure 145.4). There is a wide differential diagnosis for these imaging findings, including all of the provided options; however, careful analysis of the angiographic images (Figures 145.5, 145.6, and 145.7) suggests AV shunting and venous congestion as the most likely etiology in this patient.

2. **C.** Sagittal maximum intensity projection image from a CT angiogram (Figure 145.5) shows arterialized flow in the straight sinus. Right vertebral artery injection shows a tentorial dural arteriovenous fistula, with arterial supply primarily from a meningeal right P1 segment branch (artery of Davidoff–Schechter) draining directly into the straight sinus. Lateral DSA from the external carotid artery injection more clearly shows early venous drainage into the straight sinus from a dAVF (Figure 145.7). On ECA injection, there was also arterial supply from the right ascending pharyngeal artery (not shown).

3. **C.** The artery of Davidoff and Schechter is a dural branch arising from the P1 segment, the P1–2 junctions, or the proximal P2 segment of the posterior cerebral artery. It is usually not identified on angiography except when enlarged in the setting of a dural AVF, as in this case (Figure 145.6), or vascular tumors such as a meningioma.

4. **C.** All of these cause bilateral thalamic lesions, except cocaine which typically involves bilateral globus pallidi.

Comment

The differential diagnosis for bilateral thalamic lesions is broad ranging from toxic/metabolic, infectious as well as vascular causes. Vascular causes include arterial infarction (Percheron), deep cerebral venous thrombosis, atypical posterior reversible encephalopathy syndrome (PRES), and vascular malformations. Tentorial dAVF is an uncommon and an often overlooked cause of bithalamic edema, as cross-sectional imaging findings in these cases are usually extremely subtle, noting that thalamic edema from venous congestion may be the only finding. Patchy areas of restricted diffusion or enhancement due to venous ischemia and/or blood products may also be present. CT angiography may show increased vascularity, with increased number, size, or tortuosity of vessels, which can also be a clue to the diagnosis of a dAVF. An arterialized venous structure may also be evident, which strongly suggests the presence of AV shunting, as was seen in this case.

dAVFs are believed to be acquired lesions that typically arise as a consequence of dural venous sinus thrombosis. As a result, a collateral network of vessels develops, including enlargement of normally present microscopic arteriovenous shunts within the dura. As arteriovenous shunting increases, venous hypertension develops. Approximately 10% to 15% of DAVMs are associated with intracranial hemorrhage, which is usually intraparenchymal or subarachnoid. dAVFs that drain strictly to the dural venous sinuses are not usually associated with hemorrhage.

In cases of tentorial dAVFs, it is our experience that partial or complete thrombosis of the straight sinus is usually present with thalamic venous edema/ischemia, potentially representing the underlying cause of the fistula. Presenting symptoms can include thalamic dementia, with progressive cognitive dysfunction that includes deficits in executive function, attention, memory, and disorientation. Aphasia, ataxia, or focal neurologic deficits may also be present. Patients may be started on anticoagulation for incomplete diagnosis of dural venous thrombosis, which could potentially put them at higher risk of venous hemorrhage in the setting of elevated venous pressures from the fistula. In some circumstances, patients may also undergo invasive biopsy if the signal abnormalities in the thalamus are mischaracterized as a tumor. Vascular imaging should be considered in all patients who present with bilateral thalamic edema, especially in the older age groups in which dAVFs are more common. In this patient, successful Onyx embolization of the meningeal right P1 segment branch (artery of Davidoff–Schechter) was performed with significantly decreased filling of the fistula and improvement in symptoms.

REFERENCES

Cox M, Rodriguez P, Mohan S, et al. Tentorial dural arteriovenous fistulas as a cause of thalamic edema: 2 cases of an important differential diagnosis to consider. *Neurohospitalist.* 2021;11(1):33-39.

Hegde AN, Mohan S, Lath N, Lim CC. Differential diagnosis for bilateral abnormalities of the basal ganglia and thalamus. *Radiographics.* 2011;31(1):5-30.

Roman NIS, Rodriguez P, Nasser H, et al. Artery of Davidoff and Schechter: a large angiographic case series of dural AV fistulas. *Neurohospitalist.* 2022;12(1):155-161.

Neuroradiology: THE REQUISITES. 4th ed. pp 3, 148-149.

CASE 146

Ruptured Mycotic Aneurysm

1. **C.** Angiographic images reveal a ruptured 4 × 3 mm infectious aneurysm arising from the distal left M4 parietal branch, with mild irregularity of the branch just before aneurysm (Figures 146.2 and 146.4). The peripheral location of the aneurysm is suggestive of a mycotic aneurysm, which was subsequently coiled (Figure 146.5). Note two additional small aneurysms arising from the proximal right M4 branch (Figure 146.3). The patient was found to have *Streptococcus constellatus* endocarditis involving the VSD patch (site of prior VSD repair), which was the cause in this patient. Hypertensive hemorrhages are usually located in the basal ganglia, and there was no nidus or AV shunting to suggest an AVM.

2. **B.** The most common location of intracranial mycotic (infectious) aneurysms is the peripheral branches of the middle cerebral artery (M2 and beyond) in 75%–80% of cases, reflecting the embolic origin of these lesions. Unlike berry aneurysms, mycotic aneurysms preferentially affect distal branches rather than branch points around the circle of Willis.

3. **D.** Up to 25% of cases may have more than one intracerebral mycotic aneurysm. They are friable and have a greater propensity to bleed than other aneurysms.

4. **A.** The vast majority of mycotic aneurysms originate from left-sided bacterial endocarditis. All other options are correct.

Comment

Mycotic aneurysms comprise an important subtype of potentially life-threatening cerebrovascular lesions and are estimated to account for 0.7%–5.4% of all intracranial aneurysms. The advent of antibiotic therapy has substantially decreased the occurrence of endocarditis in the developed world; however, endocarditis still persists due to the increasing use of prosthetic valves, intravenous drug abuse, and degenerative valve diseases. The vast majority of mycotic aneurysms are seen occurring in the setting of left-sided bacterial infective endocarditis, although these can also be secondary to fungal and viral (rarely) etiologies. *Streptococcus viridans* and *Staphylococcus aureus* are the most common pathogens accounting for up to 90% of all cases.

A mycotic aneurysm results from an infectious process that involves the arterial wall. These aneurysms may be caused by a septic embolus that causes inflammatory destruction of the arterial wall, beginning with the endothelial surface. Infected embolic material also reaches the adventitia through the vasa vasorum. Inflammation then disrupts the adventitia and muscularis, resulting in aneurysmal dilation. Typically, intracranial aneurysms secondary to bacteremia are located in peripheral branches of the middle cerebral artery (M2 and beyond), while those secondary to fungemia are often more proximal involving the long segments of intracranial vessels. Intracranial mycotic aneurysms can be evaluated with CT/CTA, MRI/MRA, or DSA which remains the gold standard.

Aneurysms may be asymptomatic prior to rupture. Ruptured aneurysms present with subarachnoid hemorrhage or intracerebral hemorrhage, as in this case. Most cases are treated emergently with a 6-week course of IV antibiotics. While ruptured aneurysms should be immediately secured via either surgical or endovascular approaches, unruptured mycotic aneurysms may be treated empirically with antibiotics and followed by serial angiographic imaging. If the aneurysm increases in size or remains unchanged, intervention is indicated. Even with aggressive multimodal treatment, prognosis remains poor with a mortality of up to 30% for unruptured mycotic aneurysms, which increases to 80% for ruptured intracranial mycotic aneurysms.

REFERENCES

Ducruet AF, Hickman ZL, Zacharia BE, et al. Intracranial infectious aneurysms: a comprehensive review. *Neurosurg Rev.* 2010;33(1):37-46.

Wajnberg E, Rueda F, Marchiori E, Gasparetto EL. Endovascular treatment for intracranial infectious aneurysms. *Arq Neuropsiquiatr.* 2008;66(4):790-794.

Neuroradiology: THE REQUISITES. 4th ed. pp 5, 183.

CASE 147

Paraneoplastic Autoimmune (Limbic) Encephalitis

1. **B.** There is a near-symmetric T2/FLAIR hyperintense signal in bilateral mesial temporal lobes (Figure 147.1 and 147.2), with associated mild cortical thickening, no diffusion restriction (Figure 147.3), and patchy enhancement (Figure 147.4), which is most compatible with autoimmune (paraneoplastic) limbic encephalitis.

2. **C.** The most common locations of involvement are the mesial temporal lobes and limbic system. Involvement is most commonly bilateral (60%), although often asymmetric. Basal ganglia involvement is also common.
3. **B.** Paraneoplastic autoimmune encephalitis is classically associated with small cell carcinoma of the lung, and anti-Hu is the most commonly identified antibody.
4. **C.** As a general rule, antibodies targeted to intracellular antigens are more frequently associated with an underlying tumor.

Comment

The term "autoimmune limbic encephalitis" generally refers to a group of closely related antibody-mediated inflammatory CNS disorders, typically involving the limbic system with overlapping clinical and neuroimaging features and are ultimately differentiated by the specific antibody subtypes driving the underlying immune-mediated attack to CNS. It can be divided broadly into two groups: paraneoplastic limbic encephalitis where antibodies are present against intracellular antigens, and nonneoplastic autoimmune limbic encephalitis where antibodies are against extracellular antigens, usually with better outcomes.

In approximately 60% of cases of paraneoplastic limbic encephalitis, antineuronal antibodies are present such as the *anti-Hu antibody* in small cell lung cancer (the most common malignancy associated with paraneoplastic syndrome), the *anti-Ta antibody* in testicular cancers, and *anti-NMDA NR1* in ovarian teratomas. In this patient, the serum paraneoplastic panel was mostly negative except for elevated *AChR antibody* and was presumed to have atypical autoimmune encephalitis.

Typical imaging findings of autoimmune limbic encephalitis include T2 hyperintensity and swelling of the mesial temporal lobes sometimes with patchy enhancement. On PET scans, FDG avidity can be seen. The primary differential is herpes simplex encephalitis that can be distinguished by a typical clinical presentation and the presence of hemorrhage in the temporal lobes, with classic sparing of the basal ganglia. Other differentials include status epilepticus, neurosyphilis, and infiltrative gliomas. When limbic encephalitis has hypothalamic involvement, inflammatory conditions such as neurosarcoidosis or lymphocytic hypophysitis should also be considered.

Paraneoplastic limbic encephalitis may present with a change in mental status, personality changes, seizures, and memory impairment. On pathologic evaluation, nonspecific inflammatory changes and cellular infiltrates are identified without the presence of a tumor or viral inclusions. Treatment of the primary malignancy may result in improvement of the neurologic symptoms. Most forms of autoimmune encephalitis respond to immune therapies, although powerful immune suppression for weeks or months may be needed in difficult cases.

REFERENCES

Carter BW, Glisson BS, Truong MT, et al. Small cell lung carcinoma: staging, imaging, and treatment considerations. *Radiographics*. 2014;34(6):1707-1721.
Gozzard P, Woodhall M, Chapman C, et al. Paraneoplastic neurologic disorders in small cell lung carcinoma: a prospective study. *Neurology*. 2015;85(3):235-239.
Kelley BP, Patel SC, Marin HL, Corrigan JJ, Mitsias PD, Griffith B. Autoimmune encephalitis: pathophysiology and imaging review of an overlooked diagnosis. *AJNR Am J Neuroradiol*. 2017;38(6):1070-1078.
Lancaster E. The diagnosis and treatment of autoimmune encephalitis. *J Clin Neurol*. 2016;12(1):1-13.
Neuroradiology: THE REQUISITES. 4th ed. pp 2, 81-82.

CASE 148

Drug-Induced Hypophysitis—Immune Checkpoint Inhibitor–Induced Hypophysitis

1. **D.** There is diffuse pituitary gland hypertrophy with irregular thickening of the pituitary infundibulum (Figure 148.2), and diffuse enhancement (Figure 148.3) in keeping with an immune checkpoint inhibitor (ICI)–induced hypophysitis. This patient had stage 4 melanoma and became symptomatic after the third dose of ipilimumab.
2. **A.** Hypophysitis is one of the well-known adverse effects of ICIs.
3. **D.** The management of ICI-induced hypophysitis includes discontinuation of immunotherapy, initiation of corticosteroids, and long-term supplementation of deficient hormones. The imaging findings, as well as clinical manifestations usually normalize following cessation of ICI therapy and/or corticosteroid treatment, as was seen in this patient (Figure 148.4). Ipilimumab was stopped, and the patient was started on dexamethasone 4 mg daily with clinical improvement in 5–6 hours. Synthroid was also started at the same time.
4. **A.** On imaging, hypophysitis secondary to ICI is usually accompanied by subtle and nonspecific findings. It develops relatively quickly without bony remodeling of the sella, as in this case. There is inflammatory cell infiltration with a relatively low T2 signal (Figure 148.1) compared to pituitary macroadenomas with hypertrophy and enhancement of the pituitary gland and infundibulum and loss of the normal posterior pituitary bright spot. Despite the involvement of the infundibulum, diabetes insipidus is not seen. It is reported that imaging can be normal in up to 50% of patients. A high degree of clinical suspicion is necessary, and a normal MRI does not exclude the diagnosis.

Comment

Autoimmune hypophysitis is a rare complication of immune checkpoint inhibitors (ICIs), a class of drugs that block immune checkpoints by releasing T cells to attack cancer cells. There are two major classes of ICI including monoclonal antibodies to cytotoxic T-lymphocyte-associated protein 4 (CTLA-4), and programmed death 1 receptor and ligand (PD-1 and PD-L1) which have been used for advanced melanoma, renal cell carcinoma, lung cancer, and many other cancers. As a side effect, these can cause an excessive immune response due to the infiltration of activated T-cells into various organs. Hypophysitis occurs when there is an inflammation of the pituitary gland caused by the anti-CTLA-4 antibody ipilimumab, as was seen in this case. It presents with nonspecific symptoms, e.g., fatigue, headache, weakness, visual changes, and/or endocrinopathies. The diagnosis is confirmed clinically when there is ≥1 pituitary hormonal dysfunction, such as hyposecretion of corticotropin or thyroid-stimulating hormone (TSH). This patient had a low trending TSH and acutely presented with headache after the third cycle of ipilimumab.

The overall fatality rate with ICI-induced hypophysitis is very low (2%), but the associated endocrine toxicity is very high (>91%). It is often irreversible and requires long-term hormone replacement.

Autopsy studies have revealed near-complete destruction of the anterior lobe of the pituitary gland caused by extensive necrosis and fibrosis and lymphocytic and necrotizing hypophysitis.

MRI is the imaging modality of choice, but a negative study does not exclude the diagnosis. Positive cases demonstrate glandular hypertrophy with irregular thickening of the infundibulum, and diffuse enhancement, as in this case. All patients show an improvement in clinical and radiological findings following the withdrawal of ICI, including high-dose steroids with or without hormonal supplementation. This patient also responded well to dexamethasone with a resolution of imaging findings but remained on a long-term thyroid replacement therapy (levothyroxine).

REFERENCES

Carpenter KJ, Murtagh RD, Lilienfeld H, et al. Ipilimumab-induced hypophysitis: MR imaging findings. *AJNR Am J Neuroradiol.* 2009; 30(9):1751-1753.
Garon-Czmil J, Petitpain N, Rouby F, et al. Immune check point inhibitors-induced hypophysitis: a retrospective analysis of the French Pharmacovigilance database. *Sci Rep.* 2019;9(1):19419.
Kurokawa R, Ota Y, Gonoi W, et al. MRI findings of immune checkpoint inhibitor-induced hypophysitis: possible association with fibrosis. *AJNR Am J Neuroradiol.* 2020;41(9):1683-1689.
Nada A, Bhat R, Cousins J. Magnetic resonance imaging criteria of immune checkpoint inhibitor-induced hypophysitis. *Curr Probl Cancer.* 2021;45(1):100644.
Neuroradiology: THE REQUISITES. 4th ed. pp 10, 358.

CASE 149

Spontaneous Subperiosteal Hematomas of the Orbit

1. **B.** This patient underwent a biopsy of a suspicious rectal mass under anesthesia in the Trendelenburg position. When the patient awoke from anesthesia, she complained of bilateral eye pain and was noted to have bilateral proptosis, periorbital edema, and conjunctival injection. On examination, there was near complete loss of vision bilaterally. Coronal (Figure 149.1) and axial (Figure 149.2) unenhanced CT images showed biconvex hyperdense masses within the superior orbits. Coronal T1-weighted with fat saturation (Figure 149.3), coronal short T2 inversion recovery (Figure 149.4), axial T1 (Figure 149.5), and fat-suppressed axial T2-weighted (Figure 149.6) images from unenhanced MRI of the orbits showed similar biconvex T1 and T2 hyperintense masses within the subperiosteal region, which inferiorly displaced the superior rectus muscle complex, extraconal fat, and optic nerves. These imaging findings were most consistent with spontaneous bilateral subperiosteal orbital hematomas.
2. **F.** Spontaneous, nontraumatic subperiosteal hematomas are rare but have been reported in the setting of systemic diseases that are associated with bleeding diatheses (especially liver disease), in association with acute sinusitis, with sudden elevations of intracranial venous pressure, severe vomiting, severe coughing, during child birth, weight lifting, scuba diving, and rarely, in the setting of anesthesia and interventional procedures. In this patient, the hematomas were ascribed to a combination of increased central venous pressure (from prolonged positioning in the Trendelenburg position), which was transmitted through the valveless venous system into the orbit leading to rupture of the subperiosteal venous plexi.
3. **D.** The superior orbit is the most common location as the frontal bone contributes the greatest surface area to the orbit and the periosteal attachment in this location is relatively loose. The management of patients with spontaneous subperiosteal hematomas associated with significant vision loss includes high-dose steroids and emergent surgical decompression of the hematomas, as was performed in this patient.

Comment

Spontaneous subperiosteal hematomas are often bilateral and may present with eye pain, periorbital swelling, diplopia, and vision loss from compression of the optic nerve within the orbital apex or optic canal. Examination reveals poorly reactive pupils, proptosis with inferior displacement of the globes, periorbital ecchymoses, chemosis, and/or exotropia with limitation of supraduction.

Subperiosteal hematomas develop between the bony orbit and the periosteum because of abrupt changes in venous pressure which is transmitted through the valveless venous system in the orbit, leading to rupture of the bridging subperiosteal veins. Connective tissue disorders (as in this case) are thought to weaken the periosteal attachment to the bone, thereby limiting the ability of the periosteum to tamponade.

Subperiosteal hematomas are typically well-defined biconvex high-attenuation masses on CT, and MR signal intensity characteristics vary depending on the age of the blood products. On imaging, these can be distinguished from other intraorbital hematomas based on their anatomic location and the manner in which they displace adjacent structures.

The management of patients with spontaneous subperiosteal hematomas associated with significant vision loss includes high-dose steroids and emergent surgical decompression. In patients in whom visual acuity is not affected or is improving, surgery can be deferred. In these cases, close observation with high-dose steroids and follow-up until complete resolution of the hematomas occurs may be appropriate. This patient underwent emergent bedside upper and lower canthotomy which partially restored the patient's vision. On follow-up, there was an increase in the size of these hematomas consistent with ongoing hemorrhage with a worsening mass effect on the superior muscle complexes and optic nerves. The patient was subsequently taken for surgical decompression, which confirmed active bleeding within large bilateral subperiosteal hematomas. Two weeks after surgical decompression, the patient regained full baseline visual function.

REFERENCES

Crawford C, Mazzoli R. Subperiosteal hematoma in multiple settings. *Digit J Ophthalmol.* 2013;19(1):6-8.
Devenney-Cakir B, Selouan R, Branstetter BF, Melhem E, Loevner LA. *Neurographics.* 2015;5(2):64-67.
Leovic D, Zubcic V, Kopic M, et al. Posttraumatic subperiosteal orbital hematoma. *J Craniomaxillofac Surg.* 2011;39(2):131-134.
Neuroradiology: THE REQUISITES. 4th ed. pp 4, 167-171.

CASE 150

Rhombencephalosynapsis

1. **D.** The skull is brachiturricephalic in shape (Figures 150.1 and 150.2) with a dysgenetic corpus callosum (Figure 150.3) and an absence of the septum pellucidum (Figure 150.6). There is a small volume posterior fossa with flattening of the midbrain and pons, and nonvisualization of the vermis with midline fusion, consistent with rhombencephalosynapsis (RES). The patient was shunted for hydrocephalus with a right frontal ventriculostomy catheter in situ.
2. **G.** All of these can be seen in association with RES. Agenesis of the posterior pituitary has been reported, but the posterior pituitary gland was normally seen in this patient (Figure 150.3).
3. **D.** Dandy–Walker malformation and Joubert syndrome. Joubert anomaly is also known as vermian aplasia with molar tooth configuration. In this condition, there is a variable degree of cerebellar vermian agenesis, and the cerebellar hemispheres abut each other but are not fused.
   Dandy–Walker malformation is characterized by the triad of vermian hypoplasia, cystic dilatation of the fourth ventricle, and enlarged posterior fossa with torcular-lambdoid inversion. In Chiari 2 malformation, the cerebellar vermis

is normally formed, but the tonsils and vermis are displaced inferiorly through the foramen magnum.

4. **D.** Observation of a normal cavum septum pellucidum (CSP) is an important normal landmark in the second and third trimester prenatal ultrasound. In most cases, nonvisualization of the CSP on prenatal sonography is associated with anomalies such as agenesis of the corpus callosum, schizencephaly, septo-optic dysplasia (SOD), holoprosencephaly, chronic hydrocephalus, and acquired fetal brain injury. Since optic nerve hypoplasia and endocrine anomalies cannot be ruled out completely on prenatal imaging (ultrasound and fetal MRI), in utero differentiation between isolated absent septum pellucidum and SOD is not possible. Other options are correct.

Comment

Rhombencephalosynapsis is a rare cerebellar malformation of an unknown etiology, characterized by agenesis or hypogenesis of the cerebellar vermis. There is a fusion of the cerebellar hemispheres (single-lobed cerebellum), with a variable fusion of other posterior fossa structures, including the cerebellar peduncles, dentate nuclei, and colliculi. In the cerebellar hemispheres, the orientation of the folia is disorganized. They are usually transverse in configuration, extending across the midline without intervening vermis, MRI typically shows an absent or severely hypoplastic vermis, with a fusion of the cerebellar hemispheres, as seen in this case. There is usually posterior pointing of the fourth ventricle with a diamond or keyhole appearance. It either occurs as an isolated anomaly (rare) or as part of wider cerebral malformation with variable degrees of neurological impairment,

depending on the extent of associated supratentorial anomalies. The associated supratentorial anomalies include partial or complete absence of the septum pellucidum, a hypoplastic anterior commissure, ex vacuo enlargement of the ventricular system related to surrounding volume loss of the brain parenchyma, and fusion of the thalami. Hypertelorism and migrational anomalies have also been reported with this condition.

Joubert's syndrome, another dysplasia of the posterior fossa contents, is characterized by severe hypoplasia or aplasia of the cerebellar vermis. It has a characteristic imaging appearance, including a "bat-wing" configuration of the fourth ventricle, as well as a horizontal orientation of the superior cerebellar peduncles. Unlike rhombencephalosynapsis, the cerebellar hemispheres are apposed in the midline but are not fused. Associated supratentorial anomalies are uncommon.

REFERENCES

Chemli J, Abroug M, Tlili K, et al. Rhombencephalosynapsis diagnosed in childhood: clinical and MRI findings. *Eur J Paediatr Neurol.* 2007; 11(1):35-38.

Hosseinzadeh K, Luo J, Borhani A, Hill L. Non-visualisation of cavum septi pellucidi: implication in prenatal diagnosis? *Insights Imaging.* 2013;4(3):357-367.

Truwit CL, Barkovich AJ, Shanahan R, Maroldo TV. MR imaging of rhombencephalosynapsis: report of three cases and review of the literature. *AJNR Am J Neuroradiol.* 1991;12(5):957-965.

Weaver J, Manjila S, Bahuleyan B, et al. Rhombencephalosynapsis: embryopathology and management strategies of associated neurosurgical conditions with a review of the literature. *J Neurosurg Pediatr.* 2013; 11(3):320-326.

Neuroradiology: THE REQUISITES. 4th ed. pp 8, 280-283.

Index of Cases